PERIPHERAL NEUROPATHIES

DEVELOPMENTS IN NEUROLOGY

Volume 1

PERIPHERAL NEUROPATHIES

Proceedings of the International Symposium on Peripheral
Neuropathies held in Milan, Italy on June 26-28, 1978.

Editors:

N. CANAL

and

G. POZZA

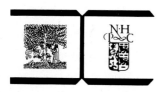

1978

ELSEVIER/NORTH-HOLLAND BIOMEDICAL PRESS
AMSTERDAM · NEW YORK · OXFORD

Published by:
Elsevier/North-Holland Biomedical Press
335 Jan van Galenstraat, P.O. Box 211
Amsterdam, The Netherlands

Sole distributors for the U.S.A. and Canada:
Elsevier North-Holland Inc.
52 Vanderbilt Avenue
New York, N.Y. 10017

ISBN for this volume: 0-444-80079-4
ISBN for the series: 0-444-80078-6

Library of Congress Cataloging in Publication Data

International Symposium on Peripheral Neuropathies,
    Milan, 1978.
    Peripheral neuropathies.

    (Developments in neurology ; 1)
    Bibliography: p.
    Includes index.
    1. Nerves, Peripheral--Diseases--Congresses.
2. Neurologic manifestations of general diseases--
Congresses. 3. Axonal transport--Congresses. I. Ca-
nal, N. II. Pozza, Guido. III. Title. IV. Series.
RC409.I57 1978   616.8'7'07   78-9951
ISBN 0-444-80079-4

PRINTED IN THE NETHERLANDS

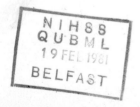

PREFACE

This volume is the Proceedings of the Symposium on Peripheral Neuropathies held on June 26-28, 1978 at the University of Milan.

The initial idea was to devote the entire meeting to the metabolic and genetic neuropathies, but then we thought it more interesting and complete to divide the Symposium into different "Main Themes" in order to enlarge the interest in peripheral neuropathies and also in other scientific branches. In this way, pharmacologists and anatomists, orthopaedists, diabetologists and nephrologists have discussed, together with neurologists, subjects such as axonal transport, neuropathies in chronic renal failure, compression neuropathies and diabetic neuropathies.

Naturally we did not completely forget our initial purpose and an entire session was devoted to the metabolic and genetic neuropathies.

We also had a good number of contributions on basic problems in peripheral nerve pathology which were of such an outstanding quality to be grouped in another special Session.

The volume includes almost all the invited lectures presented at the Symposium and some of the free communications which were more strictly related to the chapters of the book.

The Editors would have liked to have been able to include all the 100 and more communications, of excellent quality, but this would have brought us to considerably exceed the number of pages agreed upon with the Publishers.

The Organizers gratefully acknowledge the support given by FIDIA Research Laboratories.

N. Canal and G. Pozza

CONTENTS

COMPRESSION NEUROPATHIES

Peripheral Neuropathies
N. Canal and G. Pozza, eds.
© 1978 Elsevier/North-Holland Biomedical Press

SENSORY ACTION POTENTIALS AND BIOPSY OF THE SURAL NERVE IN NEUROPATHY

FRITZ BUCHTHAL AND FRIEDRICH BEHSE

Institute of Neurophysiology, Laboratory of Clinical Neurophysiology and Research Laboratories of the Rigshospital, section 4112, Copenhagen, Denmark 2100.

ABSTRACT

In 167 consecutive patients with various types of neuropathy the amplitude of the sensory potential and the maximum conduction velocity along the sural nerve were compared with conduction in other sensory nerves and related to nerve biopsy. Electrophysiological findings in the sural nerve were similar to those in the superficial peroneal and the median nerve, though the distal segment of the median nerve was normal in 20% of the patients when it was abnormal in the sural nerve. Quantification of histological findings was a more sensitive method than the electrophysiological study in that two-thirds of 33 patients with normal electrophysiology in the sural nerve showed slight loss of fibres or signs of remyelination in teased fibres. Of the 95 nerves from which teased fibres were obtained, maximum conduction velocity was abnormal in 43. In 18 nerves slowing in conduction was due to axonal degeneration: the velocity was as to be expected from the diameter of the largest fibres in the biopsy ("proportionate slowing"). In nine nerves slowing was severe and more marked than to be expected from loss of the largest fibres ("disproportionate slowing"); these nerves showed paranodal or segmental demyelination in more than 30% of the fibres. In 16 nerves from patients with neuropathy of different ætiology, among these three from patients with diabetic neuropathy, neither loss of fibres nor demyelination could explain the moderate slowing. When an incidence of teased fibres with demyelination over a length of 10 mm of the nerve is extrapolated to 140 mm of the nerve, 50% of the fibres would have no myelin defects (either de- or remyelination).

The cause of the slowing is possibly a functional defect in the excitable membrane of the nerve.

Finally the limitations are discussed and minimal requirements are suggested for the electrophysiological diagnosis of a peripheral neuropathy with discrete clinical symptoms and signs.

INTRODUCTION

Experimental and clinical science advances as much by the development and application of new techniques as by new theories. In the field of peripheral neuropathy the progress in techniques lies essentially in the quantification of morphological and electrophysiological findings. The progress in theory was inspired by the concept that neuropathies can be divided into two types: One with extensive demyelination and marked reduction in conduction velocity primarily affecting the Schwann cell. Another larger group is characterized by axonal degeneration and little or no demyelination. Slowing in conduction is less than in nerves with extensive demyelination. This concept, originally based on findings in experimental neuropathy, has greatly stimulated work in the field. It was, however, soon recognized that a neuropathy with extensive demyelination is nearly always associated with marked loss of fibres[1,2,3,4]. In our material of 85 nerves from which teased fibres were obtained, segmental demyelination without fibre loss was present in two nerves. Moreover, signs of paranodal demyelination were found in axonal neuropathy, possibly indicating involvement of the Schwann cell secondary to the involvement of the axon[5,6]. To suggest demyelination as the underlying pathology for slowing in conduction encounters difficulties when slowing is of the order of 30 to 40%. This degree of slowing occurs in axonal neuropathy in the absence of segmental or paranodal demyelination.

Based on electrophysiological and biopsy findings in 167 patients with neuropathy (Table 1) we shall adress two problems, the one concerns the relation between morphometric findings in the sural nerve, conduction velocity and amplitude of the evoked potentials. The other problem concerns the early recognition of neuropathy. This problem has attracted interest because of growing awareness of possible toxic agents in the environment.

Table 1[7]
167 PATIENTS WITH POLYNEUROPATHY

Acquired neuropathy of different ætiology	No. of patients	Hereditary neuropathy	No. of patients
Diabetic	12	Peroneal muscular atrophy	
Postinfectious	14	neuronal type	19
Alcoholic	38	hypertrophic type	10
Postgastrectomy	6	*neuronal "plus"	9
Paraneoplastic	4	Spino-cerebellar ataxia	3
Collagen disease	3	Hered. liability to	
Uræmic	2	pressure palsies	10
Lead intoxication	9		
Hepatic	1		
B_{12}Malabsorption	1		
Acute interm. porphyria	1		
Unknown	25		

*Peroneal muscular atrophy of the neuronal type plus involvement of the central nervous system.

METHODS

The method of stimulation and recording has been described[8,9,10]. Fig. 1 shows the sites of recording in the median and sural nerves and the site of the biopsy of the sural nerve and Fig. 2 shows the position and dimensions of the near-nerve electrode at an optimal distance from the sural nerve. Electronic averaging of 500 to 2000 responses was used to estimate amplitudes of less than 3 µV (lower limit 0.02 µV) and to record the conduction velocity of the fastest and of the slow components.

Biopsy: 3 to 5 cm of the sural nerve were removed in toto and prepared for light and electron microscopy and for preparation of 50 to 70 teased fibres as described[12,13,14,15]. In each biopsy the transverse endoneurial area was measured. Moreover, the total number and size distribution of myelinated fibres and of groups of three or more regenerating fibres ("clusters") were determined within an area of 0.4 to 0.6 mm^2, sampled from all fascicles.

4

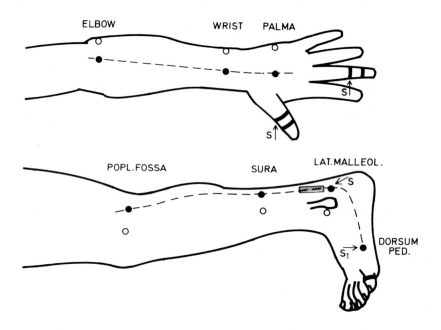

Fig. 1. Placement of the near-nerve (●) and remote (o) needle electrodes to record from different segments of the median and sural nerves. S, stimulating cathode (surface or needle). S_1, cathode to stimulate the sural nerve. "Sura" denotes the site of recording 12 to 14 cm proximal to the lateral malleolus. The shaded area shows the 3-5 cm long segment of the sural nerve taken in toto as biopsy[11].

In addition, we counted sites with clumps of myelin and determined the incidence of degenerated fibres and of bands of Büngner in electron micrographs. In teased fibres the incidence of fibres, of segments with segmental and paranodal demyelination, of remyelination and of regenerated fibres was determined.

RESULTS

   The most frequent histological abnormality that changes nerve conduction and amplitude of the sensory potentials is loss of myelinated fibres. The amplitude of the potential recorded via needle

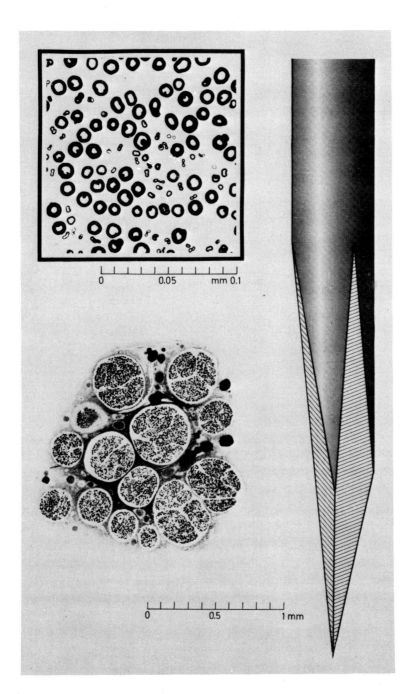

Fig. 2. Recording electrode (right) at an optimal distance from the
sural nerve (left) to ascertain that the action currents from
the fibres of all fascicles are about equally represented when they
reach the leading-off surface of the electrode. Above, left, cross-
section through the sural nerve at a 10 times higher magnification
(courtesy of Professor Annelise Rosenfalck).

electrodes from the sural nerve increases with the number of large myelinated fibres [11,14,18,7]. Since loss of large fibres was equally prominent in nerves with axonal degeneration as in those with demyelination[15], the question arises whether the type of pathology can be predicted from the degree of slowing in conduction. We have tried to answer this question by determining whether and when the slowing in conduction in a given sural nerve from a patient with polyneuropathy could be predicted from the largest fibres found in the biopsy of the same nerve. The prerequisite for the prediction of the maximum conduction velocity is the fact that conduction velocity varies proportionally with the diameter of the nerve fibre[16]. The fastest component of the sensory potentials was related to the myelinated fibres of largest diameter in the histogram of diameter of the same nerve as shown in Fig. 3. In the human sural nerve the maximum conduction velocity was 4.3 (S.D. 0.3) times the fibre diameter. Findings in nerves with purely axonal degeneration showed that the conversion factor was the same for fibres of more than 7 μm in diameter[11,17].

To calculate conduction velocity from the diameter of the largest fibres, we have assumed that at least 10 fibres must be present to give a response distinguishable from noise when 500-2000 responses are averaged. This assumption is based on the relation between amplitude of the sensory potential and number of large myelinated fibres in the sural nerve[11,14,17,18].

When slowing in maximum conduction velocity deviates by less than 20% from that to be expected from the fibres of largest diameter, it can be explained by axonal loss and demyelination does not slow the maximum conduction velocity. The scatter of 20% is derived from findings in controls[14,18].

From counts of myelinated fibres and from quantitation of abnormalities in teased fibres axonal degeneration was shown to be the dominating pathology in 20 sural nerves from patients with alcoholic neuropathy[19,14]. The incidence and extent of paranodal and segmental demyelination (0.3%) and remyelination (20%, compared with 5-20% in controls) was unimpressive[14]. This was the case even when fibre loss was insignificant and when the neuropathy had lasted for only a few weeks. When present at all, myelin damage was distributed over multiple sites of a given fibre

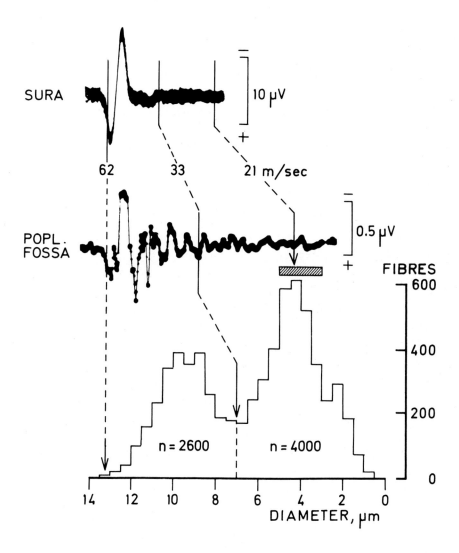

Fig. 3. Components of the sensory potential and distribution of diameters of myelinated fibres in a normal sural nerve. Above and middle: The nerve was stimulated maximally at the lateral malleolus and the potential was recorded 15 cm (sura) and 50 cm (fossa poplitea) proximally to it. The dashed lines connect components conducted at the same velocity and point to the corresponding fibre diameter in the histogram below (6600 fibres). Note that the diameter of the fibres is plotted from right to left[11,17].

in one third of the fibres, interpreted to be secondary to beginning axonal degeneration[56]. Axonal degeneration was also the main
pathology in 19 biopsies from patients with the neuronal type of
peroneal muscular atrophy[15], in Friedreich's ataxia[20], in three of
four patients with paraneoplastic neuropathy, in patients with
rheumatoid neuropathy, polyarteritis nodosa, hepatic neuropathy,
acute intermittent porphyria[7] and in lead neuropathy[21].

In alcoholic neuropathy, in the neuronal type of peroneal muscular atrophy, in paraneoplastic neuropathy, in lead neuropathy
and in lead-exposed men the recorded conduction velocity was equal
to the velocity expected from the fibres of largest diameter, i.e.
the slowing in conduction could be explained by axonal degeneration (Fig. 4). A decrease in conduction velocity from the normal
53 m/s to 30 m/s (to 55% of normal) could be due solely to loss
of the largest fibres. Not unless the recorded sensory conduction
velocity was disproportionally slower than expected or - when no
biopsy was available - not unless the velocity was slowed to less
than 60% of normal is it justified to assume causes other than
axonal degeneration for the diminution in conduction velocity.

A reduction in amplitude and conduction velocity is also seen
in regenerating fibres. This is illustrated by the recovery of
the sensory potential after section and suture of the nerve[23].
The sensory potential of regenerating nerve is characterized by
30 to 50 components of low amplitude. Five months after suture
of the median nerve at wrist, when the first response could be
distinguished, the cumulative amplitude, obtained by adding the
amplitude of component potentials, was 1 to 3 µV, the fastest
component was conducted at 10 to 25 m/s, the slowest at 2 to 3 m/s.
40 months after suture, when tactile sensibility had become normal,
the potential was still split-up in 20 to 30 components, the
cumulative amplitude was normal as was the maximum conduction
velocity. The velocity of the slowest components was still markedly diminished (Fig. 5). Fig. 6 shows the time course of recovery
of the cumulative amplitude of the sensory potential recorded
just proximal to the site of the end-to-end suture at wrist.
The left plot shows the much faster recovery after a transient
compression of the ulnar nerve at the elbow, that presumably has
caused segmental demyelination[23].

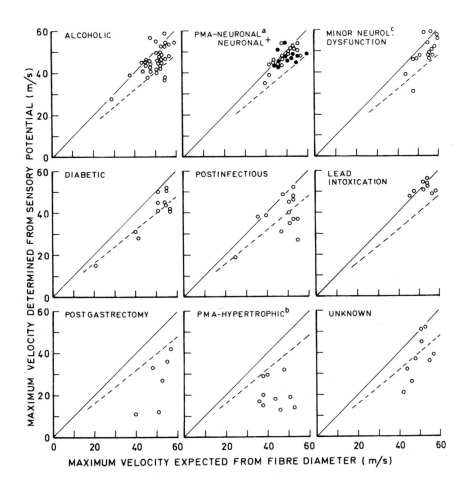

Fig. 4. Maximum conduction velocity determined from the sensory
potential of the sural nerve (ordinate) as a function of the velocity expected from the diameter of the largest myelinated fibres
(abscissa) in polyneuropathies of different ætiology. The full
line indicates equality between the recorded and the expected velocity. Loss of large fibres can explain the slowing in conduction
when the recorded velocity is within 20% of that expected from
fibre diameter (dashed line lower limit of normal range).
a: Peroneal muscular atrophy of the neuronal type and of type
neuronal plus (Table 1).
b: Peroneal muscular atrophy of the hypertrophic type.
c: Nerves from patients with discrete (uncertain) clinical symptoms and signs in neuropathy of unknown ætiology[22,7].

In the biopsy regeneration is indicated by an incidence of
three or more closely packed small myelinated fibres ("clusters")
and in teased fibres by the occurrence of fibres in which all
internodal segments are shorter than in normal fibres of the same
diameter. The degree of regeneration differs in different types
of neuropathy. Thus, in the neuronal type of peroneal muscular
atrophy the number of the largest fibres was diminished whereas
the number of small fibres was as in controls, because their
loss was compensated by regeneration[15]. In the hypertrophic type
of peroneal muscular atrophy[15] and in alcoholic[14] and diabetic[24]
neuropathy the number of small fibres was diminished because of
lack of regeneration. When the histology suggests purely axonal
degeneration components may occur conducted at extremely slow
rates side by side with components conducted at a near normal or
moderately slowed rate.They must be attributed to regeneration.
This is illustrated in Fig. 7, which shows the sensory potentials
of the sural nerve in a patient with discrete signs and symptoms
of neuropathy. The patient was a 45-year-old woman who complained
of weakness in the legs for the past 14 months. The family history
was negative and the glucose tolerance test and vitamin levels of
B_{12} and B_6 in blood were normal. The force was graded as being
normal, there was no wasting, tendon jerks in the legs were weak
to absent, and tactile, vibrational and postural sensibility were
normal. The maximum conduction velocity and the amplitude of the
sensory potential were normal in the sural nerve, the only abnormality being components conducted at 3 to 9 m/s that do not occur
in normal nerve. The sensory conduction velocity along the distal
segment of the posterior tibial nerve was slowed to 78% of normal
and the amplitude of the sensory potential recorded at the medial
malleolus was diminished to 8% of normal. The biopy of the sural
nerve showed a diminished number of large fibres (1400, normal
range 1650-3300) and an increased incidence of clusters of regenerating fibres (63, normal range 0-38). Teased fibres were not
obtained.

When slowing of the fastest components is to more than 60% of
normal, the sensory potential does not give a clue as to whether
the late components are originally fast components or are due to
conduction along immature remyelinating fibres. There is experi-

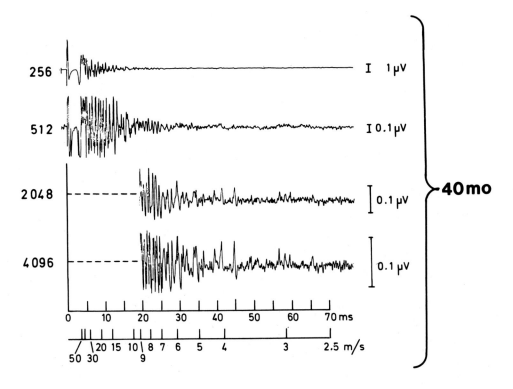

Fig. 5. Sensory potential evoked by maximal stimuli to the proximal phalanx of digit III and recorded at wrist, proximal to the site of suture of the median nerve. The recording was obtained 40 months after suture, when the cumulative amplitude and tactile sensibility were normal and the maximum sensory conduction velocity 80% of normal. The upper scale below the traces indicates the latency, the lower scale the conduction velocity. The figures to the left denote the number of responses that were averaged. The patient was 20 years old at the time of the suture[23].

mental evidence that demyelination is associated with slowing in conduction and may lead to block of nerve fibres. The muscle weakness in the absence of wasting in idiopathic poly-radiculo-neuropathy is due to block in conduction of demyelinated fibres[1,2,25,26]. The rapid recovery in muscle force is compatible with remyelination rather than with regeneration after axonal loss.

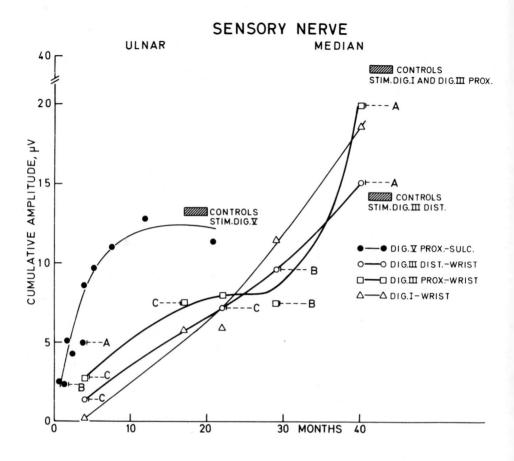

Fig. 6. Recovery of the cumulative amplitude of the sensory potentials recorded just proximal to the suture of the median nerve at
wrist (right) compared with the recovery of the sensory potential
recorded proximal to the elbow (left) after transient compression
of the ulnar nerve at the elbow. The patients were 20 and 33 years
old. A: Normal tactile sensibility. B: The patient could distinguish light touch (0.3 g) from pin-prick but was unable to localize the stimulus. C: The patient perceived touch as an uncharac-
teristic stimulus and was unable to distinguish touch from pin-
prick and to localize the stimulus.
The curves were drawn by eye[23].

Teased fibres are the only way to quantitate abnormalities in
the myelin sheath[28,29,30]. In evaluating myelin defects one must
consider that some abnormalities occur in controls[14]. Thus, in the

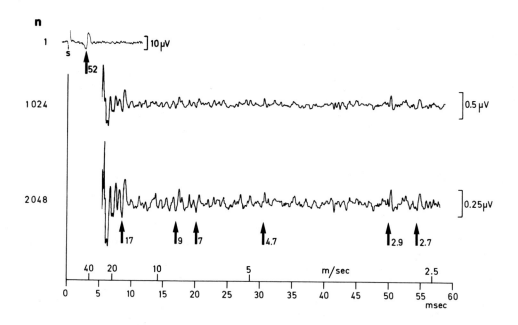

Fig. 7. Slow components conducted at 2.7-9 m/s (arrows) as the only electrophysiological abnormality in the sural nerve of a patient with discrete clinical signs and symptoms of neuropathy of unknown ætiology. The potential was evoked by maximal stimuli at the lateral malleolus and recorded at midcalf. The upper trace shows the potential, recorded by a single sweep, conducted at a maximum speed of 52 m/s. The lower traces show slow components after averaging of 1000 and 2000 responses (36°C).

seven controls we have analyzed (15 to 54 years old), rows of mye-linated segments occurred in up to 20% and solitary intercalated segments in up to 10% of the teased fibres. Segmental and parano-dal demyelination were not encountered (Fig. 8). Segmental demye-lination was found in 45 nerves of 167 patients with neuropathy. It usually occurred in less than 10% of teased fibres except in the hypertrophic type of peroneal muscular atrophy[15], in the neu-ropathy after gastrectomy[14] and in one patient with neuropathy of unknown ætiology[7]. In these conditions segmental demyelination was present in 30 to 100% of the fibres. Paranodal demyelination occurred in a quarter of the nerves, the incidence rarely exceed-ing 15%. We have obtained teased fibres from 9 nerves of patients

with diabetic neuropathy[24]. Segmental and paranodal demyelination
were rare: Segmental demyelination occurred in 8 of 141 teased
fibres from 2 nerves and paranodal demyelination in 17 of 198
teased fibres from 3 nerves. Both were present when the neuropathy
was of short duration. Since axonal degeneration was present in
all nerves, also in those from patients with the shortest duration
of the neuropathy, demyelination and axonal degeneration seem to
proceed side by side rather than demyelination being secondary to
axonal degeneration.

Segmental remyelination was increased above the level of controls in 33 nerves but only in 5 did more than half of the fibres
show this abnormality. The most frequent abnormality, seen in half
the nerves, is paranodal remyelination, i.e. solitary intercalated
segments. They occurred in half the nerves, twice the incidence in
controls.

In this connection the question arises whether findings obtained
over 10 mm of 50 teased nerve fibres are representative for the
120 to 150 mm of the 100 to 3500 fibres over which conduction velocity was determined[7]. Teased fibres were obtained from 3-5 different fascicles. This probably compensates for the differences in
myelin abnormalities in different fascicles.

The incidence of fibres with myelin abnormalities did not increase proportionately with the length over which the fibres were
teased. Thus, in 16 nerves of patients with slowing that could
not be explained by loss of the largest fibres, the incidence of
normal fibres, of fibres with myelin abnormalities and of myelin
defects per fibre (including remyelination) obtained over 5 mm of
teased fibres was compared with that obtained over 10 mm of teased fibres[5]. When the length of nerve teased was 10 mm, the incidence of abnormalities was 30% higher instead of doubled. By
extrapolation Mr. Steenstrup found (unpublished) that the incidence of fibres with myelin damage increases from e.g. 20% in
10-mm-long teased fibres to 50% over a 130-mm-long portion of the
nerve, i.e. with this assumption half of the fibres do not have
segments with myelin abnormalities[7].

It is unlikely that the diminished conduction velocity in demyelinating neuropathy is due to selective loss or block of the fastest fibres. This would result in a shortening of the duration of

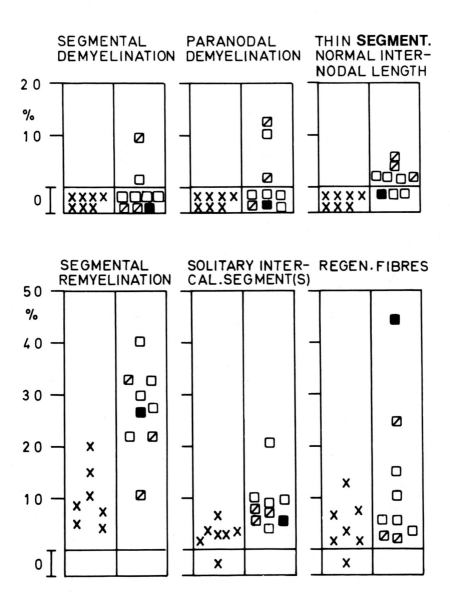

Fig. 8. Incidence of fibres with myelin abnormalities and of regenerated fibres among teased fibres from sural nerves of controls
(X) and of patients with diabetic neuropathy of different types:
sensory (□), sensory-motor (■), multiple mononeuropathy (▨)[24].

the sensory potential. In fact, the slowed potentials were prolonged. Nor can the decreased conduction velocity be due to selective slight slowing of conduction in the fastest fibres (9 to 14 μm
in diameter) because this would result in an increased amplitude.
In fact, the amplitude was decreased. Therefore either all components of the potential are conducted at a diminished velocity, or
the fastest fibres are slowed such that they contribute or give
rise to components throughout the range of velocities represented
in the prolonged potential. Slowing in conduction per se causes
an increased temporal dispersion and thereby a diminished amplitude. Reconstruction of the compound sensory potential from its
components showed that an amplitude of less than 40% of normal
could not be accounted for solely by temporal dispersion[8,10].

The relation of histological abnormalities to slowing in conduction was evaluated in the 43 nerves with slowing from which teased
fibres were obtained (Fig. 9). In 18 nerves slowing was moderate
and was due to axonal loss; demyelination occurred in less than
3% of teased fibres. Conversely, in 9 nerves, axonal loss could
not explain the marked slowing; demyelination was seen in many
teased fibres and could account for the marked slowing.

There remain 16 nerves (37%), among these three from diabetic
neuropathy, in which slowing could be explained neither by fibre
loss nor by the incidence of demyelination present in at most 20%
of the fibres. Remyelination occurred as frequently in nerves with
as in those without slowing. With remyelination included in the
incidence of myelin defects, the model on which the extrapolation
and the statistical calculations were based shows that so many
fibres do not have myelin defects over the length along which conduction is measured that morphologically evident defects cannot
explain the slowing in conduction. There are conditions in which
slowing occurs in the absence of structural changes: i) In the
hypoxic segment of the nerve conduction decreased to 40% of the
pre-hypoxic level[31,32], whereas it regained normal velocity proximal to the hypoxic segment, indicating that there was true slowing
before conduction was blocked (Fig. 10)[32]. Presumably hypoxia prolonged the rate of rise of the nodal action current. ii) In experimental diabetes[34,35] and in galactosæmia[36] slowing in conduction has been found in the absence of fibre loss or other struc-

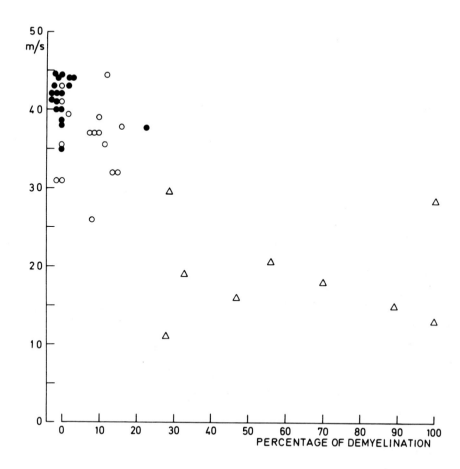

Fig. 9. Maximum sensory conduction velocity as a function of the incidence of segmental and paranodal demyelination in teased fibres of 43 sural nerves with slowed conduction from the lateral malleolus to midcalf: ●18 nerves in which slowing in conduction was as to be expected from the diameter of the largest myelinated fibres. Δ 9 nerves with a high incidence of demyelination and disproportionate slowing (p. 8). o 16 nerves with disproportionate slowing and an incidence of demyelination of 19% or less[7,22].

tural or ultrastructural changes. Some kind of a functional defect in the nerve membrane may be more common than hitherto assumed. When superimposed on the slowing due to loss of fast fibres the functional defect may explain why in nerves with proportionate slowing the recorded velocity tended to be slightly lower than that calculated from diameter. Depending on the severity of the defect, nerves in alcoholic, diabetic or postinfectious neuropathy may exhibit proportionate or disproportionate slowing.

MINIMUM ELECTROPHYSIOLOGICAL REQUIREMENTS FOR THE DIAGNOSIS OF POLYNEUROPATHY

In most patients the clinical examination can establish whether or not a patient has polyneuropathy. When the clinical investigation shows discrete abnormalities and leaves doubt the electrophysiological study and nerve biopsy or both may help to substantiate a diagnosis. It is then important to appreciate the limitations and the diagnostic significance of these studies. Even though the temperature is kept constant, there is a considerable scatter in the conduction velocity and particularly in the amplitude of the evoked responses in normal subjects matched for age. With respect to motor conduction velocity we have to consider that one large motor nerve fibre results in the measurement of a normal maximum conduction velocity even if all other fibres conduct abnormally slowly. In general, abnormalities in sensory or motor conduction in a single nerve are insufficient evidence to diagnose a systemic neuropathy. A low amplitude of the sensory potential of the ulnar nerve at wrist or mild slowing in motor or sensory conduction velocity along the ulnar nerve in the forearm may be secondary to local damage of the nerve at the elbow. Similarly, slowing along the distal sensory or motor branch of the deep peroneal nerve is a poor indicator of a systemic neuropathy since this nerve is often damaged by pressure.

The most prominent abnormality in men with increased levels of lead in the blood was a prolonged latency from the ankle to the extensor digitorum brevis muscle[21]. This turned out to be due to pressure by the metal-lined safety shoes rather than to a subclinical lead neuropathy. For the same reason, electromyographic signs of partial denervation in the extensor digitorum brevis muscle (diminished number of motor units or fibrillation potentials or both) are unreliable signs of systemic disease.

The nerve biopsy can give information as to the nature and the severity of pathological changes; only rarely can it contribute to elucidate the ætiology (amyloid neuropathy, metachromatic leucodystrophy, hereditary neuropathy with liability to pressure pal-

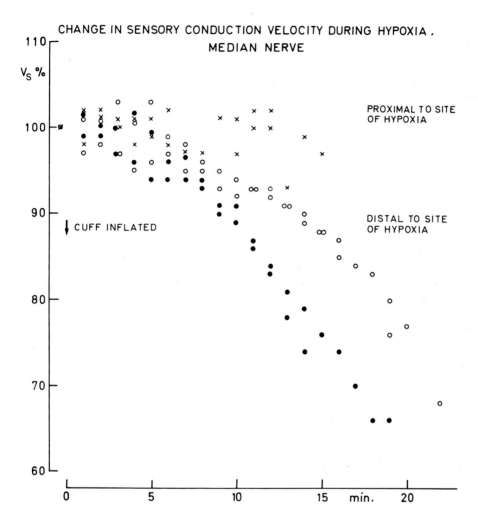

CHANGE IN SENSORY CONDUCTION VELOCITY DURING HYPOXIA.
MEDIAN NERVE

Fig. 10. The normal maximal sensory conduction velocity (V_S) proximal to the region of hypoxia (X) for the 15 min of hypoxia (abscissa) during which a sensory potential could be discriminated outside the region of hypoxia, illustrates that the same fibres along which conduction was slowed in the hypoxic portion of the nerve conducted at a normal rate proximal to it. Thus, slowing in the hypoxic segment is not due to block of the largest fibres[33].

sies etc.). Onion-bulb formations, once thought to be specific of hypertrophic neuropathy, have been observed in neuropathies of different ætiology. An increase in the perivascular space of endoneurial vessels thought to characterize diabetic neuropathy has been found in other neuropathies as well[24]. Unless histological abnormalities are advanced, it is necessary to quantitate biopsy findings in cross-sections and among teased fibres. We have determined the total number of myelinated nerve fibres from transverse sections of the nerve in toto rather than their number per mm^2. In two-thirds of the sural nerves taken from 100 consecutive neuropathies the endoneurial area was increased above that in 10 controls. An increased endoneurial area may simulate (19% of the nerves) or erroneously accentuate (21% of the nerves) loss of nerve fibres[13].

In summary: If diabetes, uræmia and alcoholism can be excluded and the patient shows discrete neurological symptoms and signs we investigate (i) the sural nerve, from the lateral malleolus to midcalf, (ii) motor and sensory conduction along the peroneal nerve from ankle to capitulum fibulae (on the contralateral leg) and (iii) motor and sensory conduction along the distal segments of the median and posterior tibial nerves.

These studies we supplement by electromyography of a muscle with moderate weakness in the lower and the upper extremities (e.g. m.tibialis anterior and m.abductor pollicis brevis).

Unless we find abnormalities in conduction (velocity or amplitude) in at least two nerves and electromyographic abnormalities in at least one muscle, we consider the electrophysiological study inconclusive. One or the other of these patients may non the less have a neuropathy which only can be demonstrated by quantified biopsy findings.

ACKNOWLEDGEMENTS

We are indebted to the Departments of Neurology of the Rigshospital and of the Municipal and County Hospitals, Copenhagen, for referring patients under their care. The sural biopsies were skillfully performed by the staff of the Department of Neurosurgery, Rigshospital, Copenhagen. We thank Mr. S. Stenstrup of the Institute of Physics II for calculating the incidence of nerve fibres with myelin abnormalities with increasing fibre length.

The work was supported by grants from the Michaelsen Foundation, Copenhagen and the Muscular Dystrophy Associations of America, New York.

REFERENCES

1. Gilliatt, R.W. (1966) Proc. Roy. Soc. Med., 59, 989-993.

2. Gilliatt, R.W. (1973) in New Developments in Electromyography and Clinical Neurophysiology, Desmedt, J.E. ed., S. Karger, Basel, vol. 2. pp. 2-18.

3. Dyck, P.J., Gutrecht, J.A., Bastron, J.A., Karnes, W.E. and Dale, A.J.D. (1968) Mayo Clin. Proc., 43, 81-123.

4. Thomas, P.K. (1971) Proc. Roy. Soc. Med., 64, 295-298.

5. Dyck, P.J., Johnson, W.J., Lambert, E.H. and O'Brien, P.C. (1971) Mayo Clin. Proc., 46, 400-431.

6. Hopkins, A. (1970) J. Neurol. Neurosurg. Psychiat., 33, 805-816.

7. Behse, F. and Buchthal, F. (1978) Brain, 101, 473-493.

8. Buchthal, F. and Rosenfalck, A. (1966) Brain Res. (Amsterdam), 3, 1-122.

9. Behse, F. and Buchthal, F. (1971) J. Neurol. Neurosurg. Psychiat., 34, 404-414.

10. Buchthal, F. and Rosenfalck, A. (1971) Brain, 94, 241-262.

11. Buchthal, F., Behse, F. and Rosenfalck, A. (1975) in Peripheral Neuropathy, Dyck, P.J., Thomas, P.K. and Lambert, E.H. eds., W.B. Saunders, Philadelphia, vol. 1., pp. 442-464.

12. Behse, F., Buchthal, F., Carlsen, F. and Knappeis, G.G. (1972) Brain, 95, 777-794.

13. Behse, F., Buchthal, F., Carlsen, F. and Knappeis, G.G. (1974) Brain, 97, 773-784.

14. Behse, F. and Buchthal, F. (1977) Ann. Neurol. 2, 95-110.

15. Behse, F. and Buchthal, F. (1977) Brain, 100, 67-85.

16. Gasser, H.S. and Erlanger, J. (1927) Amer. J. Physiol., 80, 522-547.

17. Behse, F., Buchthal, F. and Rosenfalck, A. (1973) in Studies in Neuromuscular Diseases, Kunze, K. and Desmedt, J.E., eds., S. Karger, Basel, pp. 229-231.

18. Buchthal, F. and Behse, F. (1977) Brain, 100, 41-66.

19. Walsh, J.E. and McLeod, J.G. (1970) J. Neurol. Sci., 10, 457-469.

20. McLeod, J.G. (1971) J. Neurol. Sci., 12, 333-349.

21. Buchthal, F. and Behse, F. (1978) Brit. J. Industr. Med., accepted for publication.

22. Buchthal, F. and Behse, F. (1978) in Contemporary Clinical Neurophysiology, Cobb, W.A. and van Duijn, H.J., eds., Electroenceph. Clin. Neurophysiol. Suppl. 34, pp. 373-383.

23. Buchthal, F. and Kühl, V., in preparation.

24. Behse, F., Buchthal, F. Carlsen, F. (1977) J. Neurol. Neurosurg. Psychiat., 40, 1072-1082.

25. Kaeser, H.E. and Lambert, E.H. (1962) Electroenceph. Clin. Neurophysiol., Suppl. 22, 29-35.

26. McDonald, W.I. (1963) Brain, 86, 481-500.

27. Rasminsky, M. and Sears, T.A. (1972) J. Physiol. (London), 227, 323-350.

28. Fullerton, P.M., Gilliatt, R.W., Lascelles, R.G. and Morgan-Hughes, J.A. (1965) J. Physiol. (London), 178, 26P-28P.

29. Gutrecht, J.A. and Dyck, P.J. (1966) Mayo Clin. Proc., 41, 775-777.

30. Takahashi, K. (1908) J. Comp. Neurol., 18, 167-197.

31. Caruso, G., Labianca, O. and Ferrannini, E. (1973) J. Neurol. Neurosurg. Psychiat., 36, 455-466.

32. Nielsen, V.K. and Kardel, T. (1974) Acta Physiol. Scand., 92, 249-262.

33. Behse, F. and Buchthal, F. (1975) 21st Scand. Congr. Neurol., Abstract, p. 4.

34. Sharma, A.K. and Thomas, P.K. (1974) J. Neurol. Sci., 23, 1-15.

35. Sharma, A.K., Thomas, P.K. and De Molina, A.F. (1977) Diabetes, 26, 689-692.

36. Sharma, A.K., Thomas, P.K. and Baker, R.W.R. (1976) J. Neurol. Neurosurg. Psychiat., 39, 794-802.

BASIC PROBLEMS IN
PERIPHERAL NERVE PATHOLOGY

Peripheral Neuropathies
N. Canal and G. Pozza, eds.
© 1978 Elsevier/North-Holland Biomedical Press

FACT AND FANCY IN THE HISTOLOGICAL DIAGNOSIS OF DENERVATION [x]

C. COERS and N. TELERMAN-TOPPET

Department of Neurology. Brugmann Hospital, Brussels University

Myopathic changes of the muscle fibers occur frequently in chronic denervation [1,2,3] and may lead to misdiagnosis particularly within the group of
limb girdle muscular atrophy (fig. 1), many cases of which, formerly considered as muscular dystrophy had to be included within the group of spinal
muscular atrophy [4]. Conversely, the group atrophy pattern, considered as
the hallmark of denervation may occasionally be observed in myopathy [5]
(fig. 2).

Histochemical study of muscle biopsies has provided new morphological
criteria of denervation. A striking change, probably related to collateral
reinnervation and enzymatic conversion of reinnervated muscle fibers, has
been described as type grouping [6] (fig. 3). It seems likely that this conversion is preceded by a transitional state characterized by a blurring of the
reciprocal relationship between glycolytic and oxydative enzymes (intermediate fibers [7] and type III fibers [8]) (fig. 4). It has also been assumed that
denervated fibers undergoing atrophy became angulated and darkly stained
with oxydative enzymes, particularly NADH-TR [9]. However these changes,
although characteristic, are not specific of denervation. Type grouping is
occasionally seen in myopathy and has been related to regeneration of muscle
fibers (myopathic type grouping [10,11]). Small angular dark fibers are
numerous in facio-scapulo-humeral and in oculo-pharyngeal dystrophy and
absent in Werdnig Hoffman infantile spinal muscular atrophy [9]. Intermediate and type III fibers are found in high proportion in muscular dystrophy
particularly the Duchenne type [12] (fig. 5).

An increased collateral branching of intramuscular motor axons quantitatively estimated by a high value of the terminal innervation ratio (TIR) is
very frequent in all denervating conditions (fig. 6), but has also been
occasionally found in limb girdle and facio-scapulo-humeral muscular

---

[x] This work was supported by grants from the F.R.S.M. of Belgium and
from the Free University of Brussels.

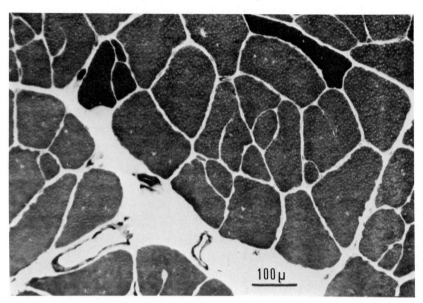

Fig. 1. Kugelberg-Welander disease ATPase. Type I fiber predominance and marked longitudinal splitting.

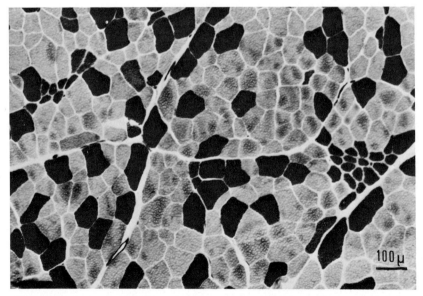

Fig. 2. Limb girdle muscular dystrophy ATPase. Two groups of small type II fibers are seen.

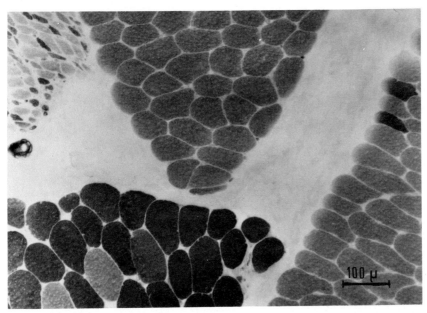

Fig. 3. Charcot-Marie-Tooth disease ATPase. Type grouping and large group atrophy.

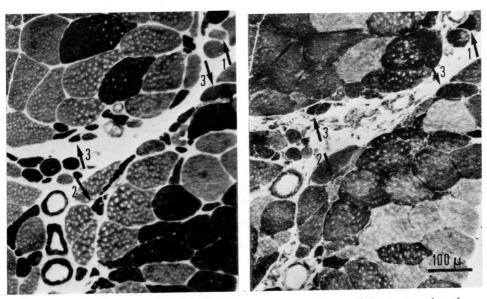

Fig. 4. Left ATPase, right NADH-TR. Serial sections. Polyneuropathy of unknown etiology, shows dark fibers of various sizes, round or angular of type I and III and small type II fibers (arrows).

dystrophy and more often in myotonic dystrophy [13].

This paper is devoted to a critical analysis of the reliability of histological data in the diagnosis of denervation, namely the group atrophy pattern, the type grouping, the small angulated dark fibers, the muscle fibers with aberrant enzymatic profile, and the terminal innervation ratio.

1. Group atrophy. The pattern of muscular atrophy was studied in 130 biopsies from various denervating conditions. Results are reported on Table 1.

TABLE 1

VOLUMETRIC CHANGES OF MUSCLE FIBERS IN DENERVATION

	No changes	Random Single fiber atrophy	Group atrophy	Uniform atrophy
Neuropathy				
clinically normal				
muscle (38)	13	22	3	0
weak muscle (51)	8	22	20	1
Charcot-Marie-Tooth				
disease (10)	1	2	7	0
Lower motor				
neurone disorders(31)	4	9	18	0

Group atrophy was found in 37 % of biopsies only and more frequently in motor neurone disorders (ALS, spinal muscular atrophy) and Charcot-Marie-Tooth disease than in acquired neuropathy. In these condition group atrophy was mostly found in biopsies from weak muscles. In other cases, volumetric changes were absent or were of the single fiber atrophy type : marked variability of fiber sizes with random distribution of the atrophic fibers, a pattern formerly considered as myopathic. On the other hand, small groups of atrophic fibers were observed in limb girdle myopathy. We found this change in 2 on 14 biopsies (fig. 2). Moreover small group atrophy pattern may also be seen in type II atrophy without overt denervation [14] (fig. 7).

2. Type grouping. Type grouping can be estimated on the basis of the greatest number of adjacent and enclosed fibers of the same enzymatic type

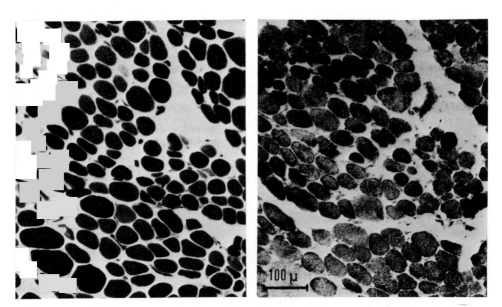

Fig. 5. Left ATPase, right NADH-TR. Serial sections. Duchenne muscular dystrophy. Impaired fiber type differenciation.

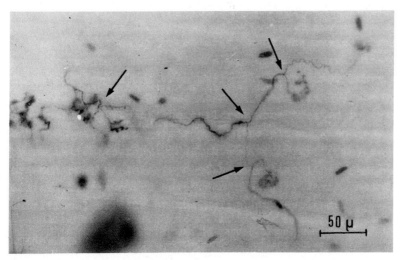

Fig. 6. Methylene blue vital staining. Charcot-Marie-Tooth disease. Collateral ramification (arrows).

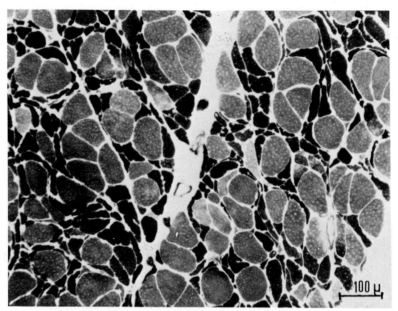

Fig. 7. ATPase. Rhumatoïd arthritis, corticotherapy. Type II atrophy with formation of groups of small type II fibers.

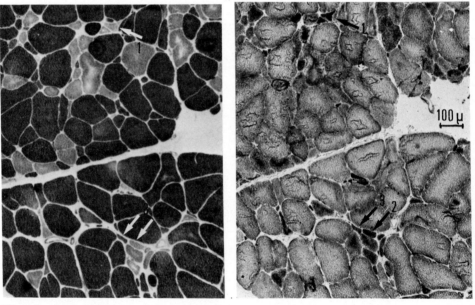

Fig. 8. Left ATPase, right NADH-TR serial sections. Limb girdle muscular dystrophy. Small dark type I and type III fibers, rounded or angulated (arrows).

found in the cross sectional area of the specimen [15] . Obviously this value is biased by the relative proportion of type I and type II fibers, and will be artificially increased for the predominant type. True type grouping can be accepted to take place only if groups of both types are observed in the biopsy, or, at least if, in addition to large groups of one type, a mozaïc pattern is present in other parts of the biopsy.

Unequivocal grouping of both fiber types is rather uncommon. It was found only in 9 on 50 biopsies from denervation, the highest incidence occured in Charcot-Marie-Tooth disease (4 on 6 cases). On Table 2 is reported the statistical analysis of quantitative data on type grouping obtained in 35 biopsies from neuropathy, 6 from Charcot-Marie-Tooth disease (CMT) and 9 from amyotrophic lateral sclerosis (ALS).

TABLE 2

TYPE GROUPING

	Contiguous fibers				Enclosed fibers			
	type I		type II		type I		type II	
	mean	SD	mean	SD	mean	SD	mean	SD
Controls	10.7	2.9	11.6	4.0	0.7	0.9	1.5	1.9
Neuropathy	20.7	27.0	16.6	15.9	11.0	24.5	5.5	16.7
CMT	74.2	68.3	62.5	60.5	63.3	72.0	46.0	59.7
ALS	10.7	7.5	18.0	7.6	1.4	2.7	4.5	4.4
Comparison t controls and neuropathy p	0.058 NS		2.386 NS		2.449 NS		5.714 0.01	
Comparison t controls and CMT p	5.838 < 0.001		5.236 < 0.001		5.502 < 0.001		6.325 < 0.001	
Comparison t controls and ALS p	0.019 NS		1.519 NS		1.019 NS		3.889 0.01	
Comparison t CMT and ALS p	2.816 < 0.05		2.221 < 0.05		2.628 < 0.05		2.117 < 0.05	

The mean value of the highest number of contiguous and enclosed type I fibers in neuropathy and ALS is not significantly different from control values. Only enclosed type II fibers are significantly more numerous. In

CMT, however, there is a highly significant increase of type grouping coefficients of both fiber types as compared to controls, and a significant increase as compared to ALS.

These data provide a quantitative basis to the statement that type grouping is anusual in neuropathy and ALS and occurs predominantly in Charcot-Marie-Tooth disease.

3. Small angular dark fibers. The presence of small fiber having a angulated outline is generally considered as indicative of denervation. According to Dubowitz and Brooke [9] these fibers, in addition to their angular shape, must be darkly staining with oxydative enzymes. In fact, an atrophic muscle fiber becomes angulated when it is closely surrounded and apparently compressed by other fibers. If there is a loss of muscle fibers and an endomyosial proliferation, the small fibers remain circular. This situation is more likely to occur in myopathy, but this is by no means always the case and when compact bundles are preserved, small fibers become angular (fig. 8). Conversely if a loss of muscle fibers and endomysial fibrosis takes place in denervation, the atrophic fibers are rounded. Therefore, an angular profile alone is irrelevant in the identification of denervated fibers.

Atrophic fibers either rounded or angulated may be darkly stained with NADH-TR. If weakly reactive with ATPase, they conform to the normal profile of type I fibers and are observed both in denervation and myopathy (fig. 4, 8). If strongly reactive for this enzyme, they fall in the category of fibers with aberrant enzymatic profile that we have classified as type III and assumed to represent a transitional state of the reinnervation of a muscle fiber by an axonal sprout of the other type preceding the type grouping [8]. An indication of the neurogenic nature of type III fibers has been obtained in type II atrophy, in which small type III fibers are more numerous when this kind of atrophy is related to denervation. This difference is significant if biopsies are compared according to a normal or an increased value of the Terminal Innervation Ratio [14]. Therefore, in type II atrophy the only histochemical evidence that denervation is taking place is the presence of small type III fibers, whether angulated or not.

From this finding and with regard to the conversion hypothesis, we have compared the proportion of muscle fibers with aberrant enzymatic profile, including small type III fibers (S III, Table 3), in denervation and in myopathy.

4. Muscles fibers with aberrant enzymatic profile. Fibers having no reciprocal relationship between ATPase and NADH-TR were labelled either type III when that had a high activity for both enzymes, or intermediate (int.) when they had a medium activity for ATPase as compared to typical type I and type II fibers. The proportion of these fibers is reported on Table 3 in control biopsies and in a variety of pathological conditions.

Fibers with aberrant profile, scarce in normal muscles, are present in variable proportion both in denervation and in myopathy (fig. 4, 5, 8), without significant difference, so that these fibers cannot be kept as a diagnostic index of peripheral nerve or motor neurone involvment. On the other hand, blurring of the reciprocal relationship between ATPase and NADH-TR appears as a non specific change that can be related not only to type conversion linked to reinnervation but to primary metabolic disorders of the muscle fiber as well [12, 16].

TABLE 3

PROPORTION OF ABERRANT FIBERS (%)

| Fiber type | Controls | | Neurop. | | CMT | | ALS | | Muscular dystrophy | | | | | |
| | | | | | | | | | Duchenne | | limb girdle | | FSH | |
	mean	SD	mean	SD	mean	SD	mean	SD	mean	SD	mean	SD	mean	SD
III	0.4	0.9	9.8	14.5	4.9	11.2	14.9	12.4	20.1	8.1	4.5	30.1	8.1	8.3
SIII	0.1	0.3	8.2	11.8	3.3	9.2	9.7	11.1	7.2	4.6	1.9	3.1	15.5	29.8
Int.	0.8	1.6	1.6	1.8	12.7	23.9	3.5	2.8	7.5	4.5	1.3	1.7	5.5	6.4

5. Terminal Innervation Ratio (TIR). The importance of collateral ramification of intramuscular motor axons can be estimated by the TIR, that is, the number of muscle fibers innervated by a given number of axons [17]. TIR measurements in various neuromuscular disorders are reported on Table 4.

The mean value of TIR is significantly increased in all denervating conditions under study, even in biopsies from clinically normal muscles in neuropathy, and remains normal in Duchenne dystrophy. Moreover a TIR exceeding 1.26 (mean of controls + 3 SD) is found in 83 % of all denervating condition including 70 % of clinically normal muscles in neuropathy, whereas it stays within normal limits in all cases of Duchenne dystrophy. It seems likely that the high values obtained in 1 limb girdle and 3 facio-scapulo-humeral syndromes correspond to cases of spinal muscular atrophy with myopathic changes of the muscle fibers [18].

TABLE 4

TERMINAL INNERVATION RATIO (TIR)

	mean TIR	Signifiance		Number of biopsies with	
				increased	normal
		t	p	TIR	TIR
Controls	1.11 ± 0.05				
Neuropathy		7.840	<0.001		
clinically normal muscle	1.43	4.018	<0.01	26	11
weak muscle	1.78			40	1
ALS	1.66	3.222	<0.005	16	2
CMT	2.16			12	0
Spinal muscular atrophy	2.27			6	0
Muscular dystrophy					
Duchenne	1.12	0.8575	NS	0	19
limb girdle	1.16			1	14
FSH	1.25			3	5

CONCLUSION

Both group atrophy and type grouping are reliable index of denervation but much less specific and sensitive than an increased Terminal Innervation Ratio.

These muscle fiber changes are found in a limited number of biopsies from denervating conditions, particularly the type grouping pattern, and they are occasionally observed in myopathy, whereas the TIR is increased in the majority of biopsies from denervation, even in clinically normal muscles, and remains normal in practically all cases of myopathy.

Other changes, namely small angulated dark fibers and impaired fiber type differenciation, are misleading since they are found both in denervation and myopathy, and cannot be taken as evidence of denervation if other data suggesting this possibility are not avaliable.

Small fibers of both types may become angulated in all kinds of muscular atrophy, provided there is neither loss of muscle fibers nor endomysial proliferation. Small fibers strongly reactive to ATPase and NADH-TR, either angulated or rounded may indeed represent a state of enzymatic conversion in the process of denervation-reinnervation, but may also be the expression of primary metabolic disturbance of the muscle fiber, since they are present in myopathic muscles as well as in denervated muscles.

REFERENCES

1. Haase, G.R. and Shy, G.M. (1960) Brain, 83, 631-637.

2. Drachman, D.B., Murphy, S., Nigham, N.P. and Hills, J.R. (1967) Arch. Neurol., 16, 14-24.

3. Mumenthaler, M. (1970) in Muscle Diseases, Walton J.N. et al eds., Excerpta Medica, Amsterdam, International congress series n° 199, pp. 585-598.

4. Walton, J.N. (1973) in Clinical Studies in Myology, Kakulas B. ed., Excerpta Medica, Amsterdam, International congress series n° 295, pp. 429-438.

5. Dastur, D.K. and Razzak, Z.A. (1973) in Clinical Studies in Myology, Kakulas B. ed., Excerpta Medica, Amsterdam, International congress series n° 295, pp. 186-191.

6. Brooke, M.H. and Engel, W.K. (1966) Arch. of Physic. Med. Rehabil., 47, 99-121.

7. Morris, C.J. (1970) J. Neurol. Sci., 11, 129-136.

8. Telerman-Toppet, N. and Coërs, C. (1971) Pathol. Eur., 6, 50-55.

9. Dubowitz, V. and Brooke, M.H. (1973) Muscle Biopsy, a Modern Approach, in Major Problems in Neurology, W.B. Saunders Company Ltd ed., vol. 2.

10. Karpati, G., Carpenter, S., Melmed, C. et al (1974) J. Neurol. Sci., 23, 129-161.

11. Carpenter, S., Karpati, G., Heller, I. et al (1978) Neurology (Minneap), 28, 8-17.

12. Coërs, C. and Telerman-Toppet, N. (1977) Arch. Neurol., 34, 396-402.

13. Coërs, C., Telerman-Toppet, N. and Gérard, J.M. (1973) Arch. Neurol., 29, 215-222.

14. Telerman-Toppet, N. and Coërs, C. (1975) J. Neurol. Sci., 25, 449-461.

15. Jennekens, F.G.I., Tomlinson, B.E. and Walton, S.N. (1971) J. Neurol. Sci., 14, 245-257.

16. Coërs, C., Telerman-Toppet, N., Gérard, J.M. et al (1976) Neurology (Minneap), 26, 1046-1053.

17. Coërs, C. (1955) Acta Neurol. Belg., 55, 741-866.

18. Coërs, C. and Telerman-Toppet, N. (1978) To be published.

Peripheral Neuropathies
N. Canal and G. Pozza, eds.
© 1978 Elsevier/North-Holland Biomedical Press

HUMAN AND ANIMAL NEUROPATHIES STUDIED IN EXPERIMENTAL NERVE TRANSPLANTS

ALBERT AGUAYO, SUZANNE PERKINS, IAN DUNCAN AND GARTH BRAY
Department of Neurology, The Montreal General Hospital and McGill University,
Montreal, (Canada).

ABSTRACT

Schwann cell behaviour can be investigated in experimental nerve grafts
where Schwann cells in the grafted nerve segments survive and myelinate axons
regenerating from the proximal stump of the host nerve. By selecting host and
donor nerves, it is possible to create different combinations of axons and
Schwann cells from normal and abnormal nerves. Thus, Schwann cells from human
patients and allogenic mice have been transplanted into nerves of immunesuppressed mice and studied by quantitative ultrastructural and radioautographic
techniques. The results of these experimental nerve grafts indicate that: (a)
there is a primary failure of Schwann cells to form and sustain myelin in
Trembler and quaking mice, (b) the abnormal persistence of Schwann cell proliferation which is found in Trembler nerves also occurs when Trembler Schwann
cells are transplanted into normal nerves, (c) normal myelination influences
the calibre of axons, (d) transplanted human Schwann cells can myelinate mouse
axons , (e) myelination is deficient in transplants from the sural nerve of
a patient with Charcot-Marie-Tooth neuropathy.

INTRODUCTION

The normal function of a peripheral nerve depends on the concurrent action
of neuronal processes (axons) and sheath cells (Schwann cells and fibroblasts).
Axons can influence Schwann cell proliferation[1,2] and differentiation[3,4,5,6]
while the Schwann cells may exert metabolic and trophic influences on axons[7].
The role of fibroblasts in nerve is still poorly understood but recent information suggests these cells play a more important and complex role than
hitherto recognized[8,9].

The interdependencies between axons and sheath cells are also reflected
in the pathogenesis of certain neuropathies. Quantitative histologic analysis
of the distribution of segmental demyelination and axonal degeneration in sural
nerve biopsies has indicated that axonal abnormalities may cause a failure of
Schwann cells to sustain myelin in some neuropathies while changes in the

Schwann cells themselves are responsible in others[10]. In the present report we review the results of studies in which the technique of nerve grafting was applied to the question of whether axons or Schwann cells are primarily responsible for the pathogenesis of certain demyelinating neuropathies.

METHODS

The nerve graft technique is based on the observation that transplanted Schwann cells survive and myelinate host axons regenerating from the proximal stump of the recipient nerve[5,6]. It is therefore possible to combine axons and sheath cells from different animals, strains of animals, or species, and to assess the contribution of axons, Schwann cells and systemic factors to the development of a neuropathy.

For nerve grafting, a segment approximately 5 mm in length is removed from the donor nerve and immediately transplanted between the cut ends of the recipient mouse sciatic nerve at the mid-thigh level. Grafts are secured to the host nerve stumps by 10-0 nylon sutures. For allotransplants (grafts between genetically dissimilar individuals of the same species), the grafts were segments of whole sciatic nerves while single fascicles of human sural nerves obtained from biopsy or limb amputations were used as xenografts (transplants between different species). To prevent rejection of allo-and xenogenic nerve grafts antilymphocytic serum (ALS) was administered subcutaneously to the host animal in doses of 0.5 ml twice weekly beginning on the day of transplantation. This antiserum was prepared by injecting rabbits with a suspension of 10^9 living thymocytes[11]. At various intervals after grafting, host animals were sacrificed by systemic perfusion of aldehyde fixative. The grafted segments and the proximal and distal stumps of the regenerated nerve were examined by quantitative phase and electron microscope techniques and , in certain instances, by radioautography[12].

RESULTS

Transplantation of Peripheral Nerves from Mutant Mice

There are major alterations in axon-Schwann cell relationships in the nerves of Trembler (Tr) and quaking (qk) mutant mice. The Tr mutant has a dominantly-inherited neuropathy[13] characterized by the presence of abnormally-thin myelin sheaths and slow conduction in peripheral nerves[14], changes which have been considered to resemble those of human hypertrophic neuropathies[15]. In qk mice,

a recessively-inherited mutation[16], there is generalized hypomyelination of
the central and peripheral nervous systems[17]. The deficit in myelination is
present in newborn Tr mice while in qk mice the initial stages of myelin
formation appear to proceed normally until the first month of life. In addition
to the failure of myelination, there is also evidence of myelin breakdown in
Tr and qk mouse nerves; in Tr mice, segmental demyelination is prominent soon
after birth, while in qk nerves it is only found in animals older than one
month. In both mutants, but to a greater extent in Tr than in qk mice, demyelination coincides with an abnormal enhancement of Schwann cell multiplication
and an increase in the number of Schwann cells[12,18,19]. These abnormalities
are confined to the Schwann cells of myelinated nerves while Schwann cells in
the unmyelinated C-fibers are normal in structure and number[12]. Axonal diameters are reduced in Tr nerves but the total number of axons is normal in
both mutants[12].

The pathogenesis of the Tr and qk neuropathies was investigated in allo-
grafts of nerves from adult mice. Three types of nerve graft were prepared
(Fig.1): Type I, control grafts; nerve segments from C57BL/6J mice were grafted
into sciatic nerves of mice of the same strain but from a different litter. Type
II, mutant mouse nerves into normal nerves; segments from Tr or qk nerves were
grafted into sciatic nerves of C57BL/6J mice. Type III, normal grafts into
mouse mutants; segments from C57BL/6J nerves were grafted into sciatic nerves
of Tr or qk mice. In all regenerated grafted nerves examined 2 to 4 months
after grafting, the morphology of the donor was reproduced in the graft
while distal stumps of the host nerve always resembled proximal stumps.

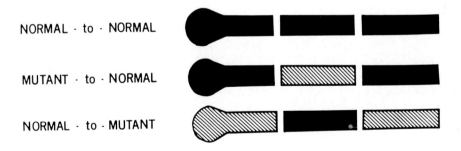

NORMAL · to · NORMAL

MUTANT · to · NORMAL

NORMAL · to · MUTANT

Fig.1. Schematic representation of nerve grafts used to study neuropathies of
Tr and qk mouse mutants. Type I (top): normal sciatic nerve segments are transplanted into sciatic nerves of normal mice. Type II (middle): A nerve from the
mutant is transplanted into a normal mouse nerve. Type III (bottom): A segment
of normal nerve is transplanted into a mutant.
(Black= normal nerves; Hatched= nerves from mutant mice)

40

In regenerated grafted nerves of Type I, the graft and distal stumps contained well-myelinated fibers. Type II animals showed normal proximal and distal stumps (recipient nerves) but fibers within the graft were deficient in myelin. The results of Type III experiments were the reverse of those seen in Type II grafts: regenerated fibers were normally myelinated in the grafted segment in contrast to the deficiency of myelination in the proximal and distal stumps of the same regenerated nerve[12,20] (Fig.2)

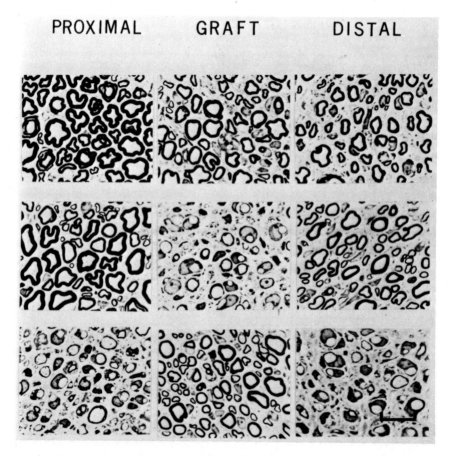

Fig.2. Phase micrographs of mouse sciatic nerve grafts at 3 different cross-sectional levels 2 months after grafting. Top row (Type I): normal into normal grafts demonstrate numerous myelinated fibers at all three levels. Middle row (Type II): after grafting a Tr mouse nerve into sciatic nerve of a normal mouse the proximal and distal stumps of the regenerated nerve are well myelinated while fibers within the grafted segment of the same nerve lack myelin or are hypomyelinated. Bottom row (Type III): normal nerve transplanted into Tr nerves results in a normal myelination of the grafted segment which contrasts with the abnormal appearance of the recipient nerve stumps. (Bar = 15 μm) (Reproduced with permission of Nature[20]).

The axon diameters of fibers in the proximal and distal stumps of Type III experiments (Trembler ——▶ normal ——▶ Trembler) resembled uninjured Tr nerves and were thinner than normal, but in the grafted portion where Tr axons were ensheathed by normal Schwann cells, axon diameters were normal; converse results were obtained in Type II (normal-Trembler-normal) experiments [12].

Radioautographic investigations of Schwann cell multiplication in 10-week-old grafts of normal or Tr Schwann cells transplanted into normal nerves demonstrated persistently high labelling indices in the regenerated nerves which contained transplants from the mutant; labelling indices were not elevated in grafts from normal animals and in the proximal and distal (normal) host nerve stumps [12,21]. The high labelling indices in normal-Trembler-normal (N-T-N) grafts resembled those in the intact Tr nerves. Thus, although Tr Schwann cells ensheathed normal axons in the regenerated N-T-N nerve graft, their increased rates of proliferation persist as in the intact nerve of the Tr mutant. Presumably myelin breakdown products are the stimulus for the continued proliferation of Tr Schwann cells [12].

The demonstration that the peripheral nerve abnormalities which characterize the neuropathies in Tr and qk mice are fully reproduced by transplanting their Schwann cells into normal nerves while the changes in the nerves of these mutants are locally corrected by grafts that contain normal Schwann cells is direct proof of a primary Schwann cell disorder in these genetically-determined neuropathies.

Transplantation of Human Schwann Cells into Immunesuppressed Mice.

On the basis of results of the investigations of neuropathies in mutant mice, it was subsequently determined that Schwann cells from human nerve segments transplanted into immunesuppressed mice will ensheath and myelinate axons regenerating from the host animal nerve [22].

Soon after the grafting of single fascicles from control human nerves, the nerve fibers in both the donor graft and the recipient distal stump undergo Wallerian degeneration but there is no rejection of human xenografts in the immunesuppressed animals. By 10 weeks after grafting, axons have grown from the proximal stumps through the graft and into the distal stumps and many myelinated fibers are seen at both these levels.

When myelination by mouse and human Schwann cells was compared by determining myelin lamellae/axon circumference ratios (ML/AC) in electron micrographs, it was found that although myelination of the mouse axons by mouse Schwann cells approximated normal values by two months, equivalent myelination of mouse axons by human Schwann cells in the graft was accomplished only by 6 months

42

after transplantation (Fig.3). These differences in the myelination of mouse
axons by human and mouse Schwann cells may be due to peculiar axon-Schwann cell
interactions in the xenografts, true species-related differences in the speed
of myelination or to experimental conditions affecting the grafts.

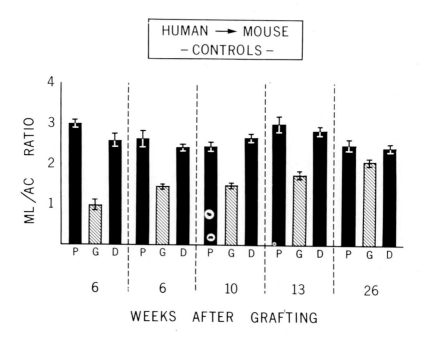

Fig.3. Myelination of mouse axons by human Schwann cells. Normal human Schwann
cells were transplanted into normal mice and ML/AC ratios determined in cross-
section electron micrographs. The ML/AC ratios in the grafted segments (G) are
lower than in proximal (P) and distal (D) stumps at 6,10 and 13 weeks after
grafting but are similar at 26 weeks.
Solid bars = myelin formed by mouse Schwann cells. Hatched bars = myelin
formed by human Schwann cells. (M ± SEM).

Because normal human and mouse Schwann cells are morphologically identical,
it was necessary to prove that, in xenografted nerves, the Schwann cells within
the grafted segment of the regenerated nerves actually originated from the
human nerve and had not migrated from the stumps of the recipient mouse nerves.
Although the possibility of Schwann cell migration has been found unlikely for
nerves regenerating in continuity[5,6,12] it is conceivable that Schwann cells

could behave differently in xenografts. The exact origin of Schwann in the graft was determined by discontinuing immunosuppression of the host mice at variable intervals after the transplantation of the human nerve grafts. In addition, two weeks after the discontinuation of ALS, host mice received an intravenous dose of 10^8 lymphoid cells from the spleen and lymph nodes of syngeneic mice hyperimmunized against human tissue[23]. This immune cell transfer was used to abrogate xenograft acceptance in the recipient animal. The earliest signs of xenograft rejection were observed 8 days after immune cell transfer (approximately 3 weeks after stopping ALS administration). Initial signs consisted of mononuclear cell infiltration of the grafted segments. At latter stages Schwann cells of myelinated and unmyelinated fibers were surrounded, penetrated and eventually replaced by mononuclear cells[22]. Perineurial fibroblasts were also rejected in the graft. During the acute phase of rejection, some axons became totally denuded of Schwann cells and were surrounded only by the basal lamina. The basal lamina, presumably because of weak antigenicity, appears to have been spared by the immune response. Schwann cells and fibroblasts in the proximal and distal stumps of the grafted nerves were not rejected. During graft rejection many fibers in the distal stump remained myelinated indicating that the continuity of their axons was preserved across the graft. Some axons were damaged, presumably within the graft, because a variable number of fibers underwent Wallerian degeneration in the distal stumps of the nerves containing the rejected grafts. The extent of the axonal damage during xenograft rejection varied from involvement of few axons in some animals to extensive axonal breakdown in other animals and may represent a "bystander", secondary effect of the immune response[24].

This method for the identification of the exact origin of Schwann cells in the grafted segment of regenerated xenografts also helps to document many morphologic features of cell-mediated immune response directed against sheath cells (Schwann cells of both myelinated and unmyelinated fibers as well as against fibroblasts) rather than against myelin itself as in most allergic neuropathies[25]. This study would not be possible during primary rejection of nerve grafts because, in such cases, the immunologic response is directed against all cellular components (sheath cells and axons alike) within the graft[26,27]. After the discontinuation of ALS the mice permitted to survive the period of xenograft rejection for over two months showed that the segments of nerve corresponding to the site of the graft were myelinated again. In these animals which had recovered their immunologic competence, it appears that the mouse axons were re-ensheathed by the animal's own Schwann cells which

44

presumably had migrated from the nerve stumps. This migration of Schwann cells
into areas lacking sheath cells may have been facilitated and guided by the
axons and basal lamina which survived graft rejection.

Transplantation into Mice of Nerve Segments from a Patient with Charcot-
Marie-Tooth Disease

A sural nerve biopsy was obtained from a 52 year old man with a dominantly-
inherited form of Charcot-Marie-Tooth (CMT) disease known to have affected
three generations of his family (Fig.4). Single fascicles from the biopsy

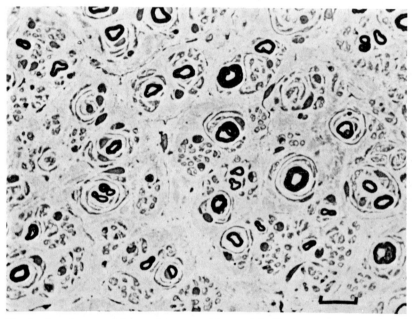

Fig.4. Sural nerve biopsy from a patient with Charcot-Marie-Tooth (CMT) disease
demonstrates deficient myelination and many "onion bulbs". (bar = 15 μm)

were transplanted into 17 immunesuppressed mice and studied from 6 weeks to 6
months after transplantation. These regenerated CMT grafts were compared with
18 control xenografts of sural nerve fascicles from the amputated leg of a 63
year old man with peripheral vascular disease. Although grafts and distal stumps
of the control xenografts were well myelinated by 6 weeks after transplantation,
a marked deficit of myelination was observed in the CMT grafts at all times
studied (Fig.5). By 3 months after transplantation, the density of myelinated
fibers in control grafts was nearly 10 times that of the CMT grafts (Fig.6).
Approximately 80% of axons with diameters greater than 1 μm were myelinated in
control grafts while in CMT grafts only 20% of such axons were myelinated.
These differences were not due to a failure of innervation of the CMT grafts by
mouse axons because the total density of axons in both the CMT and control grafts

were similar (Fig.6). By 6 months after transplantation the incidence
of large axons that were not myelinated was 7% in controls and nearly 60% in
CMT grafts. No significant differences in the thickness of the myelin sheath

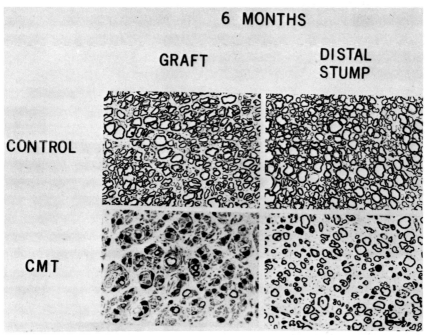

·Fig.5. Cross-sections of grafted segments and distal stumps from two regenerated
human-to-mouse nerve grafts 6 months after transplantation. Top:control sural
nerve graft.Bottom: Charcot-Marie-Tooth (CMT) disease transplant. The control
nerve is well myelinated at both levels while the CMT graft contains only a
few myelinated fibers and shows some concentric arrangement of Schwann cell
processes suggestive of an "onion bulb" formation. (bar = 15 μm)

(ML/AC ratios) of control and CMT grafts were found at 3 or 6 months after
transplantation. These experiments indicate that Schwann cells from the CMT
nerve have failed to myelinate mouse axons as effectively as Schwann cells from
control human nerves. Low grade rejection, poor vascularization and a lack of
innervation of the graft have been suggested as possible sources of error in
the interpretation of findings in xenograft experiments[28]. However, a low grade
rejection of xenografts by incomplete immunesuppression is unlikely because
such rejection would be easily detectable if myelin deficient CMT Schwann cells
were being replaced by host Schwann cells capable of normal myelination[12].

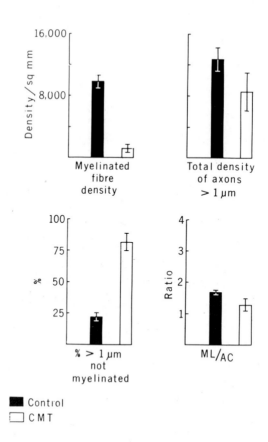

Fig.6.Three months after transplantation the density of myelinated fibers in control grafts is nearly 10 times that in CMT grafts but the density of axons with diameters greater than 1 µm is not statistically different between CMT and control grafts. For control grafts, the proportion of large axons that are not myelinated is only 20% while in the CMT grafts approximately 80% of these axons have no myelin. The relative thickness of the myelin sheath (ML/AC) is similar in both types of graft. (Values are expressed as M ± SEM;n=3 nerves each)

Inadequate vascularization of the graft would not explain the striking differences in myelination between control and CMT grafts. Finally, the results of axonal counts demonstrate that differences in CMT and control grafts are not due to a lack of innervation by axons from the host but result from a deficiency in myelination by the CMT cells.

The results in the CMT grafts closely resemble changes in the original nerve biopsy of the patient and those obtained after transplantation of nerve from the mouse mutant Trembler into normal mouse nerves[20]. Although the results of xenograft transplantation indicate that abnormalities in Schwann cells also play a major role in CMT neuropathy, additional axonal influences have not been excluded as definitely as in the Tr mutant mouse where normal Schwann cells have been grafted into the nerves of the affected host animal.

CONCLUSIONS

It is known that normal myelination depends on interactions between axons and sheath cells as well as more general environmental and nutritional influences. Unfortunately, our understanding of the biologic mechanisms involved in normal myelination as well as in the processes that lead to demyelination is hampered by the difficulty in delineating the specific role of each of these nerve components. Techniques are now available which may permit a more direct examination of axon and Schwann cell interdepencies. Neurons and Schwann cells can be segregated and recombined to study cell proliferation and myelin formation in vitro[1]. The nerve grafting method provides an additional in vivo approach. Both the cultured and the grafted Schwann cells are amenable to morphologic, radioautographic and biochemical studies which were often impossible while the cells were still part of the original nerve. The recent demonstration of the feasibility of transplanting central nervous system glia from optic nerves into peripheral nerves [29,30] provides another potential approach for studies of the mechanisms involved in myelination. Future work should establish the precise indications and limitations of these new experimental methods.

ACKNOWLEDGEMENTS

We thank Margaret Attiwell, Sandra Harrington, Jack Kasarjian, Jane Trecarten and Wendy Wilcox for valuable assistance and Drs. Patricia Kongshavn, Keisuke Mizuno and Emile Skamene for advice and help.

This work was supported by grants from the Canadian Medical Research Council, Muscular Dystrophy Association and Multiple Sclerosis Society and the American Dysautonomia Foundation.

REFERENCES

1. Wood, P. and Bunge, R.P. (1975) Nature 256: 662-664.
2. Aguayo, A.J., Peyronnard, J.M., Terry, L.C., Romine, J.S. and Bray, G.M. (1976) J. Neurocytol. 5: 137-155.

3. Weinberg, H. and Spencer, P. (1975) J. Neurocytol. 4: 395-418.

4. Weinberg, H. and Spencer, P. (1976) Brain Res. 113: 363-378.

5. Aguayo, A.J., Epps, J.S., Charron, L. and Bray, G.M. (1976) Brain Res. 104: 1-20.

6. Aguayo, A.J., Charron, L. and Bray, G.M. (1976) J. Neurocytol. 5: 565-573.

7. Varon, S.S. and Bunge, R.P. (1978) Ann. Rev. Neuroscience, Annual Reviews Inc. Palo Alto, California, pp.327-361.

8. Thomas, P.K. and Olsson, Y. (1975) in Peripheral Neuropathy, P.J. Dyck, P.K. Thomas and E.H. Lambert, eds., W.B. Saunders, Philadelphia, pp.168-184.

9. Bunge, R.P. and Bunge, M.B. (1978) J. Cell Biol. (in press).

10. Dyck, P.J., Johnson, W.J., Lambert, E.H. and O'Brien, P.C. (1971) Mayo Clin. Proc. 46: 432-436.

11. Levey, R.H. and Medawar, P.B. (1966) Proc. Nat. Acad. Sci. USA 56: 1130-1137.

12. Aguayo, A.J., Bray, G.M. and Perkins, S.C. (1978) Ann. N.Y.Acad. Sci. (in press).

13. Falconer, D.S. (1951) J. Genet. 50: 192-201.

14. Low, P.A. and McLeod, J.G. (1975) J. Neurol.Sci. 26: 565-574.

15. Ayers, M.M. and Anderson, McD. (1973) Acta Neuropath. 25: 54-70.

16. Sidman, R.L., Dickie, M.M. and Appel, S.H. (1964) Science 144: 309-311.

17. Samorajski, T., Friede, R.L. and Reimer, P.R. (1970) J. Neuropath. Exp. Neurol. 31: 352-369.

18. Perkins, S. , Mizuno, K., Aguayo, A.J. and Bray, G.M. (1977) Neurology 27: 377.

19. Perkins, S., Aguayo, A.J. and Bray, G.M. (1977) Clin. Res. 25: 709.

20. Aguayo, A.J., Attiwell, M., Trecarten, J., Perkins, S. and Bray, G.M. (1977) Nature 265: 73-75.

21. Perkins, S., Bray, G.M. and Aguayo, A.J. (1978) Neurology 28: 381.

22. Aguayo, A.J., Kasarjian, J., Skamene, E., Kongshavn, P. and Bray, G.M. (1977) Nature 268: 753-755.

23. Steinmuller, D. (1970) Transpl. Proc. 2: 438-445.

24. Madrid, R.C. and Wisniewski, H.M. (1977) J. Neurocytol. 6: 103-117.

25. Arnasson, B.G. (1975) in Peripheral Neuropathy, P.J. Dyck, P.K. Thomas and E.H. Lambert, eds., W.B. Saunders, Philadelphia, pp. 1110-1148.

26. DasGupta, T.K. (1967) Surg. Gynec. Obst. 125: 1058-1068.

27. Pollard, J.G. and Fitzpatrick, L. (1973) Acta Neuropath. 23: 152-165.

28. Dyck, P.J., Lais, A.C. and Low, P.A. (1978) Neurology 28: 261-265.

29. Weinberg,E. and Spencer, P. (1978) Brain Res. (in press).

30. Aguayo, A., Dickson, R., Trecarten, J., Attiwell, M., Bray, G. and Richardson, P. (1978) Neuroscience Letters (in press).

Peripheral Neuropathies
N. Canal and G. Pozza, eds.
© 1978 Elsevier/North-Holland Biomedical Press

ALTERED RATIO BETWEEN AXON CALIBER AND MYELIN THICKNESS IN SURAL
NERVES OF CHILDREN

J. MICHAEL SCHRÖDER, JÜRGEN BOHL*
Department of Neuropathology, Institute of Pathology, Hospitals
of the Johannes Gutenberg University, Langenbeckstraße 1,
6500 Mainz, West Germany

ABSTRACT

Maturation of myelin sheaths in normal sural nerves of children
proceeds more slowly than axon growth. This asynchronous
development of axons and myelin sheaths results in a statistically significant change of the ratio between axon caliber and
myelin thickness during normal development. Therefore, myelin
thickness of individual nerve fibers must be related to the size
of the axons as well as to the age of the individuals studied.
Abnormalities of the relationship between myelin thickness and
axon diameter (primary hypomyelination of large, or small, or all
fibers) were clearly identified in cases with metachromatic
leukodystrophy, KRABBE's, DEJERINE-SOTTAS', COCKAYNE's and
SANFILIPPO's disease, and in children with malignant neoplasms.
A striking reduction of axon diameters was seen in a unique case
with congenital, total absence of central and peripheral myelin.
On the other hand, in GM_2 gangliosidosis and ceroid lipofuscinosis no such disturbances were detected despite storage of
pathologic material in Schwann cells.

INTRODUCTION

In normal peripheral nerves, most investigators have found a
direct rectilinear correlation between myelin thickness and axon
diameter. Alterations of the ratio between axon caliber and
myelin thickness may occur following various pathologic conditions. Disproportionately thin myelin sheaths in relation to the
size of the axons are most frequently seen following segmental

---

*Supported in part by the Deutsche Forschungsgemeinschaft, Bonn-
Bad Godesberg, West Germany (Schr 195/3)

demyelination and remyelination due to diphtheritic neuritis, experimental allergic neuritis, Marek's disease, lead and tellurium neuropathy[1,2,3,4], or primarily demyelinating human neuropathies such as metachromatic leukodystrophy[5], KRABBE's leukodystrophy[6], DEJERINE-SOTTAS' hypertrophic neuropathy, and other disorders of peripheral nerves associated with secondary segmental demyelination subsequent to certain primary axonal neuropathies such as uremic neuropathy[7,8] dominantly inherited hypertrophic neuropathy[9], and others. Paranodal demyelination followed by remyelination also results in disproportionately thin myelin sheaths of the newly formed, abnormally short, intercalated internodes[10] although this has not been confirmed experimentally late after the lesion. Disproportionately thin myelin sheaths have also been noted around large axons following long periods after nerve grafting or nerve crushing in experimental animals[11].

By contrast, disproportionately thick myelin sheaths are seen following axonal atrophy that presumably results in an inward slippage of myelin lamellae secondary to a reduction of the axon diameter. This phenomenon is seen following regeneration of supernumerary nerve fibers not achieving adequate end contacts[3,12], and in a large number of neuropathies of the axonal or neuronal type. Disproportionately thick myelin sheaths may also occur in retrograde fiber change as a result of largely reversible shrinkage of the cross sectional area with preservation of the axonal circumference[12]; yet this type of axonal deformation with a relative increase of myelin thickness has not been worked out quantitatively thus far.

The various types of defective remyelination ("secondary hypomyelination"), or "secondary hypermyelination" following different types of axonal caliber reduction (axonal atrophy, retrograde fiber change) must be distinguished from defective maturation of myelin sheaths that will subsequently be called "primary hypomyelination". In the course of studying the development of nerve fibers in sural nerves of children[13], different types of alterations of the ratio between axon caliber and myelin thickness were observed: (1) Total absence of myelin associated with abnormally thin axon diameters in a unique case with a suggested defect of myelin anabolism; (2) primary hypomyelination

of large, or all fibers in various conditions such as inborn
errors of metabolism (usually associated with secondary hypomyelination due to segmental demyelination and incomplete remyelination); and (3) primary hypomyelination of small or intermediate fibers noted in three children with malignant neoplasms.

MATERIALS AND METHODS

Materials. In a preceeding study[13], the normal development of
the ratio between axon diameter and myelin thickness was morpho-
metrically examined in sural nerves of neonates or children
without evidence of neuropathy. In addition, 10 sural nerves of
subjects at the age of 19 to 65 years with no or very limited
evidence of neuropathy were used for obtaining comparable control
data in adults. For the present study, 65 normal and pathologic
nerves of subjects at the age of 4 months before term to 20 years
of age were evaluated by similar methods for establishing pathologic conditions of the ratio between axon diameter and myelin
sheath thickness.

Methods. The sural nerves were obtained at the lower midcalf
level by autopsy or biopsy. All nerves were fixed, embedded,
stained, and evaluated by identical methods although there was
some variation of the interval between biopsy and processing the
nerve from the initial 3.9% glutaraldehyde solution with 0.1
phosphate buffer (SØRENSON) to subsequent steps of washing in
buffer, and final embedding in epoxy resin, or between death and
autopsy.

For the evaluation of nerve fibers three different methods
were applied: (1) ocular micrometer measurements at a magnification of x2000 for determining axon diameter and myelin thickness of 20 selected, well preserved nerve fibers of the large
diameter group in each nerve; (2) semiautomatic evaluation of
light microscopic photographs at x1000 by a particle size ana-
lyser, the TGZ 3 Automatic (C. ZEISS, Oberkochen) for measuring
the axonal diameter and myelin thickness of large numbers of
nerve fibers in each nerve; and (3) electron microscopic counts
of the number of myelin lamellae and measurements of the axonal
circumference of nerve fibers on photographic enlargements at
x10.000 in selected nerves. (Further details regarding the

methods applied have been presented previously[13].)

RESULTS

Ocular micrometer measurements of large fibers in a number of cases with malformations of the central nervous system (Table 1) revealed considerable deviations of some values from the normal line although others were in the range of normal controls (Fig.1). Considerable deviations were seen in two anencephalics (A in Fig.1). Their sural nerves, however, were initially fixed in unbuffered 4 % formaldehyde and not in 3.9 % buffered glutaraldehyde as all the other nerves examined. Thus, their myelinated axons appear to be artificially swollen as are the unmyelinated fibers and all other cellular components of their nerves. The number of myelinated fibers per endoneural area (fiber density) however, is definitely reduced in the nerves of both anencephalics. Two cases with trisomy 18 (T in Fig 1) showing cerebellar hypoplasia and hydrocephalus, on the other hand, revealed myelin sheaths of normal thickness in relation to the age of the individuals but unusually large axons although their sural nerves were fixed in the same solutious as all the other nerves. Calculations of the regression lines based on measurements with a TGZ 3 Automatic revealed a remarkably limited increase of the regression lines in both cases. This then appears to indicate an abnormally large size of their axons during development. Erroneous dating of the developmental age in both cases seems to be unlikely. Electron microscopy revealed some degree of artificial swelling but not to the same degree as in the two anencephalics. On the other hand, there was one case with craniorachischisis also showing unusually large axons (C in Fig. 1), but this case showed myelin sheaths that were too thick for the presumed age of development. Thus it appears likely that this case has not been adequately dated. Another case with craniorachischisis (No. 4) was within the normal range (Fig. 1b).

One case with arhinencephaly (No. 8 in Table 1) and another with hydroanencephaly (No. 7) showed abnormally thin axons despite normally developed myelin sheaths. Other hydrocephalic cases showed abnormally thin myelin sheaths (No. 6), or total absence of myelin in the sural nerve (No. 5, Fig. 3). In the latter case

TABLE 1

MEAN MYELIN THICKNESS AND AXON DIAMETER OF LARGE FIBERS

No.	AGE (months)	MALFORMATION	MEYLIN (/um)	AXON (/um)	M/A RATIO
1	-3.5	anencephaly	0.5	4.9	0.087
2	-3	"	0.6	5.7	0.098
3	-2	craniorachischisis	0.9	4.6	0.187
4	-1.5	"	0.9	2.9	0.297
5	0.03	hydrocephalus; myelin deficiency	0	3	0
6	0.1	"	0.6	4	0.158
7	0.75	" (hydranencephaly)	1.1	3.9	0.273
8	1	" ; arhinencephaly	0.9	3.6	0.258
9	1	" ; trisomy 18	0.9	5.2	0.175
10	2	" "	1.1	6.3	0.173

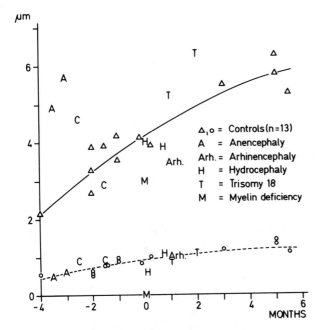

Fig. 1. Mean axon diameter (Δ) and myelin thickness (o) of 20 large diameter fibers in control cases and cases with malformations of the nervous system (see Table 1 and Text). The lines for the presumptive normal development of large axons and myelin sheaths were drawn by hand.

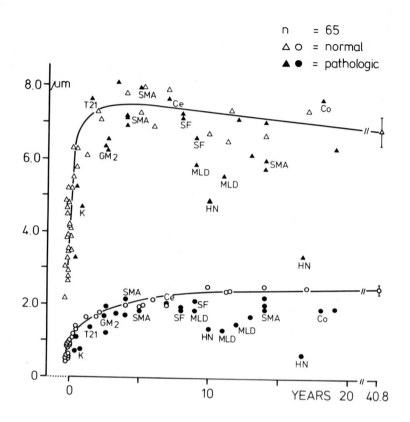

Fig. 2. Mean axon diameter and myelin thickness of 20 large diameter fibers in control cases and various pathologic conditions (for abbreviations and further details see text; T 21 = Trisomy 21). The lines for the presumptive normal development of both parameters were drawn by hand. The mean values with the standard deviations for 10 adult cases with a mean age of 40.8 years are indicated on the right side of the lines.

Fig. 3 a, b. Representative electron micrographs of promyelin fibers and Remak fibers in the sural nerve of case 5 (cf. Table 1) show an increased density of neurofilaments with very few microtubules, but neither myelin nor storage material (see Text). The nerve was obtained at autopsy, 48 hours after death. The bars indicate 1 μm.

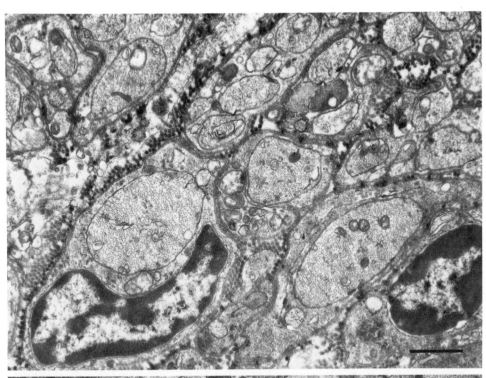

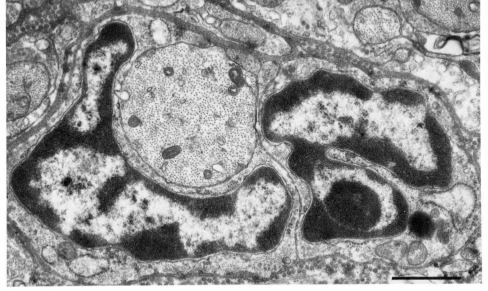

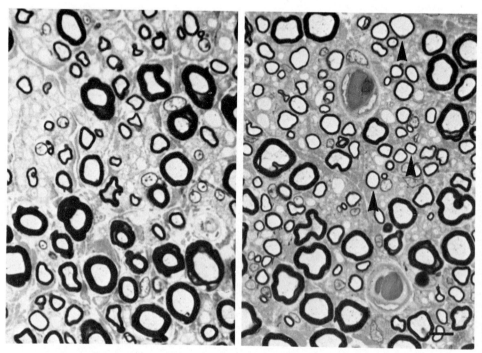

Fig. 4 a. The sural nerve of a 4-year-old boy shows nerve fibers
with normal axon diameters and myelin sheaths at this stage of
development. b. Numerous axons of small and intermediate size
are surrounded by disproportionately thin myelin sheaths
(arrowheads) in a 6-year-old boy with a metastasizing neoplasm
of high grade malignancy. No degenerating or demyelinating fibers
are apparent in this, or other areas of the nerve. The bar indicates 10 /um.

(No. 5) no myelin was detected also in the median and ulnar
nerves as well as in the supratentorial part of the central nervous system. (The lower part of the brain stem, unfortunately,
could not be studied due to inadequate sampling.) This case too
(No. 5) had abnormally thin axons as revealed by light and
electron microscopy (Fig. 5). There was a one-to-one relationship
of many axons and Schwann cells but no wrapping of cytoplasmic

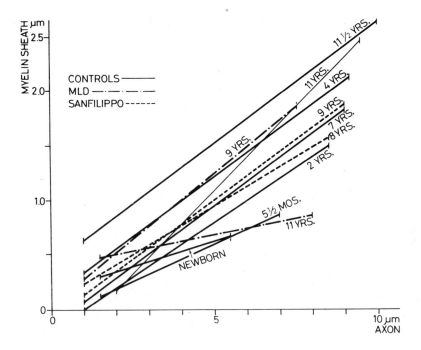

Fig. 5. Regression lines for the ratio between axon caliber
(x-axis) and myelin thickness (ordinate) for normal nerves at
various ages (thick continuous lines) and diseased nerves (thin
and interrupted lines). The age of the individuals is indicated
on the right side of the lines. The thin line for an 11-year-old
boy with a germinoma of the pineal gland shows a shift of the
inception of the line to the right side of the diagram with an
extraordinarily steep slope. (For details see Text).

processes around more than two-thirds of the axonal circumference.
Numerous axons were as large as 2 - 3 μm, that is above the minimal level at which myelination usually starts (1 μm[14,15]). The
density of neurofilaments was severely increased (approximately
500 instead of normally about 150 per μm^2). Yet there were no or

very few microtubules in axons of the pro-myelin as well as of
the Ramak type. No storage material was observed although there
were numerous filaments in the cytoplasm of some Schwann cells
(Fig. 3). There was a bilateral foot abnormality of the pes varus
variety and flexor position of both hands and fingers. The infant
died of tentorial hemorrhage at the second day post partum (CF
length: 49 cms, birth weight: 2900 gms).

Some cases studied at later stages of development showed a reduction of axon diameter and myelin thickness of the large diameter fibers if the measurements were related to the age of the
individuals (Fig. 2). This rather proportionate reduction of both
parameters was noted in one case of KRABBE's disease (K), two
cases each of metachromatic leukodystrophy (MLD) and hypertrophic
neuropathy (HN), and one case of spinal muscular atrophy (SMA).
Other cases of SMA were in the normal range. Two cases of
SANFILIPPO's disease (SF) showed a moderate reduction of myelin
thickness (Fig. 2). One case of COCKAYNE's syndrome (Co) had
disproportionately thin myelin sheaths that were too thin for the
size of the axons as well as for the age of the individual
studied. Other neuropathies were clearly in the pathological
range of measurements but the etiology remained unidentified.
There was evidence of demyelination and remyelination, or degeneration and regeneration of some fibers in COCKAYNE's syndrome
but not in the two cases with SANFILIPPO's disease. Also, one
case with GM_2-gangliosidosis (G 5) and ceroidlipofuscinosis (C e)
showed no structural evidence of neuropathy although there was
storage material deposited in the cytoplasm of Schwann cells.

The regression lines for the ratio between axon diameter and
myelin thickness as determined by measuring both values of individual nerve fibers on photomicrographs at a magnification of
x1000, revealed a prominent change only in the 11 year-old case
with MLD (Fig. 5). The regression lines for the 9 year-old case
with MLD, and for both cases with SANFILIPPO's disease were
seemingly within the normal range of their age group. Thus
measurements of large nerve fibers turned out to be more reliable
than any other method of investigation in detecting abnormalities
of nerve fiber maturation in such cases.

A developmental delay of myelination mainly of the smaller and

intermediate fiber group was noted in 3 cases with malignant
diseases, one case with a germinoma of the pineal gland dying at
the age of 135 months (11 years), one with a neuroblastoma dying
at the age of 63 months (5 years), and one with a malignant
neoplasm dying at the age of 72 months (6 years). These cases
showed normal dimensions of 20 selected large fibers, or a slight
reduction of axon diameters only. Yet some small or intermediate
axons showed unusually thin myelin sheaths (Fig. 4 b). The hypomyelination of predominantly small or intermediate fibers resulted in a change of the regression line for the ratio between axon
diameter and myelin thickness with a shift of the inception of
the regression line to the right side of the diagram. Thus the
slope of the line is steeper than in controls (Fig. 5).

DISCUSSION

   Disturbances of maturation of axons and myelin sheaths in sural
nerves of children can be detected only by careful comparison of
the dimensions of nerve fibers with adequate control data. In a
preceeding study[13] the normal development of myelinated fibers in
sural nerves has been investigated by light and electron
microscopy using three different methods of nerve fiber measurements: (1) Ocular micrometer measurements of 20 selected large
nerve fibers in each nerve; (2) evaluation of large numbers of
myelinated fibers by a particle size analyzer; and (3) precise
electron microscopic counts of the number of myelin lamellae and
measurements of the axonal circumferences. By applying these
methods selectively to a series of nerves obtained by biopsy or
autopsy three types of abnormalities have been identified that
are interpreted as developmental disturbances manifesting themselves at different age periods. The earliest abnormality is seen
in a unique case with total absence of myelin. Subsequently,
various degrees of immaturity of all fibers, or of the largest
fibers only may be seen due to inborn errors of metabolism, or
due to other, unidentified causes. And finally, primary hypomyelination of small and intermediate fibers was noted in three
children with malignant neoplasms.
   The most conspicuous case described in the present study was
the one with total absence of myelin in the sural nerve (No. 5,

in Table 1). No myelin was detected also in the median and ulnar nerves, or in the central nervous system. This nerve was from the second, maturely born male infant of a 19-year-old healthy mother with no indicative family history. The total lack of central and peripheral myelin in a mature infant indicates presumably a defective myelin anabolism although no biochemical studies verifying this assumption have been performed. The extraordinary high density of neurofilaments and the almost total absence of microtubules within the axons of the sural nerve indicate an abnormality of the neurons as well. No conspicuous accumulations of any storage material was detected in Schwann cells, and no myelin degradation products were observed in the central or peripheral nervous system. Yet many Schwann cells contained an abnormal amount of filaments as it is frequently seen in bands of Buengner long periods after Wallerian degeneration of nerve fibers. Myelin deficiency is well known in certain mouse mutants, quaking and jimpy, where a low activity of enzymes associated with myelin synthesis, the brain glycosyl transferases, has been observed[16]. In man, a prototype of a defective, or missing synthetic enzyme as an heritable disorder of anabolism has been described, a case of GM_3 gangliosidosis due to a defective N-acetylgalactosaminyl transferase[17]. In this case there was myelin splitting and inadequate myelination but not a total lack of myelin in the central and peripheral nervous system. Thus the case is unlike the present one as are all other well known disorders of sphingolipid metabolism caused by catabolic enzyme deficiencies. Contrary to other cases of congenital hypomyelination[18 - 20] the present nerve showed no evidence of neuropathy such as onion bulb formation or myelin breakdown.

A striking degree of hypomyelination of the primary and secondary type was noted in the present series of cases with metachromatic leukodystrophy (MLD), KRABBE's disease (K) and hypertrophic neuropathy (HN) (Fig. 2). This hypomyelination was usually associated with a rather proportionate reduction of axon diameters. The regression lines for the ratio between axon diameter and myelin thickness of the 9-year-old case with MLD was within the normal range whereas that of the 11-year-old was clearly abnormal (Fig. 5). In detailed studies on MLD or KRABBE's disease segmental demyelination and loss of variable numbers of axons has been well documented[5,6]. A retardation of maturation of large, seemingly intact nerve fibers in these two conditions, however, has thus far not been reckognized in these disorders by morphometric comparison of large nerve fibers with those in adequate control material of comparable age. Congenital hypomyelination in hypertrophic neuropathy, on the other hand, has been extensively discussed before[20]. In both cases of SANFILIPPO's disease thin myelin sheaths in relation to the age of the individuals, but not in relation to the size of the axons were observed. Hence, in SANFILIPPO's disease too there appears to be a delay of nerve maturation. This is most likely caused by the underlying metabolic defect since numerous Schwann cells accumulate storage material of the ganglioside type (pleomorphic bodies), occasionally also of the mucopolysaccharide type (membrane bound vacuoles approximately 1 μm in diameter).

It is of interest, on the other hand, that the representative examples of GM_2 gangliosidosis and ceroidlipofuscinosis did not show any evidence of a maturational delay of the development of either the myelin sheaths or the axons despite at least some storage material in Schwann cells.

A suggestive delay of maturation of the myelin sheaths of small and intermediate nerve fibers was noted in preliminary studies of three children dying from malignant neoplasms. There was no evidence of neuropathy as seen in cases with paraneoplastic neuropathy[21]. Two of the children were treated by cytostatics, but the one with a germinoma of the pineal gland was treated only by radiation therapy. Thus this case (Fig. 5) may support the assumption that this type of hypomyelination of small and intermediate fibers could have been caused by toxic, metabolic, or nutritional effects of the malignant neoplasms.

ACKNOWLEDGEMENT
We gratefully acknowledge the interest of Professors H. Harbauer, J. Pechstein, and J. Spranger, who arranged for the study of the biopsy material. The support of Professor W. Krücke is also appreciated.

REFERENCES

1. Webster, H. deF. (1964) In: Progr. Brain Res. 13, Mechanisms of Neural Regeneration. Edited by M. Singer and J.P. Schadé, pp. 151-172

2. Raine, C.S., Wisniewski, H., Prineas, J. (1969) Lab. Invest. 21, 316-327

3. Schröder, J.M. (1970) Proceedings of the VIth International Congress of Neuropathology, pp. 628-646 Masson et Cie: Paris

4. Lampert, P., Garrett, R., Powell, H. (1977) Acta neuropath. (Berlin) 40, 103-110

5. Webster, H. deF. (1962) J. Neuropathol. Exp. Neurol. 21, 534-554

6. Bischoff, A., Ulrich, J. (1969) Brain 92, 861-870

7. Dyck, P. J., Johnson, W. J., Lambert, E.H., O'Brien, P. C. (1971) Mayo Clin. Proc. 46, 400-431

8. Thomas, P. K., Hollinrake, K., Lascelles, R. G., O'Sullivan, D. J., Baillod, R. A. Moorhead, J. F., Mackenzie, J. C. (1971) Brain 94, 761-780

9. Dyck, P. J., Lais, A. C., Offord, K. P. (1974) Mayo Clin. Proc. 49, 34-39

10. Lubińska, L. (1961) J. comp. Neurol. 117, 275-289

11. Schröder, J. M. (1972) Brain Res. 45, 49-65

12a. Schröder, J. M. (1975) In: Studies on Neuromuscular Diseases, Proceedings of the International Symposium on Quanititative Methods of Investigations in the Clinics of Neuromuscular Diseases, Gießen, April 8-10. 1973. Editors: K. Kunze, J. E. Desmedt. Pp. 206-210. Karger: Basel

12b. Schröder, J. M., Seiffert, K. E. (1972) Zbl. Neurochir. 53, 103-118

13. Schröder, J. M., Bohl, J., Brodda, K. (1978) Acta neuropath. (Berlin), (In press).

14. Ochoa, J. (1971) J. Anat. 108, 231-245

15. Friede, R. L., Samorajski, T. (1968) J. Neuropathol. Exp. Neurol. 27, 546-570

16. Neskovic, N. M., Sarlieve, L. L., Mandel, P. (1972) Brain Res. 42, 147

17. Tanaka, J., Garcia, J. H., Max, S. R., Viloria, J. E., Kanijyo, Y., McLaren, N. K., Cornblath, M., Brady, R. O. (1975) J. Neuropath. Exp. Neurol. 34, 249-262

18. Karch, S. B., Ulrich, H. (1975) Dev. Med. Child Neurol. 17, 504-510

19. Lyon, G. (1969) Acta neuropathol. (Berlin) 13, 131-142

20. Kennedy, W. R., Sung, J. H., Berry, J. F. (1977) Arch. Neurol. 34, 337-345

21. McLeod. J.G. (1975) In: Peripheral Neuropathy, pp. 1301-1313, Ed.: Dyck, P.J., Thomas, P.K., Lambert, E.H. W.B. Saunders.

Peripheral Neuropathies
N. Canal and G. Pozza, eds.
© 1978 Elsevier/North-Holland Biomedical Press

METHODS OF EMG QUANTITATIVE ANALYSIS IN THE DIAGNOSIS OF SUBCLINICAL
POLINEUROPATHIES.

ANTONIO ARRIGO°, ARRIGO MOGLIA°,   GIORGIO SANDRINI°, FABRIZIO BERNOCCHI°;
ANTONIO PERNICE°°
° Neurological Clinic-°° Electronic Engeniery. University of Pavia (Italy).

INTRODUCTION

The data of EMGraphic tests made in our laboratory on workers in an industry
producing synthetic fibres in which carbon sulphide (CS_2) is produced and used
in various stages are presented in this paper.

From the literature it is known that this substance has a toxic effect on
different organs and apparatus. Our particular interest is in the action of CS_2
on the peripheral nervous system.

Our research concernes a group of patients in which EMG investigations were
carried out by traditional methods. Some data result of tests carried out on a small
sample of workers of another factory which uses DMF-(Dimethilformamide)- a
substance supposed to have a toxic effect on the peripheral nervous system. The
parameters of EMG signs of this group of subjects have been subjected to methods
of quantitative analysis. Our aim was to analyse critically the EMG methods of
acquiring the data and evaluating the level of reliability of those obtained
with traditional method compared to those obtained by automatic analysis.
Possible sources of data error are also considered taking into account: age of
subjects and sickness documented from collateral tests, such as chemical diabetes
and peripheral vasculopathies.

MATERIALS AND METHODS

Among the group of workers of the large industry, who are exposed to the
risks of intoxication with CS_2, we have 100 male subjects between the ages of 22
and 67. The Tibialis anterior muscles of all the subjects were examined
bilaterally with the help of an Adrian needle (of the DISA type). Bilateral
velocity of maximum motory conduction of SPE, amplitude of the distal M
responses of the muscle and distal latency were evaluated as well as classical
needle EMG examination.

Besides the electromyographic data, the following hematochemical data have
been collected and the following tests of peripheral vascular functionality have
also been carried out: Azotemia, Glycemia, Colesterol, Triglycerides,

Lipoproteins, Iodoproteins; on some subjects the glucose tolerance curve was also done.

Vascular tests: oscillography, pletizmography, rheography E.C.G.

Statistical analyses of the EMGraphic data have been done in relation to the presence of factors related to age, to chemical diabetes and to the presence of vasculopathies of the limbs using the t test between groups and the χ^2 test.

Method of Automatic Analysis

In the small industry group, where DMF is used, the data refer to five male subjects between the ages of 21 and 53.

Five male subjects of the same age group from the same factory, who were not exposed to the toxic action of DMF, were also examined.

The method described by Pinelli and Leifer (1975), subsequently improved in our laboratory, was adopted. (Arrigo and coll. 1977-78). From the Tibialis anterior muscles the activity of a single fibre is derived with the help of an EKSTED needle and through surface electrodes from all the muscles in isometric contractions, with an effort equal to 30% of the maximum possible. The potential of the fibre serves as a trigger to carry out the averaging in the phase of surface activity during a period of 36-40 seconds.

A delay constant of 5 msec. between the trigger and the point corresponding to the tracing of the surface is fixed. With respect to this point the averaging is done on a window that includes the 10 msec. preceding this point and the 26 msec. following it corresponding with a wave which is assumed to contain the contribution of the trigger itself. The fraction of energy of the signal, which is synchronous with the discharge of the trigger, is extracted from the surface signal.

The averaging operation can be stopped, either after a fixed, sufficiently large number of means or when two successive iterations give an insignificant difference between average signals. One can thus isolate the contribution of the fibre of a single motor unit to the surface signal, since one excludes the possibility of the presence of synchronous discharge from several motor units over a long period of time.

From the mean signal which we can call ASMUPs (Average Signal of Motor Unit Potentials) the following parameters can be measured: duration, amplitude, the number of phases, the number of peaks and the frequency of discharge.

In addition the energy of this signal, as well as that of the interference activity derived with the surface electrodes for periods of 500 msec., are calculated.

The M response of the Tibialis anterior, recorded from the same surface electrodes (electrodes and parameters of stimulation reported above) are then determined.

One can thus evaluate: latency, amplitude of the signals, energy of the signals of the M response.

RESULTS

The results obtained in the 100 subjects exposed to CS_2 are shown in table I,II. In table I the EMG data of the population subdivided on the basis of age of the subjects are shown.

TABLE I

< 34 YEARS [22 sub]

M Response						Fibrillation		MUAPs (π)		Max. Vol. Activity						Periph. Vascul.		Diabetis	
Max. M.C.V.		Distal L.		Distal A.						S. P.		R. I. P.		D. A.					
N	%	N	%	N	%	N	%	N	%	N	%	N	%	N	%	N	%	N	%
3	13,64	10	45,45	14	63,64	4	18,18	6	27,27	15	68,18	6	27,27	0	-	7	31,82	1	4,55

35↔45 YEARS [36 sub]

| 14 | 40 | 13 | 37,14 | 21 | 60 | 9 | 25,71 | 18 | 51,43 | 19 | 54,29 | 18 | 51,43 | 3 | 8,57 | 10 | 28,57 | 3 | 8,51 |

46↔58 YEARS [31 sub]

| 22 | 70,97 | 13 | 41,94 | 23 | 74,19 | 8 | 25,81 | 18 | 58,06 | 9 | 29,03 | 22 | 70,97 | 1 | 3,23 | 14 | 45,16 | 5 | 16,13 |

>58 YEARS [11 sub]

| 9 | 81,82 | 5 | 45,45 | 9 | 81,82 | 5 | 45,45 | 9 | 81,82 | 3 | 27,27 | 8 | 72,73 | 3 | 27,27 | 5 | 45,45 | 1 | 9,09 |

Max.M.C.V.= Maximal Motor Conduction Velocity. L.= Latency. A.= Amplitude
S.P.= Subinterference Pattern. R.I.P.= Reduced Interference Pattern.
D.A.= Discrete Activity. π= Poliphasic.

In table II the statistical analyses carried out using the t test to compare the mean values obtained in the subjects exposed with the normal means of our laboratory are shown.

Table II   T test (m.v.): Exposed sub.↔ Normal sub.

	age range			
	<34y.	35-45y.	46-58y	>58y.
Max M.C.V.	N.S.	N.S.	°	N.S.
Dist. Lat.	N.S.	N.S.	N.S.	N.S.
Prox. Ampl.	°°°	°°°	°°°	°
Dist. Ampl.	°°°	°°°	°°°	°

N.S.= p > 0.05   °=0.01< p ≤ 0.05   °°°= p ≤ 0.01

The χ^2 test gives the following results:

a) the type of voluntary activity obtained for maximum effort R.I.P. (Reduced Interference Pattern) is significant with respect to DA and SP in relation to the age of the subjects examined.

b) the over 58 age group is significant with respect to the other three groups with respect to the presence of polyphasic MUAPS of increased amplitude and/or duration.

   In table III the statistical analysis (t test) of values found in the subjects exposed to DMF with respect to the group of normal subjects studied with the method of automatic analysis of EMG is shown.

Table III   T test (m.v.): Exposed Sub. (D M F) ⟷ Normal Sub.

CASES	ASMUPs		param.		Interf.pattern	M resp.
	Ampl.	Dur.	Ph.	P.	E.P.S.	E.P.S.
1	° ° °	N.S.	° ° °	N.S.	N.S.	N.S.
2	N.S.	N.S.	N.S.	N.S.	° ° °	° ° °
3	N.S.	N.S.	N.S.	N.S.	N.S.	N.S.
4	° ° °	N.S.	N.S.	N.S.	°	° ° °
5	N.S.	N.S.	N.S.	N.S.	N.S.	°

N.S.=$p > 0.05$ °=$0.01 < p \leqslant 0.05$ °°°=$p \leqslant 0.01$ E.P.S.=Energy of the Power Spectrum. ASMUPs= Average Signal of Motor Unit Potentials.

   The tests of vascular functionality were considered to be pathological in 36 subjects. The criteria of abnormality used is the presence of at least one of these tests. On the basis of the hematochemical data and the laboratory data 10 subjects are classified as having chemical diabetes.

DISCUSSION

   From the analysis of table I one can see the relevant percent incidence of values obtained by stimulation of the nerve (M response). This is substantially in agreement with the data in the literature. Besides, one observes a high percentage of subjects which show alterations of parameters by EMG needle (fibrillations-P.U.M.-voluntary activity and maximum effort). This is not in contrast with,but rather complements,the information obtained by the technique of stimulation. As for the alterations of the peripheral vascular system,

one sees that the percent incidence increases with age. An analogous trend
seems to emerge for chemical diabetes. The statistical analysis regarding the
mean values of the parameters obtained by stimulation in the exposed subjects
compared with normal values is significant essentially for the amplitude
parameter of M responses (Table II). Such tests emphasize the necessity of an
accurate evaluation of factors related to age.

From the above data, one gets the impression that there is disagreement
between the analysing parameters within single groups expresses in percentages
and the statistical analysis of mean values. Actually, since the two types of
analysis cannot be compared, one can conclude that the two different methods
together give a more complete picture of the data, which have pathologic
significance.

As far as the subjects exposed to DMF are considered, whose EMG parameters have
been collected and evaluated by the method of automatic analysis, it is to be
emphasised that the values of the classical EMG and of the motor and sensory
conduction were within the normal range. Besides, from the analysis of table III
it is evident that at least one parameter out of those considered is significantly changed with respect to the normal values in four cases out of five.
This shows the greater sensitivity of the automatic method for detecting
probable subclinical alternatives as has already been shown in previous approaches.

SUMMARY

Our group is deeply involved in research concerning the goal of elaborating
and applying methods of authmatic quantitative EMG analysis in order to identify
cases of subclinical polineuropathies. In our opinion, in fact, for clinical
diagnostic purposes it is far more useful to define EMGraphic patterns, affor-
ding statistical evidence in early stages of peripheral nervous system involvement. In the present paper we illustrate data obtained by applying two different methods of quantitative EMG analysis to subjects exposed to the risk of
poisoning with toxic industrial substances. In the first part of the report,
methodological data and information are provided.

In the second part the results obtained are discussed in comparison with those
of the control group, having also in mind, clinical features as well as classical EMGraphic finding.

REFERENCES

1. Arrigo, A., Moglia, A., Sandrini, G., Cinquini, G. and Tanzi, F. (1977) Electroenceph. Clin. Neurophysiol., 43, 597-598.
2. Arrigo, A., Moglia, A., Sandrini, G., Cinquini, G., Tanzi, F. and Pernice, A (1978) Analisi quantitativa dell'EMG (in press).
3. Leifer, L. and Pinelli, P (1976)   3rd Int. Congress ISEK Pavia, Italy, Ed. A. Arrigo.
4. Lukas, E. (1970) Med. Lav., 61, 302-308.
5. Pinelli, P. (1977) The value of motor unit parameter measurements in current concepts in clinical neurophysiology. H. Van Duijn/D.N.J. Donker/A.C. Van Huffelen, Amsterdam.
6. Vasilescu, C. (1972) Rev. Roum. Neurol., 9, 63-71.
7. Vigliani, E.C. (1954) Br. J. Ind. Med., 11, 235-244.

Peripheral Neuropathies
N. Canal and G. Pozza, eds.
© 1978 Elsevier/North-Holland Biomedical Press

CUTANEOUS,MUSCULAR AND VISCERAL UNMYELINATED AFFERENT FIBRES : COMPARATIVE STUDY

G. SERRATRICE, N. MEI, J.F. PELLISSIER, D. CROS

C H U Timone and C N R S, I N P /1- Marseille (France)

ABSTRACT

This study compares unmyelinated afferences from skin, muscle and viscera.
Cutaneous ones are connected to high threshold nociceptors and probably to low
threshold receptors too. Muscular type IV afferences are composed of nociceptors, (55 % of units) mainly of polymodal type but non nociceptive units have
been found (45 %) and are supposed to be involved in regulatory mechanisms.
Likewise visceral C-afferences are either nociceptors or low threshold receptors
which generate homeostatic regulatory mechanisms. So the bulk of C-afferences
in each territory we considered leads to think they are not only involved in
pain and they transmit informations the evaluation of which needs further investigations.

INTRODUCTION

Unmyelinated afferent fibres (C-fibres in cutaneous and visceral nerves,type
IV fibres in muscular ones) are the most numerous of the whole afferent component. Their function in nociception is now well established. However some recent
data make one think their function is much more complex.

The purpose of this paper is to examine their putative roles in a comparative
study of cutaneous, muscular and visceral unmyelinated afferences. As a matter
of fact many points show their similarities : Firstly all histological and electrophysiological data are identical in the three territories i.e. diameter below
3 microns and conduction velocity below 2.5 m/s. Secondly everywhere it has been
investigated C-fibres have been found to be connected with free nerve endings.
Thirdly quantitative evaluations point out the bulk of C-afferences : C-fibres
density is of about 30.000/mm2 in cutaneous nerves (DYCK et al., I97I); I5.000
to 20.000/mm2 in the sensory component of muscular nerves (CROS and MEI, I978),
more than I00.000/mm2 in the cervical vagal nerve of cat. Conversely the myelinated afferent component is only of 20 % in cutaneous nerves in man (DYCK et
al., I97I), of 30 % in muscular nerves of cat (STACEY I968) and of about 20 %
in the vagal nerve (MEI, I970).

These quantitative studies alone cast doubts on functions restricted to nociception. More over recent development in both histological and electrophysiological methods now allow easier morphofunctional approaches of C-fibres in spite of their thin diameter. We intend here to give our own contribution about C-afferent fibres and to compare it to current data in this field.

UNMYELINATED CUTANEOUS AFFERENCES

Cutaneous C-fibres afferences are classically involved in nociception. The electrical stimulation of cutaneous nerves produces pain if its intensity is sufficient to excite the thinnest axons. Such experiments performed in awake animals give rise to "pseudo-affective responses" thought to be characteristics of pain. (BISHOP and HEINBECKER, 1935). In man, electrical stimulation of sural nerves generates pain only if A delta-fibres are recruited. At this stage an increase of stimulus intensity to excite C-fibres leads to an unbearable pain. (COLLINS et al.,1960).

Electrophysiological investigations in animals confirm that high threshold receptors (nociceptors) are connected to cutaneous C-afferents. Two main kinds of nociceptors are actually known : mechanical nociceptors (IGGO, 1960) and polymodal nociceptors (BESSOU and PERL, 1969). However some low threshold receptors are equally supplied by unmyelinated fibres : slowly-adapting mechanoreceptors (BESSOU et al., 1971) and thermoreceptors (review in HENSEL, 1973).

Human microneuronography is now used for more than ten years. By this way it is actually possible to record C-units activity from intact cutaneous nerves (TOREBJÖRK and HALLIN, 1970). This activity is easily correlated to perceptual changes experienced by the awake subject. This method has first confirmed the existence of polymodal nociceptor C-afferents in human skin, without to find any low threshold C-receptor. (VAN HEES and GYBELS, 1972 - TOREBJÖRK and HALLIN 1974). Since then two points can be added concerning C-cutaneous afferents physiology in man : firstly, beside numerous high threshold polymodal receptors some low threshold warm receptors exist, (TOREBJÖRK and HALLIN, 1976); secondly, activity in unmyelinated cutaneous afferents does not regularly induce pain sensation especially if a mechanical stimulus is applied (TOREBJÖRK and HALLIN 1974 - VAN HEES, 1976). Obviously because of the restricted samples obtained by microneuronography, further studies are necessary to elucidate all sensory function of cutaneous C-afferents. However it is important to point out that C-afferents discharges are not regularly correlated with pain.

On the other hand electron microscope examination permits morphological studies of unmyelinated axons.

These ultra-structural studies are generally used to make histograms of unmyelinated fibres. However these data concern only the unmyelinated component

without to compare the two populations of fibres. That is why it seems of more
interest to calculate the ratio unmyelinated/myelinated fibres from both ultrastructural and light microscopic examinations. Such studies were performed by
OCHOA and MAIR (1969) in healthy subjects and by DYCK et al. (1971) in normal
and pathological conditions. In this last work quantitative data obtained from
nerve biopsy were correlated with sensitive disturbances and with electrophysiological results of in vitro determination of compound action potentials.

The present paper deals with a comparison between the unmyelinated/myelina-
ted fibres ratio and the sensory abnormalities of several patients. The aim of
this work was to look for any pathophysiological correlations beetween clinical
conditions and morphological data. We did not in this first report systematically evaluate the A-delta component the function of which is quite identical to
C-afferents. The reason is that C-fibres largely outnumber A-delta fibres in
normal cutaneous nerves.

Material

We roughly divide our cases in three types : 1) Patients with peripheral
neuropathy and predominantly lower-limb pain. 2) Peripheral neuropathies with
distal sensory disturbances (hypesthesia) but without spontaneous pain. 3) Cases
of diabetes mellitus without clinical manifestation retained because of slow
conduction velocity discovered at a routine examination.

Pathological data are confronted to control-nerves. These nerves have been
obtained from healthy volunters or at autopsy performed in the first hour after
death.

Methods

The cutaneous nerves we studied are either the sural nerve (3 patients), on
the lateral peroneal nerve (3 patients). Controls of these two nerves have been
made. From epon-embedded nerves semi-thin and ultra-thin sections were cut and
used for optical and ultrastructural examinations. With light microscope were
performed photographs at a magnificance of 800. These photographs were used to
reconstruct the total section area and also to calculate the number of myelinated fibres and the corresponding endoneural surface. The ultrastructural examination consisted in scanning the whole surface of the section. Photographs were
randomly made so that each portion of the nerve was represented (i.e. 2 or 3
photographs per square of grid). Usually 200 to 300 slides were made per nerve
with a magnificance of 15.000. From this scattered photographs covering
$\frac{1}{5}$ th to $\frac{1}{10}$ th of the endoneural area we deduced the density of unmyelinated
axons per surface unit and built an histogram of diameters. All of the numerical
data have been obtained with aid of a computer TEKTRONIX 4051 supplied by a

graphics tablet TEKTRONIX 4956.Finally we determined in each case from both
unmyelinated fibres and myelinated fibres densities the ratio unmyelinated/mye-
linated.

Results

Firstly it is of interest to point out the results obtained in four peroneal
superficial nerve controls : Ratios unmyelinated/myelinated fibres are of/about
5 to 3 in normal subjects. They seem to decrease with age especially by loose
of myelinated fibres. On the other hand mean diameter seems to increase with
age. (table 1).

TABLE 1

CONTROLS

Patients	Age	Nerve	Endoneural/ Area	Myel.Fibres /mm2	Unmyel.Fibres/mm2	Ratio $\frac{Unmyel.}{Myel.}$
1	28	Peroneal	0,586	862I	43.235	5
2	46	Peroneal	0,430	6253	30.166	4,82
3	5I	Peroneal	0,5I0	422I	I4.250	3,37
4	53	Peroneal	0,330	7530	36.555	4,85
5	69	Sural	0,507	I4852	38.I70	2,5

The results of sural nerve counts are identical with data obtained from
superficial peroneal nerve and with results obtained by OCHOA and MAIR (I969)
and DYCK et al (I97I). In painful cases we find (table 2, n° 1 and 2) a slight
increase of the ratio due to the low density of myelinated fibres. Moreover
the histograms show a slight decrease of diameter of unmyelinated fibres. In
non-painful cases (table 2, n° 3 and 4) the ratio is very high and the histograms show a strong decrease of diameters of unmyelinated fibres. The results
in these two groups do not support the gate control theory of pain.

Examinations of two diabetic patients (cases 5 and 6) without pain nor neurological abnormalities are normal in spite of micro-angiopathy of endoneural
vessels.

TABLE 2

Patients	Age	Nerve	Endoneural Area (mm2)	Myel.fibres /mm2	Unmyel.fibres /mm2	Ratio $\frac{Unmyel.}{Myel.}$
1. MEJ.	26	Sural	0,407	5.5II	36.000	6,53
2. CHA	69	Super-ficial peroneal	0,2I0	7.595	5I.000	6,7I

3. BEO.	45	Superficial peroneal	0,560	3I6	25.882	8I
4. VAN.	36	Superficial peroneal	0,330	630	30.487	48
5. BAR.	28	Sural	0,345	6.240	28.000	4,48
6. PER.	54	Sural	0,200	4.175	I6.7I4	4

Such a ratio unmyelinated/myelinated gives a striking evaluation of both nerves populations. However several important limits are obvious : firstly it appears necessary to scan a large enough area in view of avoid an important error on unmyelinated fibres density estimation. Secondly this method is unable to distinguish autonomic efferents from unmyelinated afferences. Lastly, some difficulties frequently occur during the examination of pathological nerves: in spite of the usual criterias about unmyelinated axons, it is likely we underestimate their number.

UNMYELINATED MUSCULAR AFFERENTS

Although the unmyelinated sensory component largely outnumbers the myelinated one, thin muscular afferents have been quite poorly studied until recently. The classical views implicate them in transmission of pain impulses on the same grounds that cutaneous ones. The analysis of type IV fibres discharge shows an activation by painful stimuli for example ischemic contraction (BESSOU and LAPORTE, I958) or intra muscular injections of hypertonic Na Cl (IGGO, I96I).

We will discuss here 1) histological data, 2) Modes of activation, 3) the putative role of group IV afferents in some regulatory mechanisms.

I) Histological study

We studied the lateral gastrocnemius-soleus (L.G.C.-S) nerve of cat supplied by L6, L7 and S1 roots. In order to study dorsal root fibres only, a surgical section of the corresponding ventral roots was made. It was carefully conducted and the integrity of dorsal root ganglia cells was assessed by a post morten control. In addition, a lumbo-sacral sympathectomy was performed by a retroperitoneal approach to eliminate autonomic innervation. After 45 days the animals were killed and the L.G.C.-S. nerves removed. They were dissected from their connective sheat, fixed in glutaraldehyde IO %, then post-fixed in osmium tetroxyde, dehydrated in alcohol and embedded in epon. Semi-thin sections were cut and stained by paraphenyl ethylene diamine for optical examination. Ultra thin sections were cut and stained with lead citrate for electron-microscope study. Nerve section photographs at a terminal magnification of 700 were obtained from light microscope. From these photographs we estimated the endoneural area and

made the count and histogram of myelinated fibres. Using electron microscope
(SIEMENS Elmiskop I02) we scanned and photograph (G : I5000) an area of about
$\frac{I}{I0}$ of the total endoneural section. Overlapping photographs were voluntary made
in attempt to reconstruct a portion of nerve. Count and histogram of unmyelinated fibres were performed.

The following data were obtained from two L.G.C.-S. nerves with aid of the
same computer as above.

TABLE 3

	L.M.		E.M.		Ratio $\frac{Unmyel.}{Myel.}$
N°nerve	Total endoneural area (mm2)	Nb. Myel. fibres	Reconstructed area (mm2)	Nb.Unmyel. fibres	
2257	0.I6I	432	20.055	208	3.8
2276	0.I90	650	28.I44	407	4.2

This estimation of the unmyelinated component of muscle afferents is quite
higher than STACEY'S (1968). This author reported from two tibialis posterior
nerves a ratio $\frac{unmyelinated}{myelinated}$ of I,9 : 1 and 2 : 0. That can be explained by the
difference of bulk of the nerves, (Tibialis posterior is smaller than L.G.C.-S.
in cat) or may be by functional differences in muscles. It could also result of
Stacey's method of mapping which was not so systematic than ours. However we
cannot absolutely in our cases eliminate the persistance of any autonomic fibres since we have not examined lumbosacral sympathetic chain at autopsy.

Anyway these two studies point out the predominance of unmyelinated afferents
originating from muscle. This point contrasts strikingly with the paucity of
knowledges concerning their physiological role.

2) Mode of activation of type IV afferents

Difficulties to apply conventional recording techniques (i.e. recording of
single unit activity from nervous strands dissected of the nerve) undoubtly
explain the delay of progress in this field. In the past only IGGO (I96I) was
able to record C-unit activity in muscular nerves.

Our own study (CROS and MEI, I978) was conducted by recording single unit
activity from a micro-electrode inserted in dorsal root ganglia as described
previously (MEI, I970). By this way it is easy to record cell units activities
responding to electrical stimulation of L.G.C.-S. nerve. The latency of response permits to calculate the conduction velocity. A thin canula inserted in a

collateral of the femoral artery and was used to inject chemicals. The effects of arterial occlusions, mechanical pressure on the belly of muscle and stretch were also tested. Details of experimentations and results are summarized in the following tables :

TABLE 4

CHEMICAL STIMULI

(Icc by test is injected intra arterially)

Stimulation	Concentration	% of activated units
Na Cl	5 %	37
K cl	5 %	42
Histamine	200microgr/ml	70
Bradykinine	30microgr/ml	
5 H T P	400microgr/ml	
Ischemia		30
Pressure		75

TABLE 5

CHARACTERISTICS OF UNITS

Polymodal	25 %
Single stimulus sensitive	30 %
Silent	45 %

Our results confirm the activation of muscular group IV afferents by intra-arterial injection of algesic substances (Bradykinine, Histamine, Hypertonic Na Cl, hypertonic KCl, lactic acid.) About 55 % of fibres were activated and the half of them responded to two or more chemicals. Ischemic contraction is less constantly efficient in activation of group IV afferents. Long duration anoxia (IO') gave sustained responses in some units. A lot of responses were obtained with pressure of moderate intensity, thought not to be noxious. However some units responded only to damaging pressure. None activation was observed by stretching the muscle in the physiological range. We usually obtained low frequency discharges (about 20 c/s) of long duration (I to 3 min.) – Characteristics of type IV – fibres activation are similar to type III except of the maximal firing rate which is lower for type IV afferents.

The discussion of our results and of the current litterature leads to some comments. Much data are available from several last few years works (MENSE and SCHMIDT, I974, FRANZ and MENSE I975, FOCK and MENSE I976, MENSE I977, KUMAZAWA and MIZUMURA, I977). Most of these experiments have been conducted to test C-units sensitivity to algesic stimuli. They assess the chemo-sensitivity of numerous C-units to algesic substances and painful stimuli. However several facts

are to be pointed out : Firstly we must mention the existence of unmyelinated
fibres which are not activated by various algesic stimuli (45 % of our study).
Secondly the threshold of activation is sometime low, peculiarly to application
of moderate pressure. (IGGO, 1961 - KUMAZAVA et MIZUMURA 1977). Thirdly the
effects of stimuli supposed to be physiological mediators of muscular pain or
fatigue (KCl - lactic acid) are ambiguous : do they act as really physiological stimuli or by the way of a non specific algesic effect ? Peculiarly it
is difficult to speack of innocuous metabolic stimuli (lactate, phosphate)
because arterial blood substance concentration is unknown and because it is
impossible to eliminate an effect induced by modifications of pH or osmotic
pressure. That is why it seems actually reasonnable to keep in mind that two
kinds of receptors are connected to C-fibres : the first one is composed of
nociceptors some of them being polymodal, the second one concerns silent units
which cannot be related to a given stimulus and need further investigations
devoted to study their physiological role.

3) Functional data

In fact it seems very unlikely that such a bulk of afferences is only devoted to pain perception. Ourselves, looking for a physiological role of III and
IV afferent fibres have just began a study of calf blood flow variations measured by recording radio-activity after systemic injection of I33 Xe in cat.
Our preliminary results show modifications of the blood flow in the two hind-
limbs after activation of thin muscular afferents by chemicals. This circulatory effects depends partly of segmental dorsal root afferents since it is
very decreased after L6, L7 and S1 dorsal roots section. In the same way several
studies demonstrated that these muscular afferents activation give rise to reflex effects on arterial blood pressure and ventilation frequency (Mc CLOSKEY
and MITCHELL, 1972 - KALIA, SENAPATI et al, 1972). These effects would be to
take in account as regulatory mechanisms in adaptation to effort if activation
of some C-afferents in sustained muscular contraction was demonstrated. Likewise a work by HONG, KNIFFKI and SCHMIDT (1977), has to be quoted : it shows
that thin afferences give rise to a facilitation in the homonymous motor nuclei
neurons.

UNMYELINATED VISCERAL AFFERENTS

The functional importance of the unmyelinated sensory fibres must be reexamined in the visceral area from the recent histological and electrophysiological data.

The quantitative histological studies (AGOSTONI et al. 1957 - MEI et al.

I97I - MEI, unpublished results) have well established the predominance of afferent unmyelinated fibres in the vagal nerve. AGOSTONI et al. (1957) using a light microscope, founded 20.000 fibres of this kind in the cervical vagal trunk and only 5.000 myelinated fibres. The ultrastructural investigations shows that : 1) the sensory unmyelinated component is greater (about 40.000 according our observations), 2) the fibres diameter varies between 0,5 to 2,5 mu.m. (mean : I.I mu.m.) in the infranodose vagal nerve (MEI et al. I97I). The ratio C-fibres myelinated fibres in the visceral sensory component can even be higher; it is the case for example of the abdominal vagal nerve which contains only some hundred myelinated fibres whereas 30.000 sensory unmyelinated fibres are present at this level.

The development of the microelectrode technique (MEI, I962, I970; RANIERI et al.I973; RANIERI, I978) allow to perform a systematic study of the visceral C-afferents. The calculation of the conduction velocity of a great number of fibres is another method to analyse the nerve composition (MEI, I970).

So, it has been possible to precise the complexity of the peripheral pathway (primary afferent neuron) and peculiarly : 1) the diameter of the central pro-cess is smaller than the peripheral one; 2) the organization and the number of the fibres within the Schwann cells are different in the 2 portions of the nerves; 3) some fibres which are unmyelinated at the peripheral level, may be come progressively myelinated (DUCLAUX, MEI and RANIERI, I976); 4) the fibres originating from a same area, may follow several different pathways ; for example, the intestinal sensory fibres are situated both in splanchnic and in vagal nerves. (Fig.1)

The unmyelinated sensory fibres arise from the whole parts of viscera and not only from particular ones, as it was believed. In addition the endings are located in all the different layers : mucosa, submucosa, muscular layers, and serous membrane. That is particularly obvious for the small intestine. Thus the vagal nerves give sensory fibres to the whole gastro-intestinal tract (MEI, I970). Nevertheless the distribution of enteroceptors is not uniform : some regions, such as the sphincters of the digestive system are supplied by a higher density innervation by comparison with intestinal walls   (EL OUAZZANI and MEI I978).

Till recently, the sensory C-fibres belonging to visceral nerves were chie-fly considered as painful units like in cutaneous and muscular nerves. However this conception cannot be accepted anymore because of data obtained with the isolated fibre technique or with the microelectrode technique (see reviews by LEEK I972; PAINTAL I973; MEI I978). Actually our knowledge in visceral afferents

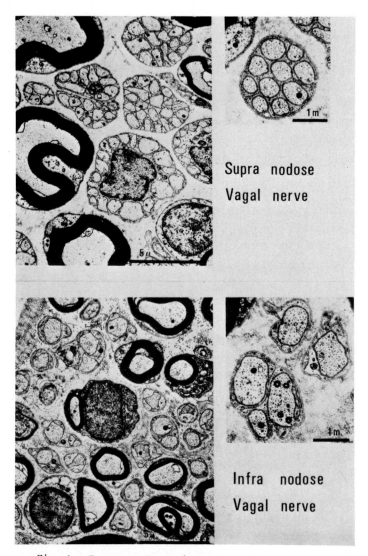

Supra nodose
Vagal nerve

Infra nodose
Vagal nerve

Fig. 1 : Transversal sections of vagal nerve in cat. The diameter of the
central process is smaller than the peripheral one. The number of axons per
Schwann cell is higher at the supra nodose level than at the infra nodose
level.

are more advanced than those concerning cutaneous or muscular nerves. Most of
sensory visceral fibres carry numerous and physiological informations. They
are produced in different specific receptors sensitive to mechanical, chemical
or thermal stimulation, although these receptors have generally the same morphological structure (free endings with more or less branchings). Of course
these enteroceptors can also produce nociceptive signals provided the stimulation is strong but they are chiefly activated by physiological events. However,
one found in the visceral territory some polymodal endings which seem mainly
scattered in the epithelium.

These recent morphological and physiological data suggest that the enteroceptors are involved in various nervous or neuro-humoral regulations (for example, the vagal intestinal glucoreceptors are implicated in the insulin release,
MEI, 1978). This fact could explain some clinical observation, for example a
better control of glucose blood level by ingestion of glucose than
by intravenously hypertonic glucose administration. The latter leads to bypass
some digestive regulatory mechanisms.

CONCLUSIONS

As previous data our results confirm the quantitative preponderance of
unmyelinated fibres in all the three territories, cutaneous, muscular and visceral. So C-fibres appear as the main sensory component of the whole organisms.

Some obvious similarities appear in the three territories. The three kinds
of receptors (i.e. mechano- thermo- and chemo-receptors), all free endings,
exist in each territory we considered. Their discharge type, slowly adapting
with low maximal discharge frequency are the same whatever their origin.

From these results three points can be discussed : The first point is that
pain is not necessarily the result of competition of impulses in thick myelinated fibres on the one hand and thin afferents (A delta and C) on the other hand
according to the gate control theory (MELZACK and WALL, 1965). The reason is
the following one : patho-clinical correlations infirm this possibility as
found by DYCK et al (1971) and by our study. Secondly some organs (i.e. viscera) have only unmyelinated afferents and if pain can be induced by some stimulations, usually they are not painful in spite of continuous discharges in
C-afferents. Finally pain is not only generate by activation of specific-recep-
tors, the bulk of nociceptive informations being more important.

In spite of these critical observations one must keep in mind nociceptive
and non nociceptive functions of unmyelinated fibres :

Nociceptive function is now well established with three types of receptors (i.e. mechano, thermo, chemoreceptors) with high threshold, slow adapting discharge and low firing rate.

Conversely non nociceptive functions are now shown. They are unequally documentated because of the differences of our knowledges in the three fields we considered.

Usually these functions are correlated with low threshold receptors, characterized by the specificity of the stimulus. Such stimulus specificity is well known in visceras for instance chemo, thermo and mechano-sensitivity. These properties explain a lot of roles in homeostatic regulations. In the skin the low threshold receptors have been more studied in animals than in man but one can think that low threshold C-receptors do exist in man. Concerning muscle only indirect evidence of such receptors is available (i.e. cardio-pulmonar adaptation to effort, and possibly segmental vascular control as homonymous reflex effect on motoneuron). But a definite investigation of these receptors has not been yet made.

REFERENCES

1. AGOSTONI, E., CHINNOK, J.E., DALY DE BURGH, M., MURRAY, J.G. (I957) Functional and histological studies on the vagus nerve and its branches to the heart, lungs and abdominal viscera in the cat. J. Physiol. (Lond.), I35, I82-205

2. BESSOU P., BURGESS P.R., PERL E.R., TAYLOR C.B. (I97I) Dynamic properties of mechanoreceptors with unmyelinated fibres. J. Neurophysiol. 34,II6-I33.

3. BESSOU P., LAPORTE Y. (I958) Activation des fibres afférentes amyéliniques d'origine musculaires. C.R. Soc. Biol. (Paris), I52, I587-I590.

4. BESSOU P., PERL R. (I969) Response of cutaneous sensory units with unmyeli-nated fibres to noxious stimuli. J. Neurophysiol., 32, I025-I043.

5. BISHOP G.H., HEINBECKER P. (I935) The afferent function of non myelinated or C-fibres. Am. J. Physiol., II4, I79-I93.

6. COLLINS, W.F., NULSEN F.E., RANDT C.T. (I960) Relation of peripheral nerve size and sensation in man. Arch. Neurol., 3, 38I-385.

7. CROS D., MEI N. (1978) Données morpho-fonctionnelles sur les fibres afférentes fines provenant du muscle gastrocnémien du chat. Communication at the 46° meeting of the French Association of Physiologists, Paris, June 22-24. Abst. in press in J. Physiol. (Paris).

8. DUCLAUX R., MEI N., RANIERI F. (1976) Etude de la vitesse de conduction dans les prolongements périphériques des divers neurones vagaux. J. Physiol. (Lond.), 260, 487-495.

9. DYCK P.J., LAMBERT E.H., NICHOLS P.C. (I97I) Quantitative measurement of sensation related to compound action potential and number and sizes of myelinated and unmyelinated fibres of sural nerve in health, Friedreich's ataxia, hereditary sensory neuropathy and tabes dorsalis. In REMOND A. (editor), Handbook of Electroencephalography and clinical Neurophysiology. Amsterdam. Elsevier. Vol. 9. pp 83-II8.

IO. EL OUAZZANI T., MEI N. (1978) Vagal thermoreceptors. (Submitted).

II. FOCK S., MENSE S. (1976) Excitatory effects of 5-hydroxytryptamine, histamine and potassium ions on muscular group IV afferent units. A comparison with bradykine. Br. Res., IO5, 459-469.

I2. FRANZ M., MENSE S. (1975) Muscle receptors with group IV afferent fibres responding to application of bradykinine. Br. Res., 92, 369-382.

I3. HENSEL H. (1973) Cutaneous thermoreceptors. In IGGO A. (editor), Handbook of sensory physiology. Berlin, Heidelberg, New York. Springer. Vol 2. pp 79-IIO.

I4. HONG S.K., KNIFFKI K.D., SCHMIDT R.F. (1977) Intra arterial injection of algesic agents into skeletal muscle : effects on the discharge of motoneurones. Proc. Int. Union Physiol. Sci. Vol.XIII, p. 329.

I5. IGGO A. (I960) Cutaneous mechanoreceptors with afferent C-fibres. J. Physiol. (Lond). I52, 337-353.

I6. IGGO A. (I96I) Nonmyelinated afferent fibres from mammalian skeletal muscle J. Physiol.(Lond.) I55, 52-53P.

I7. KALIA M., SENAPATI J.M., PARIDA B., PANDIA A. (I972) Reflex increase in ventilation by muscle receptors with non-medullated fibres. J. Appl. Physiol. 2, I89-I93.

I8. KUMAZAWA J., MIZUMURA K. (1977) Thin fibre receptors responding to mechanical, chemical and thermal stimulation in the skeletal muscle of the dog. J. Physiol. (Lond.) , 273, I79-I94.

I9. LEEK B.F. (I972) Abdominal visceral receptors. In NEIL E. (editor), Handbook of sensory Physiology, Berlin, Heidelberg, New York. Springer. Vol.3/I pp II3-I60.

20. MAC CLOSKEY D.I., MITCHELL J.M. (I972) Reflex cardio-vascular and respiratory responses originating in skeletal muscle. J. Physiol. , 224, I73-I86.

2I. MEI N. (1962) Enregistrement de l'activité unitaire des afférences vagales. Réception par microélectrodes au niveau du ganglion plexiforme. Ann. Biol. Anim. Bioch. Biophys., 2, 36I-363.

22. MEI N. (I970) Disposition anatomique et propriétés électrophysiologiques des neurones sensitifs vagaux chez le chat. Exp. Brain Res., 2, 465-479.

23. MEI N. (I978) Intestinal vagal glucoreceptors. J. Physiol. (Lond.), 225, I-22.

24. MEI N., CONDAMIN M., BOYER A. (I97I) Etude comparée des deux prolongements de la cellule sensitive vagale. C.R. Soc. Biol., I65, 237I-2374.

25. MELZACK R., WALL P.D. (I965) Pain mechanisms : a new theory. Science, I50, 97I-979.

26. MENSE S. (I977) Nervous outflow from skeletal muscle following chemical noxious stimulation. J. Physiol. (Lond.), 267- 75-88.

27. MENSE S., SCHMIDT R.F. (I974) Activation of group IV afferent units from muscle by algesic agents. Br. Res., 72, 305-3IO.

28. OCHOA J., MAIR W.G.P. (I969) The normal sural nerve in man. I Ultrastructure and number of fibres and cells. Acta Neuropath. (Berlin), I3, I97-2I6.

29. PAINTAL A.S. (I973) Vagal sensory receptors and their reflex effects. Physiol. Rev., 53, I59-226.

30. RANIERI F. (1977) Sensibilité viscerale splanchnique. Thèse de Doctorat és sciences. Marseille.

3I. RANIERI F., MEI N., CROUSILLAT J. (I973) Afférences splanchniques provenant des mécanorécepteurs gastrointestinaux et péritoneaux. Exp. Br. Res., I6, 276-296.

32. STACEY M.J. (I969) Free nerve endings in skeletal muscle of cat. J. Anat., I05, 231-254.

33. TOREBJORK H.E., HALLIN R.G. (I970) Afferent and efferent C-units recorded from human skin nerves in situ. Acta Soc. Med. Upsal., 75,277-28I.

34. TOREBJORK H.E., (I974) Afferent C-units responding to mechanical, thermal and chemical stimuli. in human glabrous skin. Acta Physiol. Scand. 92, 374-390.

35. TOREBJORK H.E., HALLIN R.G. (I976) Skin receptors supplied by unmyelina-ted (C) fibres in man. In ZOTTERMAN Y. (editor), Sensory functions of the skin in primates. Oxford. Pergamon Press. pp 475-485.

36. VAN HEES J. (I976) Single afferent C-fibres activity in the human nerve during painful and non painful skin stimulation with radiant heat. In ZOTTERMAN Y. (editor), Sensory functions of the skin in primates. Oxford. Pergamon Press.pp 503-504.

37. VAN HEES J., GYBELLS J. (I972) Pain related to single afferent C-fibres in human skin. Br. Res., 48, 397-400.

38. VAN HEES J., GYBELLS J. (I973) L'activité unitaire des fibres C enregis-trée dans un nerf cutané chez l'homme et sa relation avec la douleur. Acta Neurol. Belg., 73, 39-43.

Peripheral Neuropathies
N. Canal and G. Pozza, eds.
© 1978 Elsevier/North-Holland Biomedical Press

NERVE AND MUSCLE CHANGES INDUCED BY REPEATED LOCALIZED FREEZINGS OF
THE SCIATIC NERVE IN THE RAT

MIRA J.C. and FARDEAU M.

Research Group on Neuromuscular Biology and Pathology, (INSERM U. 153 and
CNRS ER.107), 17, rue du Fer à Moulin, 75005-Paris (France)

ABSTRACT

Localized freezings of the rat sciatic nerve repeated 2 to 5 times at monthly intervals induced a progressive increase in the number of myelinated
fibres in the distal part of the nerve (up to 220 % of the control value one
month after the last freezing). The muscle changes observed were more pronounced than those seen after a single freezing. There was a progressive increase
of type I and II_C fibres when counted 30 days after the last freezing. However
this muscle transformation was not stable.

INTRODUCTION

Despite the early observations reported by MAYER[1], VANLAIR[2] and CAJAL[3],
relatively few studies have been devoted to peripheral nerve regeneration after
repeated injuries, and the morphological and physiological results of these
observations were often conflicting ; furthermore, not many of these studies
included quantitative data (4-5-6-7-8). Similarly, muscle changes observed
during reinnervation processes have been studied by many workers, but few
reports dealt with the effects of repeated nerve lesions (9-10).

MATERIAL AND METHODS

Experiments were made on albino rats which underwent repeated localized
freezings, performed in situ on the left sciatic nerve, before it branches out
into the tibial, peroneal and sural nerves. Results were recorded at standardized levels in the nerve to the medial head of the right and left gastrocnemius muscles (RGM and LGM nerves) which divided 30-40 mm below the lesion site.

A liquid nitrogen cryode was used to perform one or more localized freezings (11). The active point of this probe was directly applied to the sciatic
nerve at three points on the same nerve circumference and quickly frozen at
about -180°C. Total duration of freezing and thawing never exceeded 30-40
seconds.

RGM and LGM nerves were removed, fixed with glutaraldehyde-osmium tetroxide
and, after dehydration, embedded in araldite. For light microscopy, 30-40 semi-
serial sections of each nerve were stained with toluidine blue.

Myelinated nerve fibre counts and measurements were made on the best 2-3
photographic prints at a magnification of x 1000. The total diameter of each
fibre was measured over the contour of its myelin sheath. These measurements

allowed the study of fibre size distribution for each nerve. In an earlier
work, the number and size of myelinated fibre populations were studied in normal unoperated rats (12). All results were comparable for both sides, and no
significant differences were observed in any mean values for the number and
size of myelinated nerve fibres. However, after every experimental lesion of
the left sciatic nerve, certain changes were observed in the number and size
of myelinated fibres of the RGM nerve, compared to normal values (13-11).

To determine the optimal period between two successive nerve injuries, a
single localized freezing was performed in several rats. The first regenerating
nerve endings were detected in the middle part of the gastrocnemius muscle
after 16-18 days, using BIELCHOWSKY-GROS silver impregnation. As a result, we
decided to separate each freezing by about three weeks.

Muscular changes induced by repeated freezings of the sciatic nerve were investigated in the medial head to the gastrocnemius muscle at standardized
levels. Cryostat semi-serial transverse sections were studied with conventional
histoensymological techniques (15). Fibre types were identified by their myosin-
adenosine-triphosphatase (ATP-ase) activity, according to the classification
proposed by BROOKE & KAISER (16). Topographical distribution of the different
muscle fibres (I, II_A, II_B) consistently defined two different zones in the
normal gastrocnemius muscle (17) (Fig. 2).

RESULTS

Repeated localized freezings were performed in two different ways. Thus,
rats in Group I underwent from 1 to 5 freezings and measurements were made one
month after the final cold injury, whereas measurements in Group II were carried out one, three, six, twelve and eighteen months after the third and final
freezing.

I. GROUP I : Nerve and Muscle changes observed one month after the last freezing.

1. Nerve changes. In the LGM regenerating nerve, the number of myelinated
fibres gradually increased after the three first freezings of the left sciatic
nerve (Figs 1,3,5). An average of 117 % was found after the first cold injury,
154 % after the second and 212 % after the third. The fourth and fifth freezings did not shw more changes : 217 % after the fourth and 218 % after the
fifth, compared to the values determined in the RGM contralateral nerve.
Simultaneously, the size of regenerating, myelinated nerve fibres was much
reduced, compared to the controls, and fibre size distribution was always uni-
modal after the final freezing. Fibre diameters ranged from 1 to 7-8 microme-
tres (Figs 7,8,9) and there again, the fourth and fifth freezings did not enhance the changes.

2. Muscle changes. One month after the first freezing, the gastrocnemius
muscle exhibited a very limited grouping of Type I fibres (17). After the second to fifth cold injuries, the changes became more pronounced. There was then
a gradual increase in the number of acid-resistant ATP-ase fibres belonging to

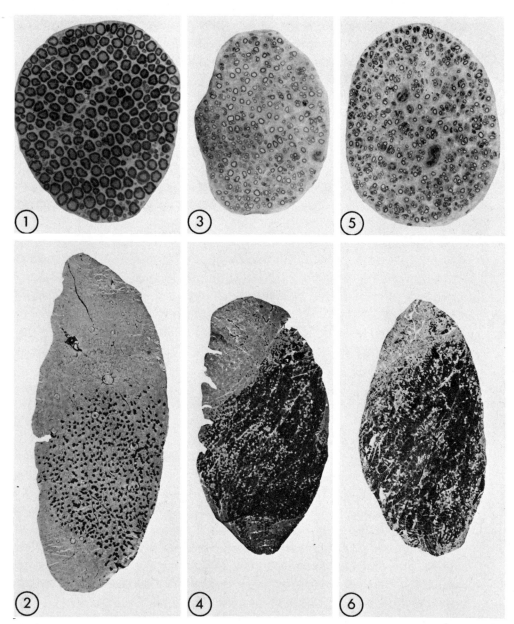

Fig. 1-6 : Transverse sections of the RGM and LGM nerves (Toluidine blue) and muscles (Myofibrillar ATP-ase, pH 4.35). Figs. 1-2 : contralateral nerve and muscle. Figs. 3-4 : one month after 2 freezings ; Figs. 5-6 : one month after 4 freezings.

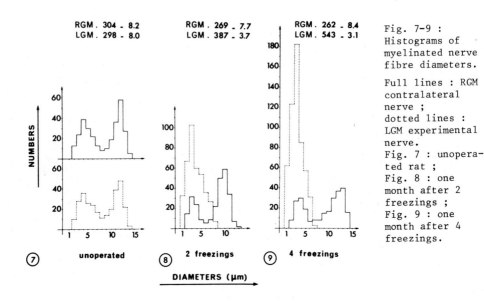

RGM. 304 - 8.2
LGM. 298 - 8.0

RGM. 269 - 7.7
LGM. 387 - 3.7

RGM. 262 - 8.4
LGM. 543 - 3.1

⑦ unoperated

⑧ 2 freezings

⑨ 4 freezings

DIAMETERS (µm)

Fig. 7-9 :
Histograms of
myelinated nerve
fibre diameters.

Full lines : RGM
contralateral
nerve ;
dotted lines :
LGM experimental
nerve.
Fig. 7 : unopera-
ted rat ;
Fig. 8 : one
month after 2
freezings ;
Fig. 9 : one
month after 4
freezings.

Types I and II_C. Type II_A and II_B fibres were only observed in a small area at the periphery of the gastrocnemius muscle.

The diameter of Type I and II_C fibres did not significantly differ from the controls. On the contrary, II_A and II_B fibres were markedly atrophic (Figs 2,4, 6). Furthermore, a few targetoid aspects were noticed amongst Type I fibres.

II. GROUP II : Nerve and Muscle changes observed 3 to 18 months after the third and final freezing.

1. Nerve changes. One month after the third freezing, the number of regenerating myelinated nerve fibres reached a mean of 212 % of the control values. Three months after the third freezing, the number dropped by about 30 %. From then on, no further variations occurred until eighteen months had elapsed (Figs 10,12,14).

However, the size distribution of the regenerating myelinated nerve fibres varied. From the third month onwards, a regular increase in fibre size was observed and fibre size distribution became bimodal (Figs 16,17,18). Eighteen

Fig. 10-15 : Transverse sections of the RGM and LGM nerves (Toluidine blue) and muscles (Myofibrillar ATP-ase, pH 4.35).Figs. 10-11 : one month after 3 freezings ; Figs.12-13 : Three months after 3 freezings ; Figs. 14-15 : six months after 3 freezings.

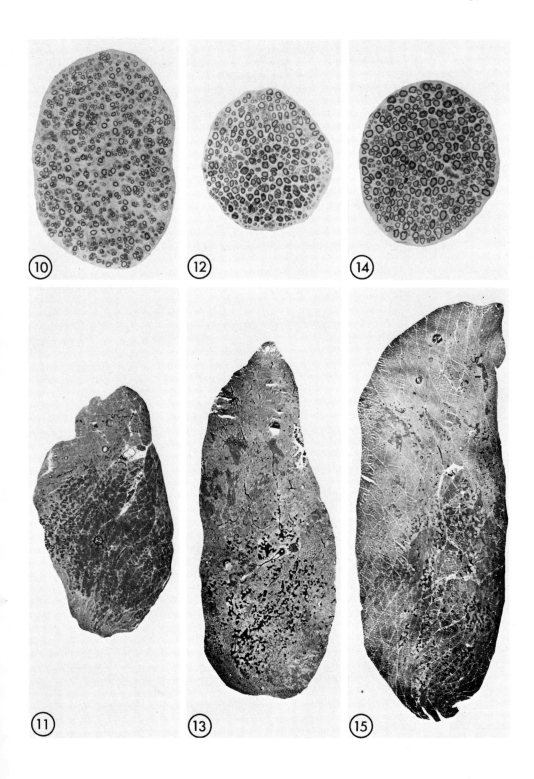

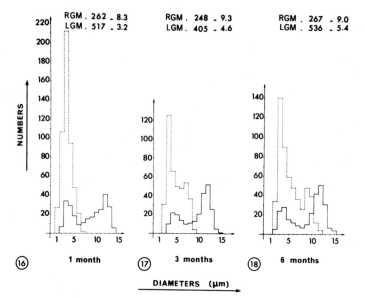

Fig. 16–18 :
Histograms of
myelinated nerve
fibre diameters.

Full lines : RGM
contralateral
nerve ;
dotted lines :
LGM experimental
nerve.
Fig. 16 : one
month after 3
freezings ;
Fig. 17 : three
months after 3
freezings ;
Fig. 18 : six
months after 3
freezings.

months after the third freezing, the mean diameter of all myelinated nerve
fibres was still very much below the control value (70 %).

2. Muscles changes. One month after the third freezing, most of the muscle
transverse area was occupied by Type I and II_C fibres. However, between the
first and third months after the third freezing, the number of Type I and II_C
fibres dropped considerably. The diameters of Type II_A and II_B fibres returned
to subnormal values. Only a restricted grouping of Type I fibres was left, and
the muscular histochemical pattern did not differ from that observed one month
after a single freezing (Figs 11,13,15).

DISCUSSION

Localized freezing was used to study the variations in the number and size
of myelinated nerve fibres as well as the muscular changes induced by repeated
nerve injuries. This technique was selected because its results are perfectly
reproducible and much more consistent than those obtained after crush or tran-
section of the nerve (11,13). Electron microscopy of the directly frozen segment
showed that the basal lamina surrounding each nerve fibre was not disrupted (18).

In previous reports, we studied quantitatively the myelinated nerve fibre
regeneration following a single freezing (11) and compared the results with
those of other nerve lesion procedures (13). After cold injury, the number of

regenerating myelinated nerve fibres returned to normal during the fourth week and increased up to a mean of 124 % during the two post-operative years. The mean diameter of all myelinated fibres gradually returned to normal at the end of the first year ; fibre size distribution became bimodal from the sixtieth day and histograms of regenerating and control nerves were superimposable at about 330 days.

After repeated freezings, there was a large increase in the number of regenerating myelinated nerve fibres observed distal to the lesion site due to the sprouting of the normal proximal end of the initial fibres. In Group I, the plateau observed from the third freezing onwards, as well as the drop in Group II in the number of myelinated fibres recorded between the first and third months after the third freezing, might be explained by the simultaneous action of central, local and/or peripheral factors, even though, at the present time, it is impossible to determine the precise part played by each of them. These limiting factors may interfere with the neuronal cell body metabolism, the nerve trunk environment and/or the capacity of the regenerating nerve fibres to make an effective connection with their former end-organs. This list is not restrictive and other as yet unidentified factors may also be involved.

Muscular changes observed after cold injuries to nerves confirmed some of the well-known facts about denervation and reinnervation processes in mammalian skeletal muscles, such as abnormal type-grouping of the fibres (9-19).

After only one freezing, this grouping remained stable from days 30 to 360. After 2 to 5 freezings, repeated every three weeks, the muscular changes observed one month after the last freezing were much more pronounced than when only one freezing was performed. These changes consisted of a gradual increase in the number of Type I and II_C fibres. Type II_A and II_B fibres remained atrophic. These observations might be explained by a quicker regeneration rate for Type I than Type II motoneurons, and by the reinnervation of initially Type II muscular fibres by axons belonging to Type I motoneurons. Type II_C fibres were considered as a transitional "flip-flop" stage between Type II (A and B) and Type I fibres (20).

However, a striking feature of this muscle transformation was its lack of stability. Thus, from three months after the third freezing onwards, the muscular histochemical pattern did not differ from the one noted after a single cold injury. In particular, the number of acid-resistant ATP-ase fibres dropped considerably and Type II_C fibres disappeared.

At the present time, there is no clear explanation for these observations. Several hypotheses may advanced, but they are not mutually exclusive. For example, one mechanism could link the histochemical type of the muscle pattern to the size of the innervating nerve fibres. Another mechanism might consist of the "recapture" of these Type II_C fibres by their original Type II motoneurons endings. This would imply a period of double-innervation for these muscle fibres. Preliminary electrophysiological observations support this hypothesis.

REFERENCES

1. Mayer, S. (1881) Z. Heilkunde, 2, 154-258.

2. Vanlair, C. (1888) Bull. Acad. roy. Sci. belges, 16, 93-110.

3. Cajal, S.R. (1928) in "Degeneration and Regeneration of the Nervous System", Oxford Univ. Press, London.

4. Duncan, D., and Jarvis, W.H., (1943) J. comp. Neurol., 79, 315-325.

5. Gutmann, E., (1948) J. Neurophysiol., 11 , 279-294.

6. Abercrombie, M., and Santler, J., (1957) J.cell.comp.Physiol., 50, 429-450.

7. Thomas, P.K., (1968) in "Research in Muscular Dystrophy", Pittman, London, pp. 413-419.

8. Thomas, P.K., (1970) J. Anat., 106, 463-470.

9. Dubowitz, V.,(1967) J. Neurol. Neurosurg. Psychiatry, 30, 99-110.

10. Bradley, W.G. and Papapetropoulos, T.A.,(1971) Nature, 236, 401-402.

11. Mira, J.C., (1977) Arch. Anat. micr. Morphol. exp., 66, 1-16.

12. Mira, J.C., (1976a) Arch. Anat. micr. Morphol. exp., 65, 209-229.

13. Mira, J.C., (1976b) Arch. Anat. micr. Morphol. exp., 65, 255-284.

14. Mira, J.C., (1978) J. Anat., (in press).

15. Fardeau, M., (1973) Ann. Anat. Pathol., 18, 7-34.

16. Brooke, M.H., and Kaiser, K.K., (1970) Arch. Neurol. (Chicago) 23, 369-379.

17. Mira, J.C., and Fardeau, M., (1978) C.R. Acad. Sci., D, 286, 1367-1370.

18. Mira, J.C., (1972) J. Microsc. (Paris) 14, 155-168.

19. Karpati, G., and Engel, W.K., (1968) Neurology (Minneap.) 18, 447-455.

20. Brooke, M.H., Williamson, E.K., and Kaiser, K.K., Arch. Neurol. (Chicago) (1971) 25, 360-366.

Peripheral Neuropathies
N. Canal and G. Pozza, eds.
© 1978 Elsevier/North-Holland Biomedical Press

FATTY ACID BIOSYNTHESIS IN RAT SCIATIC NERVE UNDERGOING
WALLERIAN DEGENERATION

ARNULF H. KOEPPEN, JOHN D. PAPANDREA AND EDWARD J. MITZEN
Research Service, V.A. Hospital, Albany, New York, U.S.A. and
Albany Medical College

ABSTRACT

Fatty acid biosynthesis was determined in fragments of normal
rat sciatic nerve and in nerve undergoing Wallerian degeneration.
Fatty acids were biosynthesized from malonyl-coenzyme A and
acetyl-coenzyme A in the presence of reduced nicotinamide
adenine dinucleotide phosphate. The predominant mechanism was
de-novo biosynthesis rather than elongation, and free palmitic
acid was the reaction product.

During Wallerian degeneration, the biosynthesis of fatty acids
increased rapidly in the distal segment of the sectioned nerve
when compared to the contralateral unoperated nerve. The enhancement reached a level of 350 percent at 25 days survival (contralateral nerve = 100 percent). Activity then declined and fell to
control values after 50 days.

INTRODUCTION

Investigators of Wallerian degeneration in the peripheral
nervous system have utilized in-vitro methods and have found
an enhanced incorporation of lipid precursors in the degenerating
nerve when compared to the contralateral unsectioned nerve[1-4].
However, we could not find a detailed study of the mechanism by
which fatty acids are biosynthesized in peripheral nervous
tissue. In this investigation, an effort was made to characterize
the biosynthesis of fatty acids in fragments of rat sciatic nerve
by incubation in a system containing either malonyl-CoA, acetyl-
CoA or both. The findings obtained with normal nerve were compared to nerve undergoing Wallerian degeneration.

MATERIAL AND METHODS

The complete incubation system contained, in final concentration and a final volume of 2 ml, sodium phosphate buffer (pH 7.0), 50 mM; KCl, 10 mM; $MgCl_2$, 1 mM; NADPH, 1 mM; malonyl-CoA, 0.1 mM; acetyl-CoA, 0.1 mM; sucrose, 0.32 M; fragments of sciatic nerve, 25-35 mm long. The incubation temperature was $37^{\circ}C$, and the reaction time was 60 min. We selected finely minced sciatic nerve rather than nerve homogenate because a comparison with numerous previous studies on Wallerian degeneration was intended. Radioactivity was introduced as either $1,3-C^{14}$-malonyl-CoA or $1-C^{14}$-acetyl-CoA.

Lipid extraction, thinlayer chromatography, gas liquid chromatography and azide decarboxylation followed standard procedures.

For the study of Wallerian degeneration, adult albino rats were anesthetized by intraperitoneal injection of sodium pentobarbital. The sciatic nerve on the right side was exposed and sectioned. Distal and proximal stumps were ligated with silk. The wound was closed in layers. After a survival of 3-50 days, the distal segment on the right and the left unoperated nerve were removed, minced and incubated as described above.

RESULTS

The pH-optimum for fatty acid labeling from $1,3-C^{14}$-malonyl-CoA was near neutrality (fig. 1). When fatty acid biosynthesis was related to the length or weight of the nerve, there was considerable variability, notably with greater length and weight (fig. 2).

Label from $1,3-C^{14}$-malonyl-CoA or $2-C^{14}$-malonyl-CoA was readily incorporated into fatty acids of nerve lipids (table 1). Acetyl-CoA label was also incorporated provided malonyl-CoA was also present. In the absence of malonyl-CoA, there was no label incorporation into fatty acids from acetyl-CoA. In contrast, label from malonyl-CoA was incorporated even when no acetyl-CoA was added. Sufficient acetyl-CoA was produced by the activity of malonyl-CoA decarboxylase. Reduced pyridine nucleotides were a requirement and NADH could not fully substitute for NADPH. Added dithiothreitol did not enhance fatty acid labeling in contrast to its known activity in brain supernatants. Neither free malonate

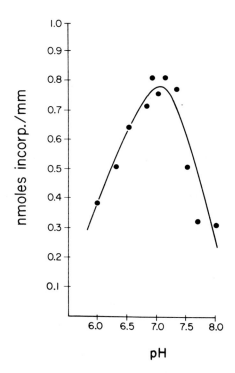

Fig. 1. pH-dependence of fatty acid biosynthesis
in normal rat sciatic nerve in-vitro. Results
expressed as nmoles malonyl-CoA incorporated/mm/hr

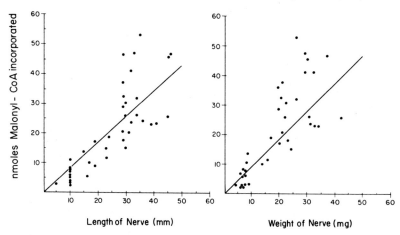

Fig. 2. Fatty acid biosynthesis in normal rat sciatic nerve
expressed on the basis of length and weight (nmoles malonyl-
CoA incorporated/hr)

TABLE 1

FATTY ACID BIOSYNTHESIS IN RAT SCIATIC NERVE IN-VITRO

Addition or Deletion	Labeled Precursor	Nanomoles Precursor Incorporated	
		per mm nerve	per mg nerve
Complete system	$1,3$-C^{14}-malonyl-CoA	0.72 ± 0.15	0.91 ± 0.24
Complete system	2-C^{14}-malonyl-CoA	0.49 ± 0.09	0.57 ± 0.07
Complete system	1-C^{14}-acetyl-CoA	0.07 ± 0.01	0.07 ± 0.01
- malonyl-CoA	1-C^{14}-acetyl-CoA	0	0
- acetyl-CoA	$1,3$-C^{14}-malonyl-CoA	0.21 ± 0.05	0.23 ± 0.09

nor free acetate could replace the respective CoA-esters in the presence of added ATP and free coenzyme A.

Palmitic acid was the fatty acid with maximum radioactivity (table 2). Decarboxylation revealed 8-15 percent of its total C^{14} in the carboxyl-group after incubation with $1,3$-C^{14}-malonyl-CoA and virtually no radioactivity after 1-C^{14}-acetyl-CoA.

The labeling of palmitic acid, the findings on decarboxylation, the dependence on NADPH and malonyl-CoA all supported a de-novo mechanism in the biosynthesis of fatty acids by peripheral nerve tissue.

Table 3 shows the relative distribution of the total fatty acid-C^{14} among the individual nerve lipids. Over 90 percent of the label was in the free fatty acids though they constituted only an estimated 1 percent of the lipid weight (cat)[5].

After nerve section, there was a rapid increase of the wet weight of the distal segment and enhanced biosynthesis of fatty acids (fig. 3). The distribution of the radioactive label did not change. Free fatty acids continued to have more than 90 percent of the total radioactivity. As the wet weight of the degenerating nerve declined again, there was a concomitant fall of fatty acid labeling (fig. 3).

TABLE 2

PERCENT DISTRIBUTION OF PEAK AREA AND RADIOACTIVITY IN TOTAL FATTY ACIDS OF RAT SCIATIC NERVE AFTER INCUBATION WITH 1, 3-C^{14}-MALONYL-COENZYME A IN-VITRO

Fatty Acid	Percent Peak Area	Percent C^{14}
12:0	0.3	0.1
14:0	1.1 ± 0.2	3.4 ± 0.9
16:0	21.7 ± 1.4	85.3 ± 0.7
16:1	3.6 ± 0.6	1.7 ± 0.6
16:2 & 17:0	0.3	0.7
18:0	8.7 ± 0.8	7.3 ± 0.8
18:1	43.1 ± 4.1	0.4
18:2	17.2 ± 6.0	0.2
20:0	0.7	0.2
18:3 & 20:1	0.9	0.1
22:0	1.2 ± 0.8	0.3
20:4 & 22:1	1.3 ± 0.1	trace
Other	0.1	0.2

S.D.; N = 3

CONCLUSIONS

Peripheral nerve biosynthesizes fatty acids in-vitro. While this observation is not new, the mechanism had not been character- ized before. Fatty acids are biosynthesized de-novo in the presence of catalytic amounts of acetyl-CoA, higher concentrations of malonyl-CoA and NADPH. In the described system, there is pre- ferential labeling of free fatty acids that normally constitute only a small portion of all nerve lipids. The subcellular localization of the biosynthetic pathway is not known but myelin

TABLE 3

PERCENTAGES OF C^{14} IN LABELED LIPIDS OF RAT SCIATIC NERVE AFTER INCUBATION WITH 1, 3-C^{14}-MALONYL-COENZYME A IN-VITRO

Lipid	Percentage of total lipid-C^{14}
Cholesteryl esters	1. 33 $\pm$ 1. 00
Triglycerides	2. 10 $\pm$ 0. 58
Free fatty acids	90. 62 $\pm$ 3. 70
Cholesterol and diglycerides	0. 73 $\pm$ 0. 32
Monoglycerides	1. 18 $\pm$ 0. 33
Phospholipids,cerebrosides, and sulfatides	3. 88 $\pm$ 2. 10

S. D. ; N = 6

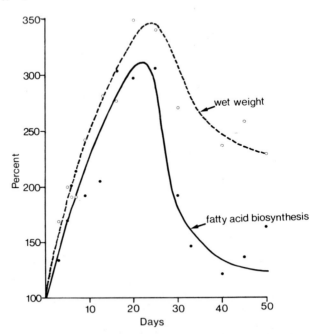

Fig. 3. Wet weight and fatty acid biosynthesis in rat sciatic nerve during Wallerian degeneration. (unoperated nerve=100 percent)

sheath and axon appear unlikely loci. The incorporation of fatty acid precursors is enhanced during Wallerian degeneration but the increase is transient. Free fatty acids and their metabolism are sensitive indicators of Wallerian degeneration and perhaps other neuropathies.

ACKNOWLEDGEMENT

Supported by medical research funds of the Veterans Administration.

REFERENCES

1. Majno, G. and Karnovsky, M.L. (1958) Neurology, 8 (suppl. 1), 88-89.
2. Kline, D., Magee, W.L., Pritchard, E.T. and Rossiter, R.J. (1958) J. Neurochem., 3, 52-58.
3. Magee, W.L., Berry, J.F., Magee, M.F. and Rossiter, R.J. (1959) J. Neurochem., 3, 333-340.
4. Pritchard, E.T. and Rossiter, R.J. (1959) J. Neurochem., 3, 341-346.
5. Berry, J.F., Cevallos, W.H. and Wade, R.R. (1965) J. Am. Oil Chem. Soc., 42, 492-500.

Peripheral Neuropathies
N. Canal and G. Pozza, eds.
© 1978 Elsevier/North-Holland Biomedical Press

NON-SPECIFIC CHOLINESTERASE (Ns.ChE) IN PERIPHERAL NEUROPATHIES

JUHANI JUNTUNEN
Department of Neurology, University of Helsinki, Helsinki, Finland

ABSTRACT

Histochemically demonstrable Ns.ChE is seen along the peripheral
nerves during their early development and it disappears along with
maturation of the peripheral neuromuscular system. In adults,
only the myoneural junctions show normally intense Ns.ChE activity.
This enzyme appears in the nerve trunks after nerve section or
disruption and it disappears after regeneration has occurred. It
also appears in the early phases of diffuse polyneuropathies; thus
it can be employed as an indicator of peripheral neuropathy. Histochemical appearance of Ns.ChE along the intramuscular nerves
probably reflects metabolic activity of the Schwann cells during
collateral sprouting, elimination of inappropriate nerves during
the early development and Schwann cell reaction during the early
stages of degeneration.

HISTOCHEMISTRY OF CHOLINESTERASES

The first demonstration of cholinesterases in nervous tissues
for about four decades ago has been followed by an extensive number of investigations in this field[12]. However, disagreement of
opinions still seem to prevail as to the significance of the different cholinesterases in the neuromuscular system. Division of
cholinesterases into specific (E.C. 3.1.1.7) and non-specific
(E.C. 3.1.1.8) cholinesterases is generally accepted, although
these groups include several substrate-specific enzymes[2]. The
histochemical demonstration of different cholinesterases is based
on the use of selective inhibitors and specific substrates of the
incubation medium[3]. Thus, by employing butyrylthiocholine iodide
as substrate and inhibiting specific cholinesterase, it is possible
to demonstrate butyrylcholinesterase, a representative of Ns.ChE[3].
The arbitrary division of the cholinesterases into these two
groups is not unequivocally supported by biochemical observations[2,10], but it has proved useful in cholinesterase histochemistry[3,4]. For practical purposes, the following method mainly

based on the Koelle thiocholine method[8] was employed to demon-
strateNs.ChE activity:

The muscle specimens were fixed at 4°C with formaldehyde (formol-
calcium 3.5%) for 12 hours. Frozen sections were cut at 30 micra
and washed in distilled water for 1-3 hours. Ns.ChE activity was
demonstrated using butyrylthiocholine iodide (Fluka AG, Buchs,
Schwitzerland) as substrate and 1:5-bis-(4-allyl-dimethyl-
ammoniumphenyl) pentan-3-one-diiodide (284C51; Burroughs &
Wellcome, London, England) as the specific inhibitor of acetylcholinesterase. Incubation was performed at 37°C and at pH 6.0
for about 3 hours after preincubation for 20 min in a solution
containing the inhibitor but not the substrate.

NORMAL DISTRIBUTION OF Ns.ChE IN THE MUSCLE

Numerous light and electron microscopic studies on the histochemical distribution of Ns.ChE in the muscle of adult animals
show that the most intense reaction is in the region of the
myoneural junctions (Fig.1d). Although there is disagreement of
opinions as to the exact localization of this enzyme, it seems to
be localized mainly in the axon terminal, the postsynaptic folds
and the terminal Schwann cells, or teloglial cells[13]. Due to the
spatial organization of the myoneural junctions in the muscle the
Ns.ChE-positive structures are seen in a longitudinal section of
the muscle as a proximal convex arch-shaped zone. Thus the intramuscular peripheral nerves representing the most distal part of
the spinal nerves are seen in a relatively narrow zone proximally to the zone of myoneural junctions.

The developing muscle shows quite a different histochemical
distribution of Ns.ChE. Intense enzyme activity is present along
the intramuscular nerves in the 16-day-old rat embryo. This
activity diminishes after the birth but still remains intense
during the early postnatal development (Fig.1a). It disappears
along with maturation of the neuromuscular system at the age of
about 3-4 weeks[13] (Fig.1c). The histochemical enchangment of
Ns.ChE activity is in agreement with the biochemical data available on the nervous cholinesterases during the development[2].

DISTRIBUTION OF Ns.ChE AFTER PERIPHERAL NERVE DAMAGE

Ns.ChE activity appears along the adult intramuscular nerves within 4 days after the nerve is sectioned and remains there, although weakened, for several months[4]. A similar pathological appearance of Ns.ChE is seen after nerve crush during degeneration (Fig.1e). Enchangement of the Ns.ChE activity occurs when the regenerating axons reach the intramuscular part of the peripheral nerves. Thereafter, normal distribution of Ns.ChE activity is reached coincidently with completed regeneration of the nerve.

Nerve section in newborn rat causes disappearance of the Ns.ChE activity from the intramuscular nerve trunks, while some activity remains in the myoneural junction. Similar disappearance of Ns.ChE activity occurs after local application of neurotubule-disrupting agents to the developing nerve[5] (Fig.1b).

The fact that some Ns.ChE activity remains in the myoneural area after the degenerating axon terminals have disappeared suggests that part of the enzyme at least is bound to the postsynaptic part of the myoneural junction, while the enzyme which is seen along the nerve trunks is located in the Schwann cells.

Thus, it is evident that Ns.ChE plays an important role in developing and regenerating nerves. Further, it is involved in the Schwann cell reaction during the early stages of nerve degeneration emphasizing the important role of the Schwann cells in the pathogenesis of peripheral neuropathies. As the nerves form increasingly collateral sproutings under pathological conditions[1], it is possible that these sproutings are responsible for the enchanged histochemical activity of Ns.ChE. On the other hand, elimination of inappropriate nerve endings in the formation of the neuromuscular connections probably accounts for the increased Ns.ChE activity during the development.

Ns.ChE AS AN INDICATOR OF PERIPHERAL NEUROPATHY

After establishing that a histochemically demonstrable Ns.ChE along the adult nerve trunks reflects degeneration of the nerve following acute mechanical trauma, experiments were performed to study whether this method could be employed in studies of diffuse toxic neuropathies[6,7]. After exposing adult rats to carbon

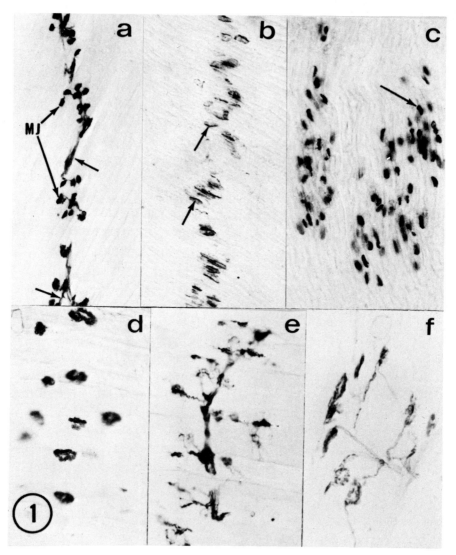

Fig.1. Distribution of Ns.ChE activity in the tibialis anterior muscle of the rat in different conditions. Magnification for Fig.1a-c: 110, for d-f: 130.

Intense Ns.ChE activity is seen in the myoneural junctions (MJ) and along the intramuscular nerves (arrows) of the developing animal (a)[5]. This neurilemmal activity disappears after disruption of the nerve (b)[5], and normal distribution of the enzyme is attained after regeneration is completed (c)[5]. Normal distribution of Ns.ChE in the adult animal (d). After nerve section, intense enzyme activity appears along the intramuscular nerve trunks within 4 days (e) Ns.ChE activity in diffuse toxic neuropathy shows clear pathological changes (f)[7].

disulphide for five months they developed signs of clinically, neurophysiologically and histologically evident peripheral neuropathy. Histochemical demonstration of Ns.ChE showed pathological distribution of this enzyme along the intramuscular nerve trunks of the tibialis anterior muscle[6] (Fig.1f). Another group of rats was fed with alcohol for about ten months, and development of alcoholic neuromyopathy was followed by electrophysiological, histological and histochemical methods[7]. It was discovered that, despite of the relatively good clinical condition of the animals at the end of the experiment, there was clear peripheral neuropathy. Histochemical demonstration of Ns.ChE appeared to be an early and sensitive indicator of neuropathy, even at stages where other techniques only show minor changes in the peripheral nerve. This technique also allows quantitation of the neuropathy more easily than many other techniques, since the activity is seen only in pathological nerves. Recent studies on the pathology of peripheral nerves emphasize the importance of histochemical techniques by which both the nerve terminals and the intramuscular nerves can be visualized[9]. The present technique may prove useful in the future due to its ability to show pathological changes in the most distal parts of the nerve, a matter of particular importance in respect to the concept of 'dying-back' mechanism in many neuropathies[11].

ACKNOWLEDGEMENTS

Supported by the Finnish Foundation for Alcohol Studies

REFERENCES

1. Diamond, J., Cooper, E., Turner, C. and Macintyre, L. (1976) Science 193, 371-377.
2. Eränkö, L. (1973) Histochemie 33, 1-14.
3. Eränkö, O. and Teräväinen, H. (1967) J. Histochem. Cytochem. 15, 399-403.
4. Eränkö, O. and Teräväinen, H. (1967) J. Neurochem. 14, 947-954
5. Juntunen, J. (1973) Z. Zellforsch. 142, 193-204.
6. Juntunen, J., Haltia, M. and Linnoila, I. (1974) Acta neuropath. (Berl.) 29, 361-369.

7. Juntunen, J., Teräväinen, H., Eriksson, K., Panula, P. and Larsen, A. (1978) Acta neuropath. (Berl.) 41, 131-137.

8. Koelle, G.B. (1951) J. Pharmacol. Exp. Ther. 103, 153-171.

9. Pestronk, A. and Drachman, D.B. (1978) Muscle & Nerve Jan/Feb., 70-74.

10. Prellwitz, W., Kapp, S. and Müller, D. (1976) J. Clin. Chem. Clin. Biochem. 14, 93-97.

11. Schoental, R. and Cavanagh, J.B. (1977) Neuropathol. Appl. Neurobiol. 3, 145-157.

12. Silver, A. (1974) The biology of cholinesterases, Norht-Holland, Amsterdam, pp 1-596.

13. Teräväinen, H. (1968) Histochemie 12, 307-315.

Peripheral Neuropathies
N. Canal and G. Pozza, eds.
© 1978 Elsevier/North-Holland Biomedical Press

NEURAL CONTROL OF GENE EXPRESSION OF SKELETAL MUSCLE FIBERS

SALVATORE METAFORA[1], ROBERTO COTRUFO[2], ARMANDO FELSANI[1], GIANFRANCO TAJANA[3], BRUNO RUTIGLIANO[4], ANTONIO DEL RIO[1], PIER PAOLO DE PRISCO[1], MARIA ROSARIA MONSURRO'[2], MARINA MELONE[2] and RICARDO MILEDI[5].

1 Laboratorio di Embriologia Molecolare, CNR; Arco Felice; Naples; ITALY.

2 Clinica Neurologica (R), 1[a] Facoltà di Medicina e Chirurgia; Naples.

3 Istituto di Anatomia Umana Normale; 2[a] Facoltà di Medicina e Chirurgia; Naples.

4 Laboratorio Internazionale di Genetica e Biofisica, CNR; Naples.

5 Department of Biophysics; University College; London; U.K.

ABSTRACT

Experimental results are presented in favour of the hypothesis that alpha-motoneurones control the gene expression of skeletal muscle; in fact, following denervation, we found significant changes in the complexity and molecular diversity of mRNA populations isolated from the ribosomal pellet of muscle homogenate, as compared with control muscles.

INTRODUCTION

Studies on the differentiation of slow and fast motor units and on the effects of denervation, direct and crossed reinnervation, block of nerve conduction, block of axonal flow, chronic electrical stimulations at various frequencies: on the properties of muscle fibers, have all led to the conclusion that alpha-motoneurones control some steps of differentiation and maintain the differentiated state of muscle fibers (1, 2).

Up to now, one of the main questions to be answered was how does the neural control operate at the muscular level. We have formulated the hypothesis that such control operates at the level of gene expression; an observation which suggested this hypothesis was that acetylcholine hypersensitivity of denervated muscles could be prevented by administration of Actinomycin D or Cicloheximide (1), drugs which inhibit the protein synthesis at the transcriptional and translational levels, respectively.

We have tried to give an answer to the above question by investigating the effects of denervation on the complexity and diversity of mRNA populations of a mammalian muscle. Our results indicate that, following denervation, there is a clear-cut change in the programme of muscle gene expression.

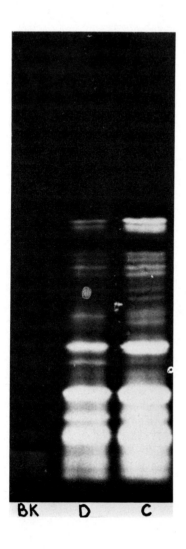

BK   D   C

Fig. 1 - Autoradiography of the electrophoretic profiles, on slabs of SDS-polyacrylamide gels, of the translation products of the incubation of muscle poly(A)$^{+}$mRNA's in a mRNA-dependent, cell free protein synthesising system, from wheat germ, in the presence of ^{35}S-methionine. Gels contained a continuous gradient of acrylamide (9% to 15%); the run was carried out from top to bottom of the figure; from top to bottom, the bands correspond to polypeptides of decreasing molecular weight. On the left side of the slab, was carried out the electrophoresis of the blank of incubation, containing all the constituents minus mRNA's; no incorporation of ^{35}S-methionine was found. In the middle, were separated the translation products of poly(A)$^{+}$mRNA's from denervated muscles; on the right side, the translation products of poly(A)$^{+}$mRNA's from control muscles. In all 3 runs, 50,000 cpm were deposited on the gel. The different proportions of the translation products of poly(A)$^{+}$mRNA's from control and denervated muscles, are self evident and indicate quantitative differences of some sequences in mRNA populations.

MATERIALS AND METHODS

All the procedures and the materials used can not be described here for lack of space and will be reported in the full paper to be published.

RESULTS AND DISCUSSION

Following purification, by affinity chromatography on oligo-DT

cellulose, of poly(A)$^+$mRNA's extracted from muscle ribosomal pellets, a big incubation of control or denervated poly(A)$^+$mRNA's
in a mRNA dependent cell free protein synthesising system from
wheat germ, in the presence of ^{35}S-methionine, was performed.[3].
Following incubation, the translation products were separated on
slabs of polyacrylamide-SDS gels; from the observation of the
autoradiography of these gels, several differences were found
between the profile obtained following incubation with poly(A)$^+$
mRNA's from control muscles and that obtained following incubation with poly(A)$^+$mRNA's from denervated muscles, as shown in
figure 1. This result, indicating quantitative differences in
some of the sequences present in mRNA populations isolated from
denervated and contralateral muscles, suggested meaningful changes in the gene expression of skeletal muscles, following denervation.

The poly(A)$^+$mRNA's, isolated from control and denervated muscles, were also used as templates to synthesize, by means of a
reverse transcriptase, the relevant complementary DNA (cDNA).
By using the radioactive cDNA thus obtained, we have kinetically
studied the molecular hybridization between homologous poly(A)$^+$
mRNA and cDNA from control and denervated muscles, as shown in
figures 2 and 3. The mathematical elaboration of the kinetic curves [4,5,6], reported in tables 1 and 2 for control and denervated mRNA populations, respectively, showed that, in control mRNA
populations, four different classes of abundance were present
(table 1), while, in denervated mRNA populations, only three
classes of abundance were detectable (table 2). In particular, the
first class of abundance found in control mRNA populations (whose
complexity was equal to 2×10^6 daltons), including 3 different sequences of 700,000 daltons, each repeated 3,200 times per diploid
genome (see also table 1), was not present as a single class in
denervated mRNA populations (table 2); therefore the most abun-

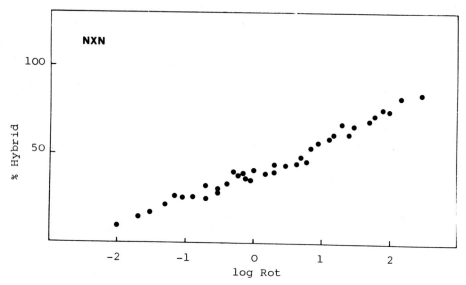

Fig. 2 – Hybridization kinetic curve of control poly (A)[+] mRNA and the homologous cDNA.

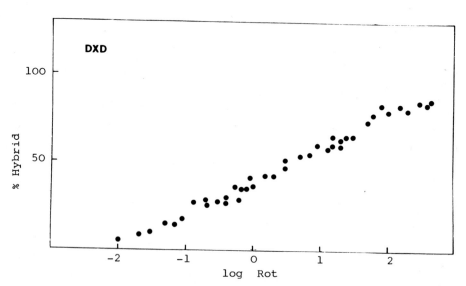

Fig. 3 – Hybridization kinetic curve of denervated poly (A)[+] mRNA and the homologous cDNA.

TABLE 1

COMPLEXITY, DIVERSITY AND ABUNDANCE OF mRNA-POLY(A)$^{+}$ POPULATION
FROM CONTROL MUSCLE

Mathematical analysis of the hybridization kinetica curve of control poly(A)$^{+}$mRNA and the homologous cDNA. Four distinct classes
of abundance were found; the first class included only 3 different
sequences of 700,000 daltons (diversity), each repeated 3,200
times (abundance)

Transition	Fraction of Hybridizable cDNA	Rot ½ (moles sec l^{-1}) Observed	Rot ½ (moles sec l^{-1}) Corrected	Base sequence Complexity(daltons)	Number of 700,000 daltons sequences	Number of copies per diploid genome	%Genome expressed
I	0.25	0.0126	0.00315	$2.000 \cdot 10^{6}$	2.9	3224	0.0002
II	0.17	0.193	0.03281	$2.090 \cdot 10^{7}$	30	210	0.002
III	0.23	3.067	0.70541	$4.490 \cdot 10^{8}$	641	13	0.05
IV	0.35	45.0	15.75	$1.000 \cdot 10^{10}$	14315	0.9	1.10
Total	1.00	—	—	$1.050 \cdot 10^{10}$	14989		1.15

Globin Standard → 1200 nucleotides ; Complexity = 420,000 daltons ; Rot ½ = 6.6014×10^{-4}

$\text{Rot } \frac{1}{2} = \frac{\ln 2}{k}$; $\begin{bmatrix} a_1 = 0.25 \\ a_2 = 0.166 \\ a_3 = 0.234 \\ a_4 = 0.35 \end{bmatrix}$; $\begin{bmatrix} K_1 = 55 \\ K_2 = 3.6 \\ K_3 = 0.226 \\ K_4 = 0.0154 \end{bmatrix}$; plateau level = 85%

dant three sequences of mRNA found in control muscles resulted
greatly reduced or absent following seven days of denervation.
It is possible to speculate that the class of abundance not detectable in denervated muscle is that normally coding for contractile proteins.

Another main difference between control and denervated mRNA
populations is the significant reduction of the total number of
different sequences per diploid genome observed following denervation, as it results by comparing tables 1 and 2.

In conclusion, experimental evidence has been given showing
that, following denervation, there is a significant change in
the program of gene expression of skeletal muscle fibers.

TABLE 2

COMPLEXITY, DIVERSITY AND ABUNDANCE OF mRNA POLY(A)$^+$ POPULATION
FROM DENERVATED MUSCLE

Mathematical analysis of the hybridization curve of denervated
poly(A)$^+$mRNA and the homologous cDNA. Only 3 classes of abundance were found; probably, the 3 sequences composing the first
class of abundance found in control muscles were greatly reduced
or absent 7 days following denervation

Transition	Fraction of Hybridizable cDNA	Rot $\frac{1}{2}$ (moles sec l^{-1}) Observed	Corrected	Base sequence Complexity(daltons)	Number of 700,000 daltons sequences	Number of copies per diploid genome	%Genome expressed
I	0.250	0.0315	0.00788	5.01 x 10^6	7.2	1042	0.0006
II	0.355	0.8350	0.2960	1.88 x 10^8	269	39	0.02
III	0.315	31.5000	12.44	7.91 x 10^9	11306	1	0.88
Total	1.000	—	—	8.10 x 10^9	11582	—	0.9

Globin Standard → 1200 nucleotides ; Complexity = 420,000 daltons ; Rot $\frac{1}{2}$ = 6.6014 x 10^{-4}

$$\text{Rot } \frac{1}{2} = \frac{\ln 2}{k} \quad ; \quad \begin{bmatrix} a_1 = 0.250 \\ a_2 = 0.355 \\ a_3 = 0.395 \end{bmatrix} \quad ; \quad \begin{bmatrix} K_1 = 22 \\ K_2 = 0.83 \\ K_3 = 0.022 \end{bmatrix} \quad ; \quad \text{plateau level} = 85\%$$

REFERENCES

1. Drachman, D.B. (1974) Ann. N. Y. Acad. Sci., 228.

2. Gutman, E. (1976) Ann. Rev. Physiol., 38, 177.

3. Roberts, B.E. and Paterson, B. M. (1973) Proc. Nat. Acad.
   Sci. USA, 70, 2330.

4. Felsani, A., Berthelot, F., Gros, F. and Croizat, B. (in press)
   Eur. J. Biochem.

5. Jacquet, M., Caput, D., Falcoff, E., Falcoff, R. and Gros, F.
   (1977) Biochimie, 59, 189.

6. Affara, N.A., Jacquet, M., Jakob, H., Jacob, F. and Gros, F.
   (1977) Cell, 12, 509.

AXONAL TRANSPORT

Peripheral Neuropathies
N. Canal and G. Pozza, eds.
© 1978 Elsevier/North-Holland Biomedical Press

THE ROLE OF CALCIUM IN AXOPLASMIC TRANSPORT IN MAMMALIAN NERVE FIBERS

S. OCHS, S. Y. CHAN, Z. IQBAL, R. WORTH AND R. JERSILD

Departments of Physiology, Anatomy and the Medical Biophysics Program, Indiana
University School of Medicine, 1100 West Michigan Street, Indianapolis, Indiana
46202, U.S.A.

INTRODUCTION

Fast axoplasmic transport was found to have a rate of 410 mm/day in the
nerves of a variety of mammalian species[1]. We recently found that Ca^{2+} is
essential for this process in cat sciatic nerve[2]. Our earlier in vitro studies[3]
and those of others[4,5], showing that axoplasmic transport was not affected when
nerves were placed in media in which Ca^{2+} was eliminated or depleted by EGTA,
have now been explained. The perineurium of sciatic nerve acts as a selective
permeability barrier and it retains the usual composition of extracellular ions,
including Ca^{2+}, within the endoneurial space when nerves are placed in an in
vitro medium depleted of this cation. When, however, we turned to the use of a
desheathed nerve preparation, the removal of Ca^{2+} from the medium was found effective in blocking axoplasmic transport in vitro.

The main results of our studies on Ca^{2+} obtained with the desheathed preparation, and additional studies on the role of Ca^{2+} in relation to axoplasmic
transport, will be presented in this review. As will be discussed, our recent
findings fit with and extend[6] the transport filament model[1] earlier put forth
to account for the mechanism of axoplasmic transport.

The desheathed peroneal nerve preparation

To assess the effect of changes in the level of Ca^{2+} on transport rather
than on processes related to synthesis, we routinely injected the L7 dorsal
root ganglia of cats with ^{3}H-leucine and allowed 2 hours in vivo for the rapidly synthesized labeled proteins to move down into the fibers of the tibial and
peroneal branches of the sciatic nerves. The nerves are then removed for de-
sheathing. The fibers of the L7 dorsal root ganglion supply the peroneal and
tibial branches close to the ganglion. Therefore, the two branches can be
readily separated by cutting their investing epineurial sheath fairly close to
the L7 ganglion, up to a distance of approximately 30 mm from the ganglion,
without severing crossing nerve fibers. The peroneal nerve is relatively un-
branched as compared to the tibial, and thus a long length of it can be readily
desheathed. This was done from 35 mm to 135 mm or more distal to the ganglion

allowing a long length of nerve to be exposed to the medium.

The sciatic nerves with their desheathed peroneal and sheathed tibial branches were then placed in flasks containing isotonic solutions of NaCl or sucrose
either with or without Ca^{2+} present and other ions added according to experimental requirements. The solutions were routinely bubbled with 95% O_2 + 5% CO_2
and kept at 38°C. After a predetermined period of an *in vitro* downflow in a
given incubation medium, axoplasmic transport was assessed by our usual technique of cutting the nerve into 5 mm lengths and counting the activity in each
segment[7]. In these experiments each branch was sectioned so that transport in
the two branches could be individually determined.

Transport *in vitro* with and without Ca^{2+} present in the medium

When a Ringer solution with a composition of 137 mM NaCl, 1.5 mM $CaCl_2$, 4 mM
KCl and 10 mM $NaHCO_3$ was used as the incubation medium, axoplasmic transport in
the desheathed peroneal branch compared favorably with that of the sheathed
tibial control (Fig. 1). Both branches showed the characteristic crest of

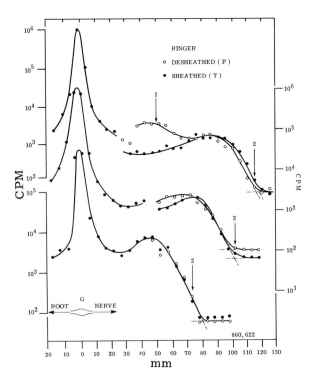

Fig. 1. Transport in Ringer in 3 sciatic nerves at 4.5, 6 and 7 hrs.
Arrow 1, nerve placed in Ringer; Arrow 2, expected normal downflow position.

activity with their fronts reaching the point expected of fast transport at the usual rate of 410 mm/day.

The general question to be settled was which components of the Ringer solution were essential to maintain transport. According to the transport filament model, the various substances synthesized in the cell bodies are considered to be bound to filaments which are moved down along the microtubules by means of cross-arms in analogy to the sliding filament theory of muscle[1]. Oxidative metabolism is the source of the energy required for the movement of the transport filaments[8]. The ATP supplied by metabolism is utilized at the cross-arms, presumably by the Ca^{2+}-Mg^{2+} ATPase found present in nerve[9]. The Ca^{2+}-Mg^{2+} ATPase is stationary or slowly moving in the nerve[9] and could be localized to the cross-arms. In our model, one would expect transport to depend critically on the activity of Ca^{2+}-Mg^{2+} ATPase. Our past experience with sheathed nerves *in vitro*, as noted above, had shown axoplasmic transport to be unaffected when Ca^{2+} was deleted from the incubation medium. However, the desheathed peroneal nerve preparation incubated in a Ca^{2+}-free isotonic solution of NaCl clearly shows an early developing profound block of transport (Fig. 2).

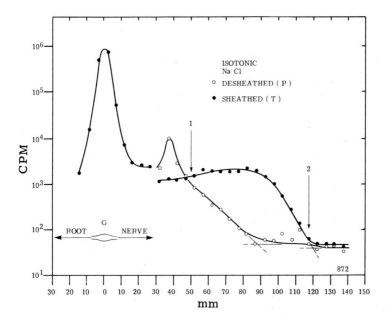

Fig. 2. Transport block in medium without Ca^{2+}. Arrow 1, nerve in Ca-free medium; Arrow 2, at normal downflow position. Total downflow time, 7 hrs.

The front of the transported activity in the desheathed nerve falls to the baseline of activity after approximately 2.6 hours of incubation. The decline in transport begins early, within 30 minutes of incubation in the Ca^{2+}-free medium. This indicates that the level of free Ca^{2+} within the fibers has changed so rapidly that mechanisms regulating the internal concentration of Ca^{2+} in the fibers are unable to supply the deficit. We will return to this point later on when discussing mechanisms of intracellular Ca^{2+} regulation. It is clearly apparent from Figure 2 that transport was little affected in the sheathed tibial nerve, in conformity with previous studies. As previously noted, this is explained by the ability of the perineurial sheath to retain the normal ionic composition of endoneurial fluid, including Ca^{2+}.

That Ca^{2+} alone can maintain transport was shown by adding concentrations of 3 to 5 mM Ca^{2+} to an isotonic NaCl solution as the incubation medium. At these concentrations of Ca^{2+} the form and rate of axoplasmic transport in the de- sheathed peroneal preparation were maintained equal to that in the sheathed tibial branch (Fig. 3). However, a 5 mM concentration of Ca^{2+} is higher than

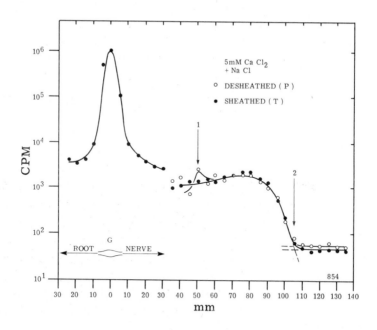

Fig. 3. Transport with Ca^{2+} added. Total downflow time, 6.2 hrs.

that present in the extracellular compartment. When a concentration of 1.5 mM Ca^{2+} was used, one more similar to extracellular fluid, the front of outflow in the desheathed nerves had a somewhat shallower slope, though it advanced to the distance expected of fast axoplasmic transport. This suggested that at this concentration of Ca^{2+}, axoplasmic transport was somewhat less than optimal. However, with a physiological concentration of 4 mM K^+ added to the incubation medium containing 1.5 mM Ca^{2+}, the shape of labeled outflow was similar to that seen with a Ringer solution or in the sheathed nerve. We conclude that such an amount of K^+ plays a facilitating role.

Further documentation that Ca^{2+} is critical in maintaining transport was obtained by the addition of 4 mM EGTA to a Ringer solution. The block of transport found with this medium was similar to that seen in a Ca^{2+}-free incubation solution. The specificity of action of Ca^{2+} was further shown by the inability of Mg^{2+} to substitute for Ca^{2+} in the incubation medium. The block of transport in a Ca^{2+}-free NaCl medium took place on an average of 2.6 hours, while in NaCl containing 5 mM Mg^{2+} block occurred at 3.5 hours[2]. Thus, while it has a weak action similar to Ca^{2+}, Mg^{2+} cannot substitute for Ca^{2+} in maintaining a normal axoplasmic transport.

Sodium chloride is not essential. An isotonic solution of sucrose containing 5 mM Ca^{2+} maintains axoplasmic transport.

Increased levels of calcium and microtubules

Higher than normal levels of Ca^{2+} can also cause a block of transport. This occurs at concentrations above 25 mM. The block was first seen at a concentration of 35 mM, occurred earlier when a 50 mM Ca^{2+} solution was used, and developed most rapidly when nerves were placed in an isotonic Ca^{2+} medium (Fig. 4).

We consider that while normally only a small amount of Ca^{2+} enters the fibers, enough enters at these high concentrations to exceed an optimum level of Ca^{2+} in the fibers. Increased levels of Ca^{2+} intracellularly may affect transport by a disassembly of microtubules, an action seen in studies of purified microtubular protein[10,11]. In the transport filament hypothesis the microtubules are viewed as the "rails" along which the transport filaments are moved. Thus, a disassembly of the microtubules could readily account for a block of axoplasmic transport. A marked loss of microtubules had been observed in rat sciatic nerve fibers with as little as 1 mM Ca^{2+} present in an incubation medium[12]. However, in those studies the nerves were transversely sectioned into lengths of 0.5 mm or so, allowing a ready access of Ca^{2+} to the interiors of the nerve fibers. In our preparations a much smaller amount of Ca^{2+} would be expected to enter the fibers through the intact axolemma. To further pursue

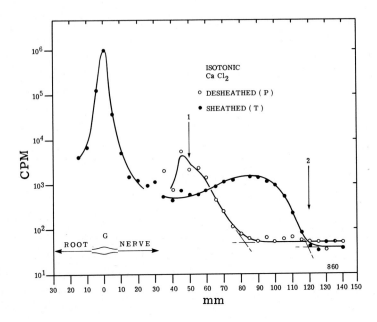

Fig. 4. Block of transport with high Ca^{2+}. Total downflow time, 7 hrs.

such a possibility, desheathed nerves were exposed to high levels of Ca^{2+} *in vitro* for 4 hours and pieces of nerve were taken and prepared for electron microscopy. The microtubules were seen to have their usual densities in the large fibers with concentrations as high as 25 mM Ca^{2+} where block of transport did not occur. At concentrations of 35 mM Ca^{2+} where block was seen, there was evidence of a loss of microtubules. The loss was more marked at concentrations of Ca^{2+} above 50 mM, but additional signs of damage were also present.

The role of microtubules in transport has been further studied by the use of a number of microtubular blocking agents. The mitotic blocking agents colchicine and the vinca alkaloids bind to the microtubule subunit tubulin and are considered to block axoplasmic transport[13,14] by causing a disassembly of the microtubules, a concept first advanced to explain the effect of colchicine on mitotic spindles in arresting cell division. The loss of microtubules seen in peripheral nerve with these various mitotic blocking agents has similarly been explained; the binding of the agent to the tubulin affects an equilibrium existing between tubulin and microtubules with a shift toward tubulin and away from the microtubules causing their disassembly. This concept has been brought into question because a block of transport has been reported with colchicine without apparent loss of microtubules[16]. For some time we have been comparing the vinca alkaloids vincristine, vinblastine and vindesine for their effectiveness in blocking axoplasmic transport *in vitro*. These agents cause a disassembly of microtubules at levels which block transport [17]. Additionally, studies made with a new type of mitotic blocking agent, maytansine (MYT), clearly show the relationship of microtubules to axoplasmic transport[18,19]. An important aspect in those studies was to relate transport in the large fibers which carry the bulk of labeled materials[7] and microtubular density after treatment with mitotic agents. Microtubular loss correlated well with the block of transport. However, the decreased number of microtubules does not in itself prove that these agents bind to tubulin with a resultant shift of tubulin from the microtubules. While we have some evidence for this possibility, the disassembly of microtubules could come about by some alternative mechanism in the intact nerve fiber which differs from the process observed when using purified microtubular protein (cf. 20).

The apparent exceptions to a relation of microtubules to transport which have been noted in the literature may be due to several factors. Assessing microtubular densities in the unmyelinated fibers which contribute little to the labeled downflow carried in the large diametered fibers is misleading. Another factor which may result in a block with a substantial fraction of microtubules remaining is that breaks occurring at intervals along the length of the microtubules could prevent the transport filaments from passing. These breaks, if relatively few, would give little evidence of disassembly in cross-sections taken for counting of microtubular densities in electron micrographs. With respect to the block seen with high levels of Ca^{2+}, an explanation other than a microtubular disassembly may be that an optimal level of Ca^{2+} is needed for the action of Ca^{2+}-Mg^{2+} ATPase[8,9] and an excess of Ca^{2+} would interfere with enzyme activity. Transport would be halted by the reduced activity of the cross-bridges due to decreased utilization of ATP.

Another possibility is that a Ca-activated protease, such as had been found in *Myxicola* giant axon[21], may be present in mammalian fibers and its activation cause a dissolution of organelles. Additionally, Ca^{2+} could block the sodium pump and the resulting increase of fiber Na^+ may have a blocking action.

The regulation of Ca^{2+} in the fibers in relation to transport

We consider that the block of axoplasmic transport seen in a Ca-free medium is brought about by a depletion of Ca^{2+} from within the nerve fibers. On the assumption that the level of free Ca^{2+} in the axoplasm of the mammalian fiber is similar to that found in cephalopod giant axons, Ca^{2+} should be present in a concentration close to 10^{-7} M[22,23]. The free Ca^{2+} concentration in the axoplasm is regulated by several mechanisms. Most important is the extrusion of Ca^{2+} by a Na^+-Ca^{2+} exchange mechanism or carrier, or by a Ca^{2+} pump in the axonal membrane[22-28]. In the giant nerve fiber a reduced Ca^{2+} efflux is seen in Na^+-deficient media indicating that a Na-Ca carrier acts as an exchange mechanism rather than being directly driven by ATP. We found that the block of axoplasmic transport in the desheathed peroneal nerve incubated in a Ca-free isotonic sucrose occurred approximately at the same time as in a Ca-free isotonic NaCl medium. This finding is not in accord with the expectations of a pure Na-Ca exchange mechanism. It is possible that an active Ca^{2+} pump mechanism similar to that of the RBC membrane[28] is present in the axolemma of mammalian nerve fibers. On the other hand, the Ca^{2+} efflux studies of Kalix[29] carried out in mammalian nerve do not appear to support the presence of a Ca^{2+} pump. Further investigation of flux characteristics of the desheathed peroneal nerve preparation with $^{45}Ca^{2+}$ is required to resolve this point.

Another mechanism which may regulate Ca^{2+} in the nerve fibers is the binding or sequestration of Ca^{2+}. Several mmoles of Ca^{2+} are sequestered in the mitochondria of giant nerve axons[22] through the activity of the respiratory chain or the hydrolysis of ATP[30,31]. Calcium sequestration may also occur in the smooth endoplasmic reticulum (ER). The cell body was shown to contain Ca^{2+} in the ER by means of a histochemical technique using pyroantimonate[32]. Calcium was found in mitochondria and in the smooth ER close to the axolemma of the giant axon with oxalate and verified as such with an X-ray EM probe[33].

Using the pyroantimonate method, we found dense staining particles, some apparently in smooth ER profiles and also some in and associated with the mitochondria. When higher levels of Ca^{2+} were present in the media of *in vitro* incubated nerves, there was an increased number of these particles. Evidence that the dense staining material represented Ca^{2+} was gained by treating the thin sections with EGTA. This removed a number of the dense-staining particles which then showed open clear spaces.

How effective sequestration may be as compared to the action of a Ca^{2+} pump in the axonal membrane in regulating the level of free Ca^{2+} in the axon is as yet unresolved. It should be noted that the block of axoplasmic transport we found in Ca^{2+}-free media began rapidly, within 30 minutes. This indicates that the sequestered stores of Ca^{2+} in the mitochondria and/or ER have such a low rate of release that they cannot supply the deficit of Ca^{2+} in the axoplasm, at least in the short term.

Metabolism and calcium regulation

A relation of oxidative metabolism to storage of Ca^{2+} in the mitochondria was also suggested in our preparation by a fall in the level of ~P to as much as 22% when transport was blocked in a Ca-free medium[2]. This amount of ~P decrease would not in itself account for the block of axoplasmic transport, since axoplasmic transport and the action potentials are not blocked until ~P falls to 50% of control levels[8]. We found that in desheathed nerves exposed to a Ca-free medium, action potentials could still be elicited for at least 2 hours after axoplasmic transport had been blocked, indicating that an adequate supply of ATP was still available to maintain the sodium pump. Since a common pool of ATP is considered to supply both the sodium pump and the transport mechanism[7], a decrease in ~P of 22% could still adequately support transport. In an earlier study made with sheathed nerves treated with oxalate, a similar 22% fall of ~P was seen with an associated block of transport[1]. Most likely in those earlier studies, a sufficient amount of oxalate had passed through the perineurium to produce an essentially Ca^{2+}-free endoneurial fluid, resulting in a block of transport and fall of ~P.

Another important relation between metabolism and Ca^{2+} has been noted in the squid axon. Addition of $NaHCO_3$ and use of a 95% O_2 and 5% CO_2 gas mixture allows CO_2 to enter the fibers with a fall in their internal pH to 6.7. This caused a decrease in the level of ionized Ca^{2+} within the axons[35]. In mammalian nerves, little difference in transport could be traced to pH changes over a range of 6-8. However, an extension of those studies is required.

A calcium-binding protein in nerve and its possible role in Ca^{2+} regulation

Another means by which Ca^{2+} could be regulated in nerve fibers is through the calcium-binding protein (CaBP) found in the cat sciatic nerves[36,37]. When $^{45}Ca^{2+}$ was injected into cat L7 dorsal root ganglia, a crest of fast transported radioactivity was seen to move down the nerve at the usual rate of 410 mm/day. This same rate had earlier been reported for $^{45}Ca^{2+}$ downflow in frog nerve *in vitro* by Hammerschlag and his colleagues when they scaled the rate up to a temperature of 37°C[5]. In our studies, the $^{45}Ca^{2+}$ was shown to be carried down in association with a 15,000 dalton protein which had earlier been found to be fast transported in nerves as a ^{3}H-leucine labeled component peak Ic fraction[38].

A careful examination of this protein by gel filtration, various other isolation techniques and equilibrium dialysis, showed it to have the properties expected of a Ca^{2+}-binding protein. It has a Ca^{2+} disassociation constant of 6.6×10^{-5} M, a value consistent with the binding characteristic known for other CaBPs and its molecular weight of 15,000 is also close to that of other CaBPs[39].

The fast transport of CaBP in nerve raises some interesting possibilities. The most attractive is that it, itself, may be the transport filament or a part of the transport filament. We can conceive it to act as muscle troponin C to regulate locally the level of Ca^{2+} and through such control, the ATPase activity on which ATP utilization and the movement process itself depends. A CaBP was found in the synaptosomes with the same molecular weight, electrophoretic mobility on acrylamide gels, and binding properties as the CaBP of the nerve[38,40]. In the nerve terminals, the CaBP could participate in translocation of components and the mechanism of release of transmitter and/or trophic materials.

SUMMARY

Our recent findings that Ca^{2+} is required to maintain axoplasmic transport and that a fast transported CaBP is present in nerve, open up new possibilities for a better understanding of the underlying mechanism. These findings are in accord with the transport filament hypothesis, and an interesting possibility is that the CaBP may be all or part of the transport filament. By locally regulating Ca^{2+} it could modulate Ca^{2+}-Mg^{2+} ATPase activity and the utilization of ATP, thus acting integrally as part of the movement process itself. Calcium at high concentrations and antimitotic agents block transport and decrease microtubular density. These findings are in accord with our transport model in which the microtubules are thought to act as the "rails" along which the transport filaments and the materials they carry are moved. Further specification of the mechanism is required.

ACKNOWLEDGMENTS

We would like to thank Jennifer A. Gallagher for her help with the preparations and Vera McAdoo for help with the electron microscopy. The assistance of the Illustrations Department at the Indiana University School of Medicine is also appreciated. This work was supported by NIH PHS RO1 NS8706 and NSF 77-24176.

REFERENCES

1. Ochs, S. (1972) Science, 176, 252-260.

2. Ochs, S., Worth, R. M. and Chan, S. Y. (1977) Nature, 270, 748-750.

3. Ochs, S. and Smith, C. (1975) J. Neurobiol., 6, 85-102.

4. Banks, P., Mayor, D. and Mraz, P. (1973) J. Physiol., Lond., 229, 383-394.

5. Hammerschlag, R., Dravid, A. R. and Chiu, A. Y. (1975) Science, 188, 273-275.

6. Ochs, S. (1978) in Nerve Repair: Its Clinical and Experimental Basis, Jewett, D. L. and McCarroll, H. R. eds., Mosby, St. Louis (in press).

7. Ochs, S. (1972) J. Physiol., 227, 627-645.

8. Ochs, S. (1974) Fed. Proc., 33, 1049-1058.

9. Khan, M. A. and Ochs, S. (1974) Brain Res., 81, 413-426.

10. Weisenberg, R. C. (1972) Science, 177, 1104-1105.

11. Shelanski, M. L., Gaskin, F. and Cantor, C. R. (1973) Proc. Nat. Acad. Sci. U.S.A., 70, 765-768.

12. Schlaepfer, W. W. (1971) Exp. Cell Res., 67, 73-80.

13. Kreutzberg, G. W. (1969) Proc. Nat. Acad. Sci., 62, 722-728.

14. Dahlström, A. (1969) Acta Physiol. Scand., 76, 33A-34A.

15. Inoue, S. and Sato, H. (1967) J. Gen. Physiol., 50, Suppl., 259-292.

16. Fernandez, H. L., Huneeus, F. C. and Davison, P. F. (1970) J. Neurobiol., 1, 395-409.

17. Chan, S. Y., Worth, R. M. and Ochs, S. (1978) Trans. Amer. Soc. Neurochem., 9, 201.

18. Ghetti, B. and Ochs, S. (1977) Soc. Neurosci. Abst. 3, 30.

19. Ghetti, B. and Ochs, S. (1978) These proceedings.

20. Wilson, L., Anderson, K. and Chin, D. (1976) in Cell Motility, Book, C., Goldman, R., Pollard, T. and Rosenbaum, J. eds., Cold Spring Harbor Laboratory, Cold Spring Harbor, pp. 1051-1064.

21. Gilbert, D. S., Newby, B. J. and Anderton, B. H. (1975) Nature, 256, 586-589.

22. Baker, P. F. (1972) Prog. Biophys. Molec. Biol., 24, 177-223.

23. Dipolo, R., Requena, J., Mullins, L. J., Brinley, F. Jr., Scarpa, A. and Tiffert, T. (1976) J. Gen. Physiol., 67, 433.

24. Blaustein, M. P. (1974) Rev. Physiol. Biochem. Pharm., 70, 33-82.

25. Brinley, F. Jr., Spangler, S. G. and Mullins, L. J. (1975) J. Gen. Physiol. 66, 223-250.

26. Baker, P. F. (1976) Fed. Proc., 35, 2589-2595.

27. Dipolo, R. (1976) Fed. Proc., 35, 2579-2582.

28. Schatzmann, H. J. (1975) Curr. Topics Memb. Transport, 6, 125-168.

29. Kalix, P. (1971) Pflügers Arch., 326, 1-14.

30. Lehninger, A. L. (1976) Biochemistry, 2nd ed., Worth Publ. Co., New York.

31. Carafoli, E. and Crompton, M. (1976) Symposia Soc. Exper. Biol., 30, 89-115

32. Stockel, M. E., Hindelang-Gertner, C., Dellman, H. D., Porte, A. and Stutinsky, F. (1975) Cell Tiss. Res., 157, 307-322.

33. Henkart, M., Reese, T. S. and Brinley, F. Jr. (1978) Abst. J. Biophys., 21, 187a.

34. Dipolo, R. (1978) Abst. J. Biophys., 21, 186a.

35. Baker, P. F. and Honerjäger, P. (1978) Nature, 273, 160-161.

36. Iqbal, Z. and Ochs, S. (1976) Soc. Neurosci. Abst., 2, 47.

37. Iqbal, Z. and Ochs, S. (1978) J. Neurochem., (in press).

38. Iqbal, Z. and Ochs, S. (1975) Soc. Neurosci. Abst., 1, 802.

39. Kretsinger, R. H. (1976) Int. Rev. Cytol., 46, 323-393.

40. Iqbal, Z. and Ochs, S. (1978) Soc. Neurosci., Abst., (in press).

Peripheral Neuropathies
N. Canal and G. Pozza, eds.
© 1978 Elsevier/North-Holland Biomedical Press   125

AXONAL TRANSPORT AND INTRACELLULAR ORGANIZATION OF SKELETAL AND
CONTRACTILE STRUCTURES IN MATURING NEURONS

MARIA FLAVIA DI RENZO and PIER CARLO MARCHISIO
Department of Human Anatomy, University of Turin, Turin, Italy

ABSTRACT

Macromolecules are rapidly transported in maturing neurons
when axons are still elongating and their terminals have not
yet formed synapses of the mature type. The transport of glycosylated molecules, notably glycoproteins, is particularly efficient in maturing neurons and their flow may be suggested to
occur also within the axolemma along the entire length of the
axon. The mechanism responsible for driving materials along maturing axons may be located in a subaxolemmal network of contractile microfilaments which has been identified by immunofluorescence microscopy in sensory and sympathetic neurons cultured
in vitro in the presence of nerve growth factor. The role of
microtubules in axonal transport is that of providing direction
of flow and anchoring points for contractile structures.

INTRODUCTION

Most mature neurons possess two types of cellular extensions,
one axon and one or several dendrites. The axon is usually a
long, slender and branched process which may reach sites at long
distance from the cell body.

Neuronal metabolism is characterized by the confinement of
the protein synthesizing apparatus in areas located around the
nucleus, i.e. in the perikaryon and large dendrites. This fact
therefore, entirely depends on the cell body for its protein need.
Such dependence of the axon on the cell body was recognized by
Cajal long time ago. It is also known that the axonal volume

may be much larger than cell body and dendrites together. Moreover, the axon may be very long. It may then be stated that large amounts of proteins must migrate into the cell body and move
along it in order to supply the needs of the whole axonal arbo-
rization.

Axonal endings form synaptic connections either with other
neurons or with effector organs. Since axonal terminals and
synaptic boutons are sites of large renewal of proteins[1], a
continuous streaming directed from the cell body to synaptic
endings is an absolute condition for the correct function of
neuronal networks. The function of purveying axons and synaptic
boutons with cell body-assembled molecules is fulfilled by the
anterograde axonal transport.

In adult neurons axonal transport occurs in two main phases.
The rapid phase of transport occurs at rate exceeding 100 mm
day^{-1} in warm blooded animals. Wide variations in the rate of
rapid transport have been reported[2]; however, the most reliable
measure of rapid axonal transport has been reported by Ochs[3,4]
in cat sciatic nerve ($>$400 mm day^{-1}). The slow phase of transport
conveys materials at a rate of 1-2 mm day^{-1} and very likely
corresponds to the bulk movement of the axoplasm cylinder[2].

In mature neurons a broad spectrum of molecules is rapidly
conveyed along axons in order to support the renewal of worn-out
structural molecules[5]. Specific synaptic functions like impulse
transmission and maintenance of synaptic recognition are based
on this type of communication between the perikaryon and the
periphery.

In maturing and regenerating neurons rapid axonal transport
plays additional roles. Primarily, the sprouting and the elongation of processes as well as their branching require a regular
supply of new building blocks which are made in the cell body
and conveyed along the growing axon. Moreover, the subtle and
still elusive phenomenon which controls the guidance of growing

axons and leads eventually to recognition of synaptic targets
is probably dependent on surface molecules which interact with
the microenvironment of different embryonic areas[6]. These signals
are most likely conveyed to growing axonal tips by rapid transport
which plays, though indirectly, a role in controlling these fundamental phenomena of neuroontogenesis.

EXEPERIMENTAL MODELS AND RESULTS

Study model for the development of axonal transport. The optic
pathway of the chick embryo has been adopted for studying the
development of axonal transport[7,8]. The choice was justified
by a wealth of informations available about the anatomy and the
ontogenesis of the avian optic pathway and by the observation
that the system is easily amenable to surgical manipulation
in ovo. In fact, since early stages, the large pigmented eyeballs
of the chick embryos represent rather closed compartments which
are easily injected with labelled precursors. The latter are
promptly taken up by retinal ganglion cells which give rise to
optic fibers. The optic nerve undergoes complete crossing at
the chiasm and its fibers mostly reach the contralateral tectum
opticum where they synapse with the neurons of the outer tectal
layers.

The administration of labelled precursors directly to the
retina allows to measure the level of local incorporation and
to study the advancement of the labelled front toward the tectum
either by liquid scintillation spectrometry[7,8] or by autoradiography[9,10]. The front migration may be followed in one pathway
(as compared to the opposite uninjected pathway which provides
an internal control) at different stages of development and at
progressive survival times.

Axonal transport in developing retinal neurons. The intraocular administration of ^{3}H-leucine in 10-day chick embryos
leads to a marked tectal asymmetry in labelled proteins after

about 2 h[7,11]. A rough estimate of the transport velocity gave a rate in the order of 100 mm day^{-1}. Autoradiography after ^{3}H-fucose administration confirmed the existence of a rapidly advancing radioactive front and also suggested that rapid axonal transport occurs since the 7th day of development namely when optic axons are still elongating and growing tips have nor yet contacted their tectal targets[10]. Crossland et al.[12], using a more sensitive autoradiographic technique after administration of ^{3}H-proline, reported similar findings and suggested that rapid axonal transport occurs in retinal neurons as early as day 5.

From the results of earlier investigations[7,11] it was inferred that the rate of axonal transport could increase progressively with the age of the embryo confirming data obtained in the newborn rabbit[13]. Such a concept derived from the observation that the wavefront of labelled proteins reached the contralateral tectum about 2 h after precursor administration at any stage considered. Obviously the length of the optic pathway increases considerably throughout development and, therefore, should the rate of transport comparably increase. We believe that a precise evaluation of the rate of transport is difficult to achieve in developing axonal bundles because of rapid remodelling occurring within short maturation periods. Better informations are obtained when the efficiency of transport is taken into account, in other words, when the relative amount of labelled materials exported by one retina to the contralateral tectum in a standard time of 6 h is considered as the transport parameter[14].

By using this parameter, it was found[14] that ^{3}H-proline labelled proteins are transported with increasing efficiency throughout development namely between day 10 and hatching time (Fig. 1). Such an increasing transport efficiency can be justified by a parallel increase of the rate of transport; however, this interpretation seems unlikely since efficiency decreases after hatching when it is known that transport rate increases: in 3 week-

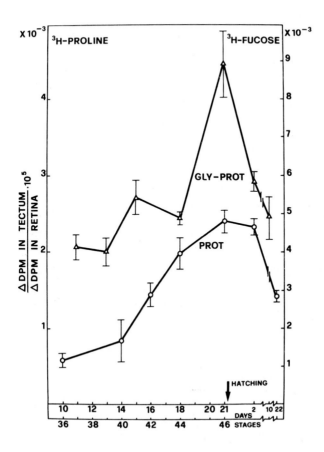

Fig. 1. Changes of the relative proportions of labelled proteins and glycoproteins transported along the optic pathway of chick embryos and recovered in the optic tecta 6 h after intraocular injection of the labelled precursor. Each point represents the mean ± SE of more than 12 embryos. From Gremo and Marchisio[14].

old chicks, when rate is close to that of adult fowls[15], efficiency is considerably lower than in embryos. These results support the idea that the relative amount of proteins which undergoes rapid somatofugal migration is proportionally much larger in the retinal neurons of the embryo than in those of hatched chicks where maturation still occurs though at a much slower rate.

Proteins flowing at a rapid rate in embryonic retinal neurons are a mixture of different polypeptides[11]. Among these proteins, glycoproteins were considered with particular attention because of their well known properties in surface recognition[16] which suggest a primary role in synaptogenesis[6].

Glycoproteins transport was studied by adopting ^{3}H-fucose as a precursor of their carbohydrate chains and following the migration of acid-insoluble radioactivity[10,14]. The following results were obtained: 1) A rapid transport of labelled glycoproteins could be demonstrated in 7-day embryos: this indicates that glycoproteins represent a predominant components of the rapidly transported protein populations of elongating axons; 2) Glycoproteins are very promptly squeezed into axons: hence they continue   slowly accumulating in the tectal terminals for at least 2 d and eventually give rise to intense labelling of the neuropile of outer tectal layers (Fig. 2); though, a considerable portion is used en route and causes durable labelling of the optic fibers; 3) The developmental pattern of glycoprotein transport efficiency is somewhat different from that of the bulk proteins (Fig. 1): instead of a continuously increasing efficiency two phases of rapid increase are found during the period of most intense synaptogenesis and between day 18 and hatching time when visual function begins.

The biphasic development of glycoprotein transport efficiency is nearly identical to that of other classes of glycosylated molecules like gangliosides and glycosaminoglycans (Di Renzo and Marchisio, unpublished results).

Thus, the rapid axonal transport of molecules mostly located in membraneous structures is also relatively more efficient in developing than in mature neurons but their transport efficiency seems to correlate better with given maturational events. The earlier phase (from day 13 to 15) is, at least chronologically,

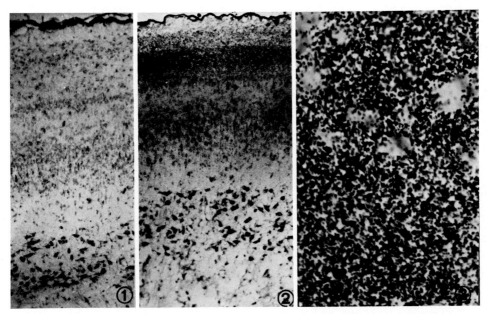

Fig. 2. Autoradiography reveals a marked accumulation of radio
activity in the outer tectal layers of 18 d chick embryos (2)
following injection of 1 μCi of ³H-fucose in the contralateral
eye. The ipsilateral tectum is unlabelled (1). Radioactivity
accumulates in the neuropile and leaves tectal cell bodies
free of silver grains (3). 1 and 2 x400; 3 x1,100.

related to maximal synaptogenesis in the tectum[17]; in the same
period critical changes have been reported in acetylcholinesterase[18] and choline acetyltransferase activity[19] as well as in
tubulin[20] and actin[21] concentrations. The following phase, lasting
from day 18 to 21, occurs along with the final maturation of
tectal synaptic connections leading to the onset of light-evoked
reflex activity in the optic pathway[22].

Neuronal cytoskeletal and contractile structures are related
to the mechanism of axonal transport. The molecular mechanism
driving axonal transport is still poorly known (for recent review

see Lasek and Hoffman[23]). The analogy between rapid axonal transport and other forms of intracellular transport[24] still supports the attribution of a primary role to cytoplasmic micro-tubules in directing axonal streaming[25,26]. However, such a role seems to be restricted to providing directionality of the move-ments and rigidity to axons in view of the cytoskeletal function, controlling maintenance and changes of the cell shape, which is now generally attributed to microtubules of most cells including neurons[27].

There is no convincing evidence that microtubules may be directly involved in providing the driving force of transport. In contrast, the energy requirements for axonal transport suggest a close functional analogy with the mechanism of muscle contrac-tion and the involvement of actin- and myosin-containing fila-mentous structures[3,4].

In order to identify the cellular topography of contractile structures in elongating axons we have recently studied the distribution of actin-containing structures in neuroblastoma cells[28,29] as well as in sympathetic and sensory neurons iso-lated from the chick embryo and induced to sprout axons in vitro by the action of NGF[30]. In axons actin is mostly localized at the very margin and close to the cytoplasmic face of the axolemma (Fig. 3, 1) while microtubules occupy the core of the axon (Fig. 3, 2). A marked amount of actin-containing structures can be found at the very edge of growth cones (Fig. 3, 3). These results confirm previous data obtained by electron microscopy which localize actin-containing microfilaments in the outer rim of axons and beneath the axolemma[31,32]. Microfilaments are most probably connected with the cytoplasmic face of the plasma mem-brane[33] and may also be anchored on microtubules[32]. Even if the

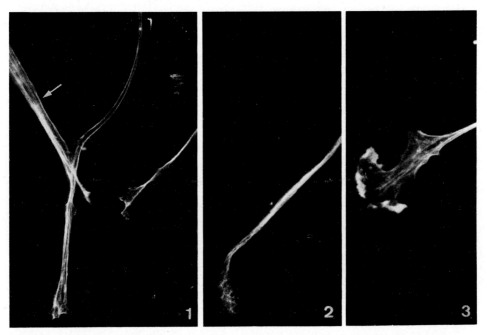

Fig. 3. Sensory ganglion cells isolated from 8-day chick embryos were cultured in vitro in the presence of 20 ng ml^{-1} NGF. Immunofluorescence microscopy, employing monospecific antibodies raised against chicken smooth muscle actin[33] and pig brain tubulin[41], reveals the peripheral location of actin containing structures in elongating axons (1) and in a growth cone (3). The arrow in (1) indicates a spindle-shaped Schwann cell. In contrast, a bundle of parallel microtubules is directed along the axis of the process (2): at the growth cone (bottom) microtubules diverge and may be individually resolved. Microtubules never reach the very edge of the growth cone which is conversely lined by actin-containing structures (3). 1 and 2 x700; 3 x1,200.

details of the organization of this subaxolemmal area are not yet known it is plausible to propose that the axonal outer rim contains channels where rapidly transported molecules are transported by a mechanism based on contractile microfilaments.

This idea receives support from autoradiographic evidence which shows that most transported materials are indeed located at the very periphery of axons[34,35]. The vehicle of transported proteins has not yet been demonstrated even if vesicles and cysternae of the smooth endoplasmic reticulum found along axons may indeed play such a role[36].

This model for transport which mostly involves subaxolemmal microfilaments does not underestimate the role of microtubules. The latter as well as neurofilaments are the most probable anchoring points for contractile microfilaments[37]. When they are destroyed by colchicine[25,26] and other mitotic drugs[14,38] anchoring points are lost and the mechanism of transport is blocked bacause the driving mechanism works ineffectively.

In embryonic axons the peculiar transport characteristics of glycosylated molecules (see above) suggest the possibility that they are first largely incorporated in the axolemma. We have proposed the hypothesis that carbohydrate-containing molecules move along the axolemma in its fluid phospholipid matrix and may reach the terminal segment by following surface lanes ("axolemmal transport")[39]. Such a surface movement rests on the concept that membrane molecules, like glycoproteins, enjoy mobility on the membrane plane and may be also modulated by the subsurface network of micofilaments[40]. In elongating axons glycoproteins, exposing their carbohydrate chains at the surface of the axon, may interact with other glycoproteins at the surface of adjacent axons or of glia cells. This interaction provides a basis for the parallel growth of axon bundles and for contact guidance toward targets.

CONCLUSION

Axonal transport is a phenomenon driving the orderly progression of cell body-assembled molecules along the axon. A proximo-
distal streaming of materials is an absolute requirement since
protein synthetic activity is confined in the cell body and proteins are needed at the terminals where functional activity and
renewal of structures take place. A retrograde transport also
occurs and its purpose is convey materials from the periphery
to the cell body.

The amount of molecules reaching the terminals is not constant
but varies according to the level of activity actually occurring
at the terminal segment of the axon. Each neuron must therefore
regulate the output of materials from the cell body in order to
comply with the needs of the peripheral compartment and the
latter must somehow inform the cell body of its needs. In our
opinion, such a regulation is operated by controlling the level
of perikaryal synthetic activity and the gating at the axonal
initial segment. This results in size control of the fraction
of synthesized materials which is shipped to the periphery.
Very little is known on how such a regulation occurs.

In maturing and regenerating neurons the normal size of the
shipped package includes materials involved in building new
structures. The extra efficiency displayed by young neurons in
driving axonal transport reflects the larger requirement of the
periphery which is engaged in building new axonal segments and
in the formation of synapses. Then, a fine control over the
efficiency of axonal transport during maturation represents a
key mechanism for timing and regulating synaptogenesis occurring
in embryonic neuronal populations.

ACKNOWLEDGEMENTS

This work was supported by Consiglio Nazionale delle Ricerche
(CNR). We are grateful to Prof. Klaus Weber, Max Planck Institute

for Biophysical Chemistry, Göttingen, West Germany, for a generous gift of antibodies against actin and tubulin.

REFERENCES

1. Droz, B. (1973) Brain Res., 62, 383-394.

2. Lasek, R. J. (1970) Int. Rev. Neurobiol., 13, 289-324.

3. Ochs, S. (1971) J. Neurobiol., 2, 331-346.

4. Ochs, S. (1972) Science (Wash.), 176, 252-260.

5. Sjöstrand, J. and Karlsson, J.O. (1969) J. Neurochem., 16, 833-844.

6. Barondes, S.H. (1970) in The Neurosciences, 2nd Study Program, Schmitt, F.O. ed., The Rockefeller University Press, pp. 747-760.

7. Marchisio, P.C. and Sjöstrand, J. (1971) Brain Res., 26, 204-211.

8. Bondy, S.C. and Madsen, C.J. (1971) J. Neurobiol.,2, 279-286.

9. Marchisio, P.C. and Sjöstrand, J. (1972) J. Neurocytol., 1, 101-108.

10. Gremo, F., Sjöstrand, J. and Marchisio, P.C. (1974) Cell Tiss. Res., 153, 465-476.

11. Marchisio, P.C., Sjöstrand, J., Aglietta, M. and Karlsson, J.O. (1973) Brain Res., 63, 273-284.

12. Crossland, W.J., Currie, J.R.,Rogers, L.A. and Cowan, W.M. (1974) Brain Res., 78, 483-489.

13. Hendrickson, A. and Cowan, W.M. (1971) Exp. Neurol., 30, 403-422.

14. Gremo, F. and Marchisio, P.C. (1975) Cell Tiss. Res., 161, 303-316.

15. Crossland, W.J., Cowan, W.M. and Kelly, J.P. (1973) Brain Res., 56, 77-105.

16. Winzler, R.J. (1970) Int. Rev. Cytol., 29, 77-125.

17. Cowan, W.M. (1971) in Cellular Aspects of Neural Growth and Differentiation, Pease, D.C. ed., UCLA University Press, pp. 177-222.

18. Filogamo, G. (1960) Archs. Biol. (Liége), 71, 159-164.

19. Marchisio, P.C. (1969) J. Neurochem., 16, 665-671.

20. Bamburg, J.R., Shooter, E.M. and Wilson, L. (1973) Bioche-

mistry, 12, 1476–1482.

21. Santerre, R.F. and Rich, A. (1976) Devel. Biol., 54, 1–12.

22. Sedlacek, J. (1967) Physiol. Bohemoslov., 16, 531–537.

23. Lasek, R.J. and Hoffman, P.N. (1976) in Cell Motility, Gold-man, R., Pollard, T. and Rosenbaum, J. eds., Cold Spring Harbor Laboratory, pp. 1021–1049.

24. Allison, A.C. (1973) in Locomotion of Tissue Cells, Ciba Foundation Symposium, 14, pp. 109–148, Elsevier.

25. Dahlström, A. (1968) Europ. J. Pharmacol., 5, 111–113.

26. Kreutzberg, G.W. (1969) Proc. Nat. Acad. Sci. U.S.A., 62, 722–728.

27. Porter, K.R. (1976) in Cell Motility, Goldman, R., Pollard, T. and Rosenbaum, J. eds., Cold Spring Harbor Laboratory, pp. 1–28.

28. Marchisio, P.C., Osborn, M. and Weber, K. (1978) Brain Res., in the press.

29. Marchisio, P.C., Osborn, M. and Weber, K. (1978) J. Neuro-cytol., 7, in the press.

30. Di Renzo, M.F., Marchisio, P.C. and Weber, K. (1977) Proc. Int. Soc. Neurochem., 6, 128.

31. Chang, C.M. and Goldman, R.D. (1973) J. Cell Biol., 57, 867–874.

32. Le Beux, Y.J. and Willemot, J. (1975) Cell Tiss. Res., 160, 1–36.

33. Weber, K., Rathke, P.C., Osborn, M. and Franke, W.W. (1976) Exp. Cell Res., 102, 285–297.

34. Hendrickson, A. (1972) J. Comp. Neurol. 144, 381–398.

35. Byers, M.R. (1974) Brain Res., 75, 97–113.

36. Droz, B., Rambourg, A. and Koenig, H.L. (1975) Brain Res., 93, 1–13.

37. Goldman, R., Pollard, T. and Rosenbaum, J. (1976) Cell Moti-lity, Cold Spring Harbor Laboratory, pp. 1–1373.

38. Marchisio, P.C., Aglietta, M. and Rigamonti, D. (1973) Experientia (Basel), 29, 1126–1127.

39. Marchisio, P.C., Gremo, F. and Sjöstrand, J. (1975) Brain Res., 85, 281–285.

40. Edelman, G.M. (1976) Science (Wash.), 192, 218–226.

41. Weber, K., Wehland, J. and Herzog, W. (1976) J. Mol. Biol., 102, 817–829.

Peripheral Neuropathies
N. Canal and G. Pozza, eds.
© 1978 Elsevier/North-Holland Biomedical Press

AXONAL TRANSPORT AND PERIPHERAL NERVE DISEASE IN MAN

STEPHEN BRIMIJOIN AND PETER JAMES DYCK

Departments of Pharmacology and Neurology, Mayo Clinic, Rochester, Minnesota
55901 (U.S.A.)

ABSTRACT

The basal content and rate of accumulation of dopamine-β-hydroxylase and
acetylcholinesterase activity against a ligature have been measured in biopsy
samples of sural nerve from normal human volunteers and patients with various
peripheral nerve diseases. Consistent reductions in the rate of accumulation of
dopamine-β-hydroxylase activity have been noted in Déjerine-Sottas disease,
peroneal muscular atrophy, and hereditary sensory neuropathy type II. Because
of the relatively normal basal levels of enzyme activity in these conditions, it
seems likely that the transport of proteins is impaired, over and above any
changes that may have occurred in the number of surviving axons and the rate of
enzyme synthesis in the cell bodies giving rise to them.

INTRODUCTION

All cells are able to support the motion of organelles and macromolecules
through their cytoplasm, but this ability is developed to a uniquely high degree
in the neuron, whose unusual geometry places key regions far away from the
sites of macromolecular synthesis. Although the mechanism is not understood,
nerve axons can propel proteins and other substances, many of them associated
with structures such as synaptic vesicles and smooth endoplasmic reticulum, at
rates of up to 400 mm/day in a distal direction[1,2]. This rapid transport appears to be concerned with delivering neurotransmitters, their synthetic enzymes, and their storage particles to nerve terminals[3,4], and with the supply
of proteins or lipids to the axonal membrane[5,6]. A nearly equally rapid retrograde transport appears to be involved in carrying trophic factors captured by
the nerve terminal back toward the cell bodies[7]. From what is known of these
functions, one would predict that axonal transport is essential to maintain the
machinery for conducting action potentials, to support the process of chemical
neurotransmission, and probably even for the continued existence of the axon.

In this laboratory, we have been investigating the question of whether
defects in the supply of essential macromolecules to distant parts of the nerve
cell are related to the development of pathology in various diseases of

peripheral nerve in man[8],[9]. The principal strategy has been to search for consistent abnormalities of transport in advanced cases of disease, with the ultimate goal of determining whether these abnormalities appear early enough in the illness to be potential links in the pathological process.

As a means of studying transport, we have capitalized on a remarkable property of this phenomenon, namely, its lack of dependence on the cell body. Since proteins continue moving in normal amounts at normal velocities in isolated lengths of axon[10], it is possible to study transport under controlled conditions in vitro. A convenient approach, which avoids the necessity of injecting labelled protein-precursors into neural tissue, has been to measure the redistribution of specific enzymes and neurotransmitters along the length of peripheral nerve samples incubated in vitro in physiologic salt solutions.

MATERIALS AND METHODS

Biopsy samples of human sural nerve, obtained under local anesthesia[11], are trimmed under a dissection microscope to remove adherent fat and connective tissue without disturbing the epineurium. These nerves are then ligated at both ends with silk thread to produce a length of 3-6 cm with no fascicles entering or leaving. The ligated nerves are incubated in bicarbonate buffered physiological salt solution containing glucose[12]. This solution is continuously bubbled with 95% O_2 - 5% CO_2 and is kept at 37°C by means of a thermostatic circulator.

At the end of an incubation period of 1-4 hours, the nerves are cut into consecutive 3-mm segments, which are homogenized in glass homogenizers containing ice-cold buffer: 0.05 M Tris HCl, pH 7.4; 0.1% (v/v) Triton X-100; and 0.2% (w/v) bovine serum albumin. Enzyme assays are performed on supernatant fractions prepared from the homogenates by centrifugation at 1000 x g for 15 min at 4°C. Dopamine-β-hydroxylase (DBH) activity is assayed by the method of Molinoff et al.[13] using tyramine as a substrate. Acetylcholinesterase (AChE) activity is measured by the radiometric method of Potter[14], with ethopropazine (10^{-4}M) added to each sample as an inhibitor of pseudocholinesterase.

From the accumulation of enzyme activity in the nerve segement immediately proximal to the distal ligature, one can calculate the distally directed flux of enzyme:

$$F = (L - C)/T$$

where 'F' is flux, 'L' is enzyme activity in the segment next to the ligature, 'C' is the overall mean activity per segment in the nerve, and 'T' is the time of incubation. This flux is closely related to the rate of synthesis of the enzyme in the cell bodies giving rise to the axons under investigation. By relating the flux of enzyme activity to the mean axonal content of enzyme activity per unit length, one can calculate the average velocity of transport of the enzyme:

$$V = (F/C) \cdot S$$

where 'V' is the velocity in mm/hr, and 'S' is the length of each nerve segment in mm.

RESULTS

When normal human sural nerves are incubated in vitro at 37°C after ligation at both ends, dopamine-β-hydroxylase (DBH) and acetylcholinesterase (AChE) activity accumulate rapidly in the 3-mm segment next to the distal ligature, and some activity also accumulates in the segment next to the proximal ligature (Fig. 1). The rate of the distal accumulation has been carefully examined as a function of time and found to be constant for several hours. The average velocities of transport in the distal direction calculated from these rates are 2.1 mm/hr for DBH activity and 1.2 mm/hr for AChE activity.

Over the last 5 years, we have examined the dynamics of DBH by this approach in more than 60 biopsy samples from patients with peripheral nerve disease. More recently, studies with AChE have been initiated. Several conditions have been identified in which the axonal content of DBH activity or the average transport velocity of this enzyme are abnormal. Among these conditions are Déjerine-Sottas neuropathy, peroneal muscular atrophy, and hereditary sensory neuropathy type II (Fig. 2). In all of the cases of Déjerine-Sottas disease studied so far, the calculated average transport velocity of DBH has been more than two standard deviations below the control mean. A t-test shows that transport velocity in this condition is highly significantly different from normal (P < 0.001). This observation is particularly interesting in the light of the measurements of basal content, which show that the Déjerine-Sottas nerves have nearly the same amount of DBH activity per unit weight as do the normal nerves (Table 1). In the case of peroneal muscular atrophy and HSN-II, there is some overlap with the normal distribution, but several cases have been found in which average transport velocity was more than two standard deviations below the control mean (Fig. 2). And a statistical analysis shows that average transport velocity in these diseases is significantly lower than normal (P < 0.005), while basal DBH activity, per mg of nerve, is slightly but not significantly reduced (Table 1). Measurements of the content and transport of AChE activity in these conditions are in progress. Preliminary results

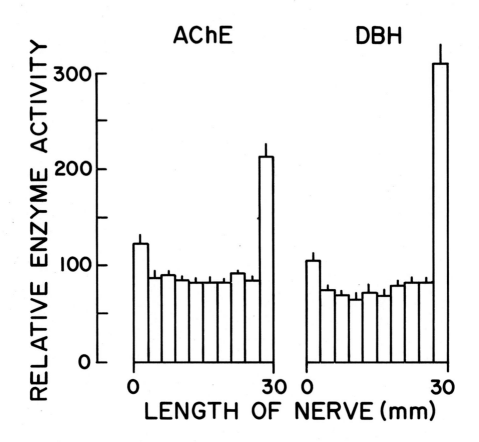

Fig. 1. Redistribution of AChE and DBH activity in doubly ligated biopsy samples of human sural nerve incubated in vitro at 37°C for 3 hr. Relative enzyme activity is shown, with the activity in each segment calculated as a percentage of the overall mean activity in the nerve from which it was derived. Means plus and minus standard errors of the means (vertical bars) represent observations on 9 nerves (AChE) and 11 nerves (DBH). The proximal ends of the nerves are to the left.

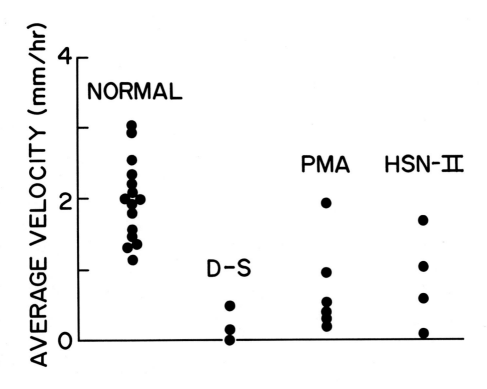

Fig. 2. Transport velocity of DBH in normal and abnormal human sural nerves in vitro. Each point represents a velocity computed from measurements on a single nerve. The normal nerves were incubated for 1-4 hr; the abnormal nerves were all incubated for 3 hr. D-S indicates Déjerine-Sottas disease, PMA indicates peroneal muscular atrophy, HSN-II indicates hereditary sensory neuropathy type II.

TABLE 1

BASAL CONTENT OF DBH ACTIVITY

Nerves	Number	Activity (pmol/mg/hr)	Significance
Normal	22[a]	107 ± 14[b]	--
Déjerine-Sottas	3	103 ± 6.1[b]	N.S.
Peroneal Muscular Atrophy	5	68 ± 12[b]	N.S.
Hereditary Sensory Neuropathy II	4	65 ± 10[b]	N.S.

[a] Includes nerves not used for transport measurements.

[b] Standard error of the mean.

suggest that abnormalities in the dynamics of this enzyme will parallel those of DBH.

DISCUSSION

A reduced average velocity of transport is not compatible with a mere reduction in the number of otherwise normal fibers. Such a loss of fibers, unaccompanied by changes in transport in the remaining fibers, would be expected to reduce the accumulation of enzyme activity against a ligature and to reduce proportionately the baseline enzyme activity per unit length of nerve. In this case, the calculated average velocity of transport would not change.

On the other hand, reductions in average transport velocity do not necessarily correspond to reductions in the true velocity with which the measured substances are moving along nerve axons. It is now clear that most substances carried by rapid axonal transport also exist in a slow moving or stationary phase, which makes an equal contribution with the moving phase to calculations of average velocity[12,15]. Thus a fall in average velocity can reflect a slowing of transport, a fall in the proportion of moving material, or both.

In trying to decide whether a reduced average transport velocity indicates an impairment of transport, it is important to consider the possibility that reduced enzyme synthesis in the cell bodies could lower the proportion of enzyme moving along the axon. Especially if the moving fraction of the enzyme were a minority of the total axonal content, impaired synthesis could lead at least initially to much larger reductions in the distally directed flux of enzyme than in the basal content. This would be reflected in a fall in calculated average transport velocity even if the true transport velocity were unaffected. We have demonstrated such an effect in the sciatic nerve of rats treated with the inhibitor of protein synthesis, cycloheximide. Although this drug does not affect axonal transport per se, it does transiently reduce the average velocity of transport of DBH by reducing the proportion of enzyme in the mobile axonal fraction[17]. Nevertheless, since little or no protein synthesis occurs in the axon itself, even stationary proteins must eventually need to be renewed by molecules transported distally from the cell body. Therefore, one would expect that chronic reductions in synthesis of a given enzyme would ultimately be reflected in reductions of the content of stationary material. Thus, at equilibrium, nerves with depressed protein synthesis should lose equal amounts of stationary and moving enzyme from their axons. In such nerves, one again would expect to calculate normal average velocities of transport.

From these considerations, it seems fairly likely that there is actually an impairment of rapid transport of DBH in sural nerves of patients with Déjerine-Sottas disease, since average transport velocity is much depressed but basal enzyme levels are normal. It is also possible that the reduced average velocity of transport in peroneal muscular atrophy and HSN-II, which was accompanied only by modest, statistically non-significant reductions in basal levels, also reflects a degree of impaired transport.

These conclusions need to be tested by experiments designed to reveal the size and velocity of the moving fraction of DBH. One possible approach is offered by the stop-flow technique[12], which utilizes cycles of local cooling and rewarming to generate migrating waves of transported material whose motion can be directly characterized. This technique is applicable in principle to any nerve and to any transported substance for which a suitable assay is available and which has a reasonable average velocity of transport. Preliminary experiments with the stop-flow technique applied to human sural nerve suggest that it will be feasible to use this approach in order to determine if axonal transport of DBH and AChE are indeed abnormal in various disorders of peripheral nerve.

Even if abnormalities in axonal transport can be established conclusively, however, the relation between these abnormalities and the neuropathology will remain uncertain for some time. It seems most likely that some abnormalities will ultimately be shown to develop secondarily during the course of the illness, for example as axons are plugged by local accumulations of abnormal neurofilaments or membranes[18]. Nevertheless, it should be recognized that even secondary impairment of transport could have serious consequences for the nerve cell. For this reason, and because primary abnormalities in axonal transport are still a potential cause of peripheral nerve disease, work should continue on this problem.

ACKNOWLEDGEMENTS

We thank Ms. Mary Jo Wiermaa for excellent technical assistance. This work was supported in part by NIH Grant No. NS 14304.

REFERENCES

1. Ochs, S. (1972) J. Physiol. Lond., 227, 627-645.

2. Grafstein, B. (1977) in Handbook of Physiology Section I. The Nervous System, Kandel, E.R. ed., Am. Physiol. Soc., Bethesda, pp. 691-717.

3. Dahlström, A. (1971) Phil. Trans. Roy. Soc. Lond. B, 261, 325-358.

4. Bisby, M.A. (1976) Gen. Pharmac., 7, 387-393.

5. Droz, B. (1975) in The Nervous System, Brady, R.O. ed., Raven Press, New York, pp. 111-127.

6. Brimijoin, S., Skau, K.A. and Wiermaa, M.J. (1978) J. Physiol. Lond. in press.

7. Stockel, K. and Thoenen, H. (1975) in Proc. 6th Int. Congr. Pharmacol., Tuomisto, J. and Paasonen, M.K. eds., Finnish Pharmacol. Soc., Helsinki, pp. 285-296.

8. Brimijoin, S., Capek, P. and Dyck, P.J. (1973) Science, 180, 1295-1297.

9. Brimijoin, S. and Dyck, P.J. (1974) in Dynamics of Degeneration and Growth in Neurons, Pergamon, Oxford, pp. 291-294.

10. Ochs, S. and Ranish, N. (1969) J. Neurobiol., 1, 247-261.

11. Dyck, P.J. and Lofgren, E.P. (1968) Med. Clinic N. Am., 52, 885-893.

12. Brimijoin, S. (1975) J. Neurobiol., 6, 379-394.

13. Molinoff, P.B., Weinshilboum, R. and Axelrod, J. (1971) J. Pharmacol. Exp. Ther., 178, 425-432.

14. Potter, L.T. (1967) J. Pharmacol. Exp. Ther., 156, 500-506.

15. Wooten, G.F. and Coyle, J.T. (1973) J. Neurochem., 20, 1361-1371.

16. Brimijoin, S. and Wiermaa, M.J. (1977) Brain Res., 121, 77-96.

17. Brimijoin, S. (1976) J. Neurochem., 26, 35-40.

18. Griffin, J.W., Price, D.L. and Spencer, P.S. (1977) J. Neuropathol. Exp. Neurol., 36, 603.

Peripheral Neuropathies
N. Canal and G. Pozza, eds.
© 1978 Elsevier/North-Holland Biomedical Press   147

CHANGES IN AXONAL TRANSPORT IN VARIOUS EXPERIMENTAL NEUROPATHIES

J.SJÖSTRAND, M.FRIZELL and B.RYDEVIK
Departments of Neurobiology, Ophthalmology, Neurology and Anatomy, University
of Göteborg, Fack, S-400 33 Göteborg (Sweden)

ABSTRACT

The acute effect of some neurotoxic compounds was examined on the rapid
axonal transport of labelled proteins in rabbit vagus nerves *in vitro*. Hexachlorophene was a potent inhibitor of axonal transport giving a total block
at 2×10^{-5}M whereas millimolar concentrations (1×10^{-3}M) of acrylamide and
2,5-hexanedione had no effect on axonal transport. At high concentration
(5×10^{-3}M), however, acrylamide caused a total block, whereas 2,5-hexanedione
had no effect.

To study the pathophysiology of nerve compression trauma, rabbit cervical
vagus nerves were subjected to graded compression *in vivo* by means of a small
compression chamber around the nerve and rapid axonal transport of labelled
proteins was followed various times after compression. A pressure as low
as 50 mmHg for 2 h acutely blocked the rapid axonal transport. Higher pressures (200 and 400 mmHg) applied for 2 h induced more long-lasting blockades.
The time required for recovery of transport was correlated to the magnitude
of the pressure applied.

INTRODUCTION

The axon and its terminals are dependent on a continuous supply of macromolecules and organelles from the nerve cell body by means of axonal transport. Previous studies have shown that the anterograde axonal transport is
partially or completely blocked under various experimental conditions such
as local ischemia or compression [1] and drug treatment [2].

Due to the apparent need of axonal transport to maintain and replenish
substances necessary for the structural and functional integrity of the axon
changed axonal transport has been proposed as a possible pathogenic factor
in various neuropathies. Although we still lack convincing examples of axonal transport as a primary cause to a specific neuropathy, there have been
several reports on disturbed axonal transport in various experimental neuropathies [3,4].

To elucidate the role of changed axonal transport in the pathophysiology of toxic and traumatic neuropathies, we have studied the rapid anterograde axonal transport of the sensory fibers of the rabbit vagus nerve under *in vitro* and *in vivo* conditions.

MATERIALS AND METHODS

Neuro-toxic effects. Cervical vagus nerves with nodose ganglia attached were removed from newly killed albino rabbits (1.5 - 2.0 kg) and were incubated as previously described [5] in a two-compartment perspex chamber containing oxygenated medium 199 (Flow, Irvine, Scotland) with the nodose ganglion in the smaller and the remainder of the nerve trunk in the larger of the two compartments (Fig. 1). A ligature was tied around the nerve 60 mm from the ganglion and 15 μl (15 μCi) of ^{3}H-leucine (L-4,5-^{3}H-leucine, 58 Ci/mmol, Radiochemical Centre, Amersham, England) were added to the medium of the ganglion compartment. The nerves were incubated for 24 h at 38,5°C in 95% O_2/5% CO_2 at a relative humidity of 96%. After six hours of incubation the medium of both compartments was replaced, *i.e.* the isotope was removed. The incubation medium of the nerve compartment, *i.e.* the nerve trunk alone, contained various concentrations of the neurotoxic drugs hexachlorophene (Sigma, U.S.A.), 2,5-hexanedione (Merck, Germany) or acrylamide (Sigma, U.S.A.) which were added to the medium at the start of the incubation.

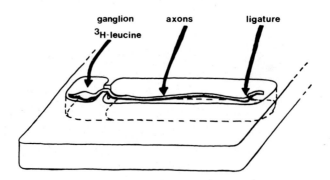

Fig. 1 The two-compartment perspex chamber for the study of axonal transport in the rabbit vagus nerve/nodose ganglion preparation *in vitro*. See text for details.

When incubation was complete, nerves were removed, cut into 5 mm pieces, and the TCA precipitable radioactivity was estimated as previously described [5]. An inhibition of axonal transport was detected as a decrease in the accumulation of radioactivity in the segment of the nerve immediately proximal to the ligature.

Nerve compression. The nodose ganglion of the vagus nerve was gently exposed and 20 μl (100 μCi) of ^{3}H-leucine in 0.9% NaCl (L-4,5-^{3}H-leucine, 58 Ci/mmol, Radiochemical Centre, Amersham, England) was injected sub-epineurially into the nodose ganglion through a 30-gauge stainless steel-needle. The fast axonal transport of ^{3}H-labelled proteins along the cervical vagus nerve was measured as described previously [6] and the effect of local graded compression in vivo was studied. The compression of the nerve trunk was accomplished by a specially designed compression chamber made by Plexiglass and rubber membranes (for details see [7, 8]). The chamber was applied around the cervical vagus nerve in vivo and connected to a pressure system. By varying the pressure in the chamber (50-200-400 mmHg) and the time of application, the nerves could be subjected to graded, controlled compression injuries.

In acute experiments (i.e. without recovery from compression) vagus nerves were compressed 2 h after labelling with ^{3}H-leucine; in others, recovery from compression of up to 14 days was allowed before the ganglia were labelled. In all experiments, the animals were killed 4 h after injection of isotope. The nodose ganglion and the cervical vagus nerve were rapidly dissected out and placed on ice. The nerve was then cut into 2.5 mm pieces and the TCA-precipitable radioactivity was measured (for details, see [6]).

RESULTS

Effect of neurotoxic drugs. In control nerves 24 h after incubation an accumulation of ^{3}H-labelled proteins was found in the 5 mm of nerve immediately proximal to the ligature, representing the rapid phase of axonal transport of the sensory vagus fibers [5]. This accumulation was expressed as a percentage of the total radioactivity in the nerve between the ligature and a point 20 mm from the nodose ganglion (Fig. 2) and was in the range of that previously found for control nerves [5].

Of the neurotoxic drugs examined, hexachlorophene at concentrations of 2×10^{-5}M and 10^{-4}M and acrylamide at a concentration of 5×10^{-3}M caused a significant reduction ($p < 0.05$) of the accumulation of ^{3}H-labelled proteins in the 5 mm nerve segment immediately proximal to the ligature (Fig. 3),

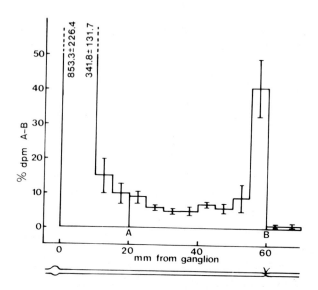

Fig. 2 Profile of ^{3}H-labelled proteins in rabbit vagus nerve-controls. Vagus nerves and attached nodose ganglia were removed and incubated *in vitro* for 24 h with a ligature at B. Labelled proteins in 5-mm segments of nerve were expressed as a percentage of the total labelled protein between points A (20 mm from the nodose ganglion) and B (the ligature). Average of three representative controls ± S.E.M.

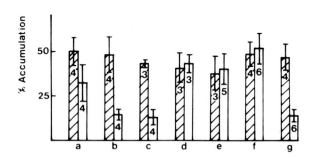

Fig. 3 The percentage accumulation (see legend Fig. 2) of ^{3}H-labelled proteins at a ligature on rabbit vagus nerves incubated *in vitro*. Each pair represents control nerves (hatched columns to the left) and nerves incubated in the presence of a) 5x10[-6]M hexachlorophene, b) 2x10[-5] hexachlorophene, c) 10[-4]M hexachlorophene, d) 10[-3]M 2,5-hexanedione, e) 5x10[-3]M 2,5-hexanedione, f) 10[-3]M acrylamide and g) 5x10[-3]M acrylamide, *i.e.* only nerve trunks and not the ganglia were exposed to the drugs. S.E.M. and the number of nerves in each experiment is indicated.

indicating a block of rapid axonal transport. Lower concentrations of hexachlorophene and acrylamide had no significant effect.   2,5-hexanedione had no effect in the concentrations used (10^{-3}M and $5x10^{-3}$M).

In the 10^{-4}M hexachlorphene-experiments, the incorporation of ^{3}H-leucine into nodose ganglia proteins was analyzed to exclude the possibility that any drug had leaked into the ganglion compartment, causing a depression of the protein synthesis. It was found that the incorporation of ^{3}H-leucine into nodose ganglion protein was not significantly different in the hexachlorophene experiments as comparted to the controls. When $5x10^{-6}$M and $2x10^{-5}$M hexachlorophene was added to the ganglion compartment only, there was no significant difference in the accumulation of ^{3}H-labelled proteins as comparted to the control nerves during the 24 h incubation. These results indicate that the inhibition of axonal transport in the hexachlorophene-treated nerves was not due to drug acting on the nerve cell bodies in the nodose ganglion.

Effects of nerve compression. In nerves which had been subjected to local compression, an acute accumulation of labelled proteins was found in the region of compression (Fig.4:b), in contrast to control (sham) experi-

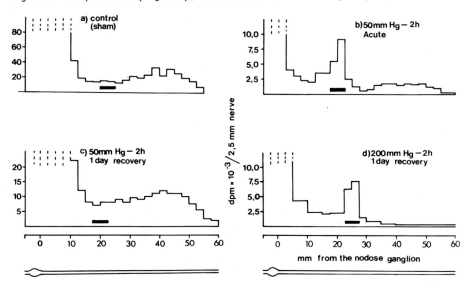

Fig. 4 The effect of nerve compression on rapid axonal transport of ^{3}H-labelled proteins in rabbit vagus nerves. The profiles demonstrate the distribution of ^{3}H-labelled material along the cervical vagus nerve 4 h after injection of ^{3}H-leucine into the nodose ganglia. a) control, sham-operated; b) compression with 50 mmHg for 2 h before killing; c) compression with 50 mmHg for 2 h, the nodose ganglion labelled one day later; d) compression with 200 mmHg for 2 h, the nodose ganglion labelled one day later. The bar indicates the site of the compression. The curves are representative, samples from 4-5 such experiments.

ments, where the chamber was applied around the nerve but not inflated with pressure air. These control experiments showed a normal transport profile (Fig. 4a), in accordance with previous studies [6]. When compression was applied for 2 hours even such low pressure as 50 mmHg caused blockage of the rapid axonal transport (Fig. 4b) which was, however, reversible within one day (Fig. 4c). The higher pressures tested, i.e. 200 and 400 mmHg, applied for 2 hours, induced a corresponding block, which was more pronounced in these nerves. Reversal of transport blockade occurred in most cases within 3 days after compression at 200 mmHg for 2 hours and within 7 days after compression at 400 mmHg for 2 hours [8]. The time required for recovery of normal transport was correlated with the magnitude of the presure applied to the nerve.

DISCUSSION

Axonal transport and neurotoxic drugs. According to Spencer and Schaumburg [9, 10] three hypotheses can be put forward concerning the pathogenesis of neuropathies induced by neurotoxic drugs, i.e. impaired metabolism of the nerve cell body, deranged axonal transport or direct toxic effect on the axons without impairing the axonal transport system. It has been proposed that the latter of these three alternatives best explains the neuropathological changes of dying-back neuropaties [9, 10] although alterations in axonal transport have been reported in acrylamide neuropathy [3] and in neuropathy induced by methyl n-butyl ketone [4]. A different mode of action may be a primary effect on the blood-nerve barrier and perineurial barrier with resulting endoneurial oedema. In an experimental study of the effects of the enzyme chymopapain an acute increase in permeability of the nerve barriers was demonstrated with no acute block of axonal transport or impulse conduction [11]. The late consequences of this barrier-breakdown was nerve fiber degeneration, intraneural fibrosis and impaired impulse conduction.

If a neurotoxic drug primarily acts due to a disturbance in the axonal transport system, it should be possible to demonstrate this effect in acute experiments. When axonal transport is studied in animals who have developed morphological changes or clinical symptoms after chronic exposure, it must be difficult to exclude that all or part of an alteration of axonal transport might be secondary to the neuropathy, especially since both degeneration and regeneration are well-known phenomenons of several peripheral neuropathies. Marked changes in axonal transport can be induced in peripheral nerves during the initial period of regeneration [12, 13].

In the present study some drugs with well-known neurotoxic properties [10,14] were tested for their ability to block rapid axonal transport of ^{3}H-labelled proteins in rabbit vagus nerves acutely exposed to the drugs. Hexachlorophene was found to be a potent axonal transport blocker giving a total block at $2x10^{-5}$M, i.e. in concentrations similar to the axonal transport blocking concentrations of vinblastine and colchicine, two well-known axonal transport blockers [5]. The pathogenesis of hexachlorophene neuropathy is not clear, but it has been proposed that it might be connected to the strong uncoupling effect on oxidative phosphorylation of the drug observed already at micromolar concentrations [15]. Since axonal transport is dependent on oxidative metabolism [16] the uncoupling effect of hexachlorophene might be one likely explanation to its axonal transport blocking effect. When the protein synthesis of the ganglia was measured in the experiments with highest hexachlorophene concentration in the nerve compartment, no significant effect was found as compared to controls, indicating that the axonal transport block was not due to inhibition of protein synthesis caused by drug leaking into the ganglion compartment during incubation.

Considering the pathogenetic relevance of the alterations in axonal transport produced by hexachlorophene, its blocking concentrations ($2x10^{-5}$M = 8 µg/ml) must be compared to hexachlorophene levels reported in blood and nervous tissue after hexachlorophene exposure. Blood-levels of 0.8 µg/ml have been found in newborn infants after repeated baths in hexachlorophene solution [17] and in severely intoxicated rats levels of 8 µg/ml in blood and 2 µg/g brain have been reported [18]. Thus the blocking concentrations of the drug on axonal transport is in the range of that found in blood of rats with severe neuropathy [18] although it is higher than the concentrations found in hexachlorophene bathed infants. It cannot be excluded that part of the neurotoxic action of hexachlorophene is due to the effects on the axonal degeneration found in sciatic nerves of mice [19] and rat optic nerve [20] after chronic exposure to the drug, might somehow be correlated to an axonal transport block. The intramyelinic vacuolization and edema found in these neuropathies [14] would be more difficult to explain as a primary effect of impaired axonal transport and have been interpreted as a direct toxic effect on the myelin. It has also been suggested that axonal degeneration following treatment with hexachlorophene is caused by the increased endoneurial pressure recorded in this neuropathy in rats [21].

2.5-hexanedione and acrylamide are both known to induce peripheral neuropathies characterized by focal axonal swellings with accumulation of neurofilaments [10]. In the present study these drugs had no blocking effect on axonal transport at a comparatively high concentration (10^{-3}M). At 5×10^{-3}M, however, acrylamide but not 2.5-hexanedione caused a total block. It seems less likely that the neurotoxic effect of these drugs primarily is due to a disturbed axonal transport, although it cannot be excluded that this mechanism might somehow be connected to the neurotoxicity of acrylamide. Alterations in axonal transport in peripheral nerves have previously been reported after chronic acrylamide exposure[3, 22]. Since these experiments were performed on animals with clinical neuropathy, it is not clear to what extent the changes in axonal transport might be primary or secondary to the neuropathological changes in the nerves. The findings that methyl n-butylketone (of which 2.5-hexanedione is a major metabolite) can cause a gradual slowing of fast axonal transport in rat peripheral nerves after chronic exposure [4] might as well be secondary to neuropathological changes of the nerves.

Our interpretation is therefore that it seems less likely that the neurotoxic effects of 2.5-hexanedione and acrylamide primarily are due to a disturbed axonal transport, although it cannot be excluded that this mechanism can contribute to the neurotoxic action of acrylamide.

Influence of compression on axonal transport. The nerve trunk comprises several tissue components: nerve fibers, intraneural blood vessels and connective tissue, and these tissue components react in different ways to compression trauma. The nerve fibers may respond with segmental demyelination after compression [23, 24] or Wallerian degeneration, depending on the magnitude of compression. The intraneural blood vessels may react to trauma with increased permeability, resulting in intraneural oedema formation [7, 25]. A longstanding oedema can be organized into an intraneural fibrotic scar.

The reaction of rapid axonal transport to graded compression trauma has been the subject of a recent investigation [8]. We have found that pressure, as low as 50 mmHg, applied for 2 hours on rabbit vagus nerves *in vivo* caused blockage of rapid axonal transport. However, normal transport profiles were found already one day after compression of this magnitude.

Compression of a rabbit nerve trunk by 50-70 mmHg interrupts intraneural microcirculation, as seen by vital microscopy [26], thus inducing ischemia of the compressed nerve segment. However, in these cases intraneural blood flow was rapidly restored when the pressure was released. Maintenance of impulse conduction and rapid axonal transport requires continuous supply of oxygen [1, 16, 27, 28, 29]. Local ischemia has been shown to block rapid axonal transport both *in vivo* and *in vitro* [1, 30]. The rapid recovery of axonal

transport to normal values in our experiments after compression by 50 mmHg
for 2 hours *in vivo* indicates that reversible ischemia of the compressed
nerve segment is the major cause of this block. This assumption is in
good agreement with results obtained in experiments on the reversibility of
axonal transport blocks induced by local ischemia *in vitro* [1, 30].

In the cases of compression by higher pressure in our experiments (200-
400 mmHg) the impairment of axonal transport was of longer duration (3-7
days). In other experiments [7] it has been shown that compression of rabbit
tibial nerves by 200 and 400 mmHg induces endoneurial oedema, in contrast to
compression by only 50 mmHg for 2 hours, where the oedema was restricted to
the epineurial layers of the nerve. Endoneurial oedema may alter the local
environment of the axons in various ways. The ionic balance of the axoplasm
may be deranged and this could possibly affect rapid axonal transport, which
is known to be influenced by alterations in ion concentration [3]. Endoneurial
oedema may also lead to increased intrafascicular pressure as shown in
experimental lead neuropathy[32] and in experimental hexachlorophene neuropathy[21]. Increased pressure in the nerve fascicles due to post-traumatic endoneurial oedema may impair endoneurial capillary circulation, leading to prolonged ischemia after the compression has been released. This might contribute to the rather slow reversal of axonal transport blocks when nerves were
compressed by the higher pressures in our experiments. A direct mechanical
effect of the externally applied pressure on the nerve fibers has also been
shown to be a factor of importance in acute nerve compression lesions [24].

SUMMARY

Rapid axonal transport of ^{3}H-labelled proteins was studied in sensory
fibers of the rabbit vagus nerve.

In vitro studies of the neurotoxic effects of some neurotoxic drugs demonstrated various degrees of axonal transport blocks. Our data indicate
that part of the acute neurotoxic action of hexachlorophene and to a lesser
extent that of acrylamide may be due to an inhibition of axonal transport
whereas this pathogenetic mechanism seems less likely for 2.5-hexanedione.

Vagus nerves were subjected to graded compression *in vivo* by means of
a "minicuff" and the influence of compression of varying magnitude on rapid
axonal transport was studied. The results indicate that blockage of axonal
transport may occur even after moderate compression trauma to a nerve.
After compression at higher pressure axonal transport block persisting up
to 3 to 7 days was seen.

ACKNOWLEDGEMENTS

This work was supported by the Swedish Medical Research Council (grants No 2226 and 5188), the University of Göteborg and the Göteborg Medical Society.

REFERENCES

1. Ochs, S. (1974) Fed. Proc. 33, 1049-1058.

2. Hansson, M. and Edström, A. (1977) J. Neurobiol. 8, 97-108.

3. Pleasure, D.E., Mishler, K.C. and Engel, W.K. (1969) Science, 166, 524-525.

4. Mendell, J.R., Saida, K., Weiss, H.S. and Savage, R. (1977) Brain Res. 133, 107-118.

5. McLean, W.G., Frizell, M. and Sjöstrand, J. (1975) J. Neurochem. 25, 695-698.

6. McLean ,W.G., Frizell, M. and Sjöstrand, J. (1976) J. Neurochem. 26, 1213-1216.

7. Rydevik, B. and Lundborg, G. (1977) Scand. J. Plast. Reconstr. Surg. 11, 179-187.

8. Rydevik, B., McLean, W.G., Sjöstrand, J. and Lundborg, G. (1978a), In preparation.

9. Spencer, P.S. and Schaumburg, H.H. (1974). Can. J. Neurol. Sci. 1, 152-169.

10. Spencer, P.S. and Schaumburg, H.H. (1977) Progr. Neuropath. 3, 253-295.

11. Rydevik, B., Brånemark, P-I., Nordborg, C., McLean, W.G., Sjöstrand, J. and Fogelberg, M. (1976) Spine, 1, 137-147.

12. Frizell, M. and Sjöstrand, J. (1974a) J. Neurochem. 22, 845-850.

13. Frizell, M. and Sjöstrand, J. (1974b) Brain Res. 78, 109-123.

14. Twofighi, J. Gonatas, N.K. and McCree, L. (1973) Lab. Invest. 29, 428-436.

15. Cammer, W. and Moore, C.L. (1972) Biochem. Biophys. Res. Commun. 46, 1887-1894.

16. Ochs, S. and Hollingworth, D. (1971) J. Neurochem. 18, 107-114.

17. Gowdy, J.M. and Ulsamer, A.G. (1976) Am. J. Dis. Child. 130, 247-250.

18. Matthieu, J.-M., Zimmerman, A.W., Webster, H. deF., Ulsamer, A.G., Brady, R.O. and Quarles, R.H. (1974) Exp. Neurol. 45, 558-575.

19. Persson, L.- Wingren. U. and Kristensson, K. (1976) Neuropath. Appl. Neurobiol. 2, 167-174.

20. Rose, A.L., Wisniewski, H.M. and Cammer, W. (1975) J. Neurol. Sci. 24, 425-435.

21. Powell, H.C., Myers, R.R., Zweifach, B.W. and Lampert, P.W. (1978) Acta Neuropath. 41, 139-144.

22. Bradley, W.G. and Williams, H. (1973) Brain, 96, 235-246.

23. Denny-Brown, D. and Brenner, C. (1944) Arch. Neurol. Psychiatry, 52, 1-19.

24. Ochoa, J., Fowter, T.J. and Gilliatt, R.W. (1972) J. Anat. 113, 433-455.

25. Olsson, Y. (1966) Acta Neuropath. 7, 1-15.

26. Rydevik, B., Lundborg, G. and Bagge, U. (1978b) In preparation.

27. Lehmann, J.E. (1937) Am. J. Physiol. 119, 111-120.

28. Bentley, F.H. and Schlapp, W. (1943) J. Physiol. (Lond.) 102, 72-82.

29. Lundborg, G. (1970) Scand. J. Plast. Reconstr. Surg. Suppl. 6.

30. Ochs, S., In: Peripheral Neuropathy, Dyck, P.J., Thomas, P.K. and Lambert, E.H. eds., Saunders, Philadelphia pp. 213-230.

31. Edström, A.(1975) Acta Physiol. Scand. 93, 104-111.

32. Low, P.A. and Dyck, P.J. (1977) Nature 269, 427-428.

Peripheral Neuropathies
N. Canal and G. Pozza, eds.
© 1978 Elsevier/North-Holland Biomedical Press

AXONAL TRANSPORT IN ACRYLAMIDE NEUROPATHY

C.G. RASOOL, Ph.D. and W.G. BRADLEY, M.A., B.Sc., D.M., F.R.C.P.

Department of Neurology, Tufts-New England Medical Center Hospital, Boston,

Massachusetts   (U.S.A.)

ABSTRACT

The axoplasmic transport of acetylcholinesterase (AChE) and choline acetyltransferase (ChAT) were studied in the sciatic nerves of normal rats and those
with neuropathy due to acrylamide by measuring the accumulation of these
enzymes proximal to single and double ligatures. Approximately 10 per cent of
the enzymes were mobile. The absolute transport rate of AChE was decreased to
287 mm/24h in acrylamide neuropathy compared with 567 mm/24h in normal nerve.
The absolute transport rate of ChAT was unchanged (176 and 170 mm/24h). The
amount of AChE activity transported in the orthograde direction in acrylamide
neuropathy was 2.03 umol/24h, which was slightly less than normal
(2.6 umol/24h). The amount of ChAT transported in acrylamide neuropathy was
0.5 umol/24h which was considerably greater than normal (0.2 umol/24h).
Specific colchicine binding by neurotubulin from acrylamide intoxicated rats
was reduced to 40 per cent of normal though the total amount of neurotubulin
appeared to be normal.

INTRODUCTION

Several pathological conditions have been associated with defects in axoplasmic transport. In neurofibrillary degeneration induced by colchicine and
other metaphase-blocking antimitotic drugs, it has been suggested that impairment of axonal tranpsort may be responsible for the accumulation of neurofilaments in the neuron cell body[1,2]. In toxic neuropathies[3] and in the
Wobbler mouse[4], it has been suggested that the axonal degeneration may be due
to impairment of axoplasmic flow, though others were unable to confirm these
reports.[5,6]. This paper describes studies on the axoplasmic transport of
acetylcholinesterase (AChE) and choline acetyltransferase (ChAT) in the
sciatic nerves of normal and acrylamide intoxicated rats.

These enzymes accumulate proximal to a nerve ligature, and are therefore
presumed to move by axoplasmic transport. Different transport rates of these
enzymes have been reported[7-10]. Double ligation experiments have indicated
that only 5-20 per cent of these enzymes are mobile[9,11,12]. We have therefore

investigated the transport of these enzymes in rat sciatic nerve using double ligature experiments.

METHODS

Young female 200 g Wistar rats were used. A toxic neuropathy was induced by administering acrylamide 200 ppm in drinking water, which produced a moderate neuropathy in 21-28 days.

AChE activity was determined by the method of Ellman et al. (1961)[13]. ChAT activity was determined by the method of Fonnum (1975)[12]. Colchicine binding was determined by the method of Morgan and Seed (1975)[14]. The nerve homogenate was centrifuged at 10,000xg for 10 min at 4°C, and the supernatant taken for assay. For determination of total colchicine binding aliquots were incubated with 2.5×10^{-5}M (3H)-colchicine (specific activity 0.05 Ci/mmol) at 37°C for 90 min. For determination of nonspecific colchicine binding, the incubation was performed in the presence of 1×10^{-3}M unlabelled colchicine. Specific colchicine binding, expressed as pmol/mg protein, was determined by deducting nonspecific from total colchicine binding.

Determination of the rate and amount of enzyme transport. Under anesthesia two ligatures were placed around the right sciatic nerve, the upper at the level of the sciatic notch and the lower at the level of the popliteal fossa. Six hours later the sciatic nerves of both sides were removed, cleaned and the enzyme activities determined in the 5 mm segment proximal to the proximal ligature and in the corresponding 5 mm segment from the contralateral control sciatic nerve. The enzyme activities were also determined in the portion of nerve between the ligatures divided into 5 mm segments, B being the most distal.

The parameters of axonal transport were determined according to the following equations:

$$\text{Apparent Transport Rate (mm/24h)} = \frac{(\text{Activity of the enzyme in ligated segment}) - (\text{Activity of the enzyme in control segment})}{(\text{Activity of the enzyme in control segment})} \times \frac{L}{h} \times 24$$

L = Length of the segment in mm

h = Time in hours after ligature

$$\text{Amount of enzyme activity transported (umol/24h)} = \text{Apparent transport rate} \times \frac{C}{L}$$

C = Average activity in control segment

L = Length of segment (mm)

The percentage of enzyme which was mobile =

$$\frac{\begin{pmatrix}\text{Activity of enzyme in} \\ \text{ligated segment B}\end{pmatrix} - \begin{pmatrix}\text{Activity of enzyme in non-ligated} \\ \text{contralateral control segment}\end{pmatrix}}{\text{(The total enzyme activity of the ligated segment)}} \times 100 \ \%$$

RESULTS

Accumulation of AChE.   There was an accumulation of AChE proximal to the proximal ligature in normal rat sciatic nerve which was linear with time up to 48 hours (Figure 1). Accumulation of AChE proximal to the distal ligature had already reached plateau by about 2 hours, and remained static there afterwards (Figure 1). This indicated that all of the mobile enzyme moving in an ortho-grade direction between the two ligatures had reached the distal ligature by 2 hours.

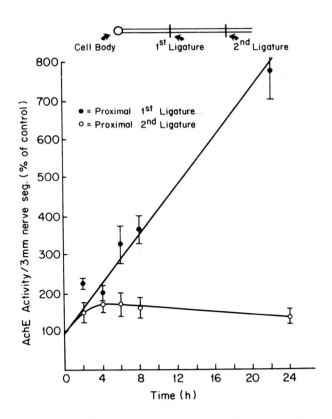

ACCUMULATION OF ACETYLCHOLINESTERASE
(AchE) IN NORMAL RAT SCIATIC NERVE

Figure 1:   The accumulation of AChE proximal to the proximal and distal ligatures in normal rat sciatic nerve.

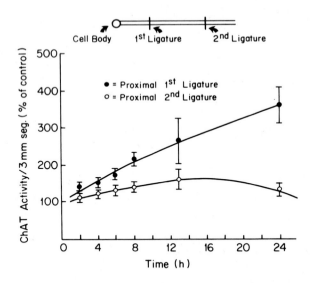

Figure 2:   The accumulation of ChAT proximal to the proximal and distal
ligatures in normal rat sciatic nerve.

in a second experiment. The specific colchicine binding was reduced to 40 per
cent of normal, while the nonspecific colchicine binding was not significantly
altered.

Polyacrylamide gel electrophoretograms of whole sciatic nerve proteins
showed no decrease in the size of the peak of neurotubulin. It therefore
appeared that the decrease in specific colchicine binding was due to some
alteration of the molecular structure of the neurotubulin in acrylamide
neuropathy.

DISCUSSION

Studies of axonal transport in disease states have produced conflicting
results. In acrylamide neuropathy abnormality of the axonal transport of
proteins was reported by Pleasure et al. (1969)[3], but Bradley and Williams

Table 1: Parameters of axoplasmic transport of AChE and ChAT in sciatic nerves of control and acrylamide intoxicated rats.

Enzyme	Treatment	Transport Time h	Apparent Transport Rate mm/24h	% of Enzyme Mobile	Absolute Transport Rate mm/24h	Amount of Enzyme Transported (umol/24h)
AChE	Control (10)	6	42.0 ± 8.2	8.1 ± 2.8	567.2 ± 191.2	2.64 ± 0.2
	Acrylamide (11)	6	30.0 ± 6.1	11.8 ± 3.9*	287.2 ± 80.1**	2.03 ± 0.3***
ChAT	Control (9)	6	8.0 ± 2.2	4.5 ± 2.3	176.3 ± 19.8	0.2 ± 0.04
	Acrylamide (12)		13.8 ± 2.1	9.0 ± 3.5*	170.0 ± 59.2	0.5 ± 0.15***

*P < 0.02   **P < 0.005   ***P < 0.001

Table 1 shows the parameters of axonal transport. The absolute transport rate of AChE in acrylamide neuropathy was reduced to approximately half the normal value. The proportion of enzyme which was mobile was significantly increased in the acrylamide intoxicated animals. The amount of AChE activity moving in an orthograde direction was slightly but significantly reduced in acrylamide intoxication.

ChAT accumulated in the segment proximal to the proximal ligature on the right sciatic nerve in a linear fashion with time (Figure 2). The accumulation of ChAT in the segment proximal to the distal ligature did not show a clear plateau, though it remained at approximately the same level from 8 to 24 hours. The rate of rise of ChAT activity was less than that of AChE.

The absolute transport rate of ChAT was unaltered in acrylamide neuropathy compared with controls (Table 1). However the percentage of enzyme which was mobile in the orthograde direction in acrylamide intoxicated animals was double the value in control animals. The amount of enzyme activity transported was increased 2½ fold in acrylamide intoxicated animals compared with controls.

Colchicine binding by neurotubulin. The total colchicine binding of sciatic nerve neurotubulin from acrylamide-intoxicated rats (expressed as pmol/mg protein) was reduced to 21.5 ± 4.9 % of the control value (P < 0.001). Table 2 shows the amount of specific and nonspecific ^{3}H colchicine bound to tubulin from acrylamide intoxicated rat sciatic nerves compared with control

Table 2:   Colchicine binding to neurotubulin from control and acrylamide
treated rat sciatic nerve supernatants.

The specific colchicine binding in control nerves was 106.0 pmol/mg protein
(89.3% of total colchicine binding), and nonspecific 12.7 pmol/mg protein
(10.7% total).   In acrylamide nerves the values were: specific binding 64.2
pmol/mg (85.1% total), and nonspecific 11.2 pmol/mg protein (14.9% total).

	Specific Binding % of Control	Nonspecific Binding % of Control
Control (3)	100.0 ± 20.0	100.0 ± 16.0
Acrylamide (3)	60.1 ** ± 7.3	88.1 * ± 17.0

**P<0.001   *0.05<P<0.1

(1973)[5] were unable to substantiate these findings.   In the Wobbler mouse
with an inherited anterior horn cell degeneration, a decrease in the slow
rate of axonal transport was reported by Bird et al. (1971)[4], but the results
of studies by Bradley and Jaros (1973)[6] indicated that the slow rate was
normal and that there was perhaps a slight increase in the faster rates of
transport.   In dystrophic mice, a decrease in the amounts of material flowing
at slower rates, and an increase in the amount moving at the faster rates was
reported by Bradley and Jaros (1973)[6] and Komiya and Austin (1974)[15].   A
reduction in axonal transport of ChAT[16] and dopamine-β-hydroxylase[17] has also
been reported in dystrophic mice.   Although there are conflicting reports on
abnormalities in axonal transport under various conditions, it seems likely
that some defect in neuronal metabolism may underlie certain neuropathic
conditions.

The results of the present studies on axoplasmic transport indicate alterations in the transport of AChE and ChAT in acrylamide neuropathy.   Our
studies confirm those of Fonnum et al. (1976)[18] showing that only approximately 10 per cent of both enzymes is mobile in normal nerve.   In acrylamide
neuropathy, the proportion of both enzymes which was mobile was significantly
increased.   In intoxicated animals, the absolute rate of transport of AChE
was reduced to about half of normal, and the amount transported reduced
slightly.   On the other hand the absolute transport rate of ChAT was unchanged
in acrylamide neuropathy compared with controls, but the amount of enzyme
transported was increased 2½ fold.

The significance of these findings in relation to the mechanism of axonal degeneration in acrylamide neuropathy is not clear. The subcellular localization of AChE and ChAT is not certain, though it is likely that AChE is associated with the smooth endoplasmic reticulum and axolemma, while ChAT may be present in the soluble fraction of the axoplasm. It appears that different elements of axonal transport can be differentially affected in toxic neuropathies.

Neurotubules are thought to play a major role in axonal transport[19-21]. Colchicine and other mitotic inhibitors bind to neurotubular protein[22] and thereby block both fast[23,24], and slow[25] axoplasmic transport.

The results of the colchicine binding experiment in acrylamide neuropathy show a reduction in specific binding to neurotubulin to 40 per cent of control levels. The degeneration and loss of axons was only mild in the nerves of the acrylamide intoxicated animals studied in these experiments. The reduction of colchicine binding was much more than could be explained by the loss of axons. Polyacrylamide gel electrophoresis of acrylamide intoxicated rat sciatic nerves showed no major change in the height of the peak due to tubulin. It therefore appears likely that the changes in specific neurotubular colchicine binding was due to some alteration of the biochemical characteristics of neurotubulin.

CONCLUSION

The present experiments suggest that alterations of neurotubulin and of axonal transport may occur in acrylamide neuropathy. The relationship between the observed changes and the cause of the axonal degeneration is not at present clear.

REFERENCES
1. Wisniewski, H., Shelanski, M.L. and Terry, R.D. (1968) J. Cell Biol., 38, 224-229.
2. Shelanski, M.L. and Wisniewski, H. (1969) Arch. Neurol., 20, 199-202.
3. Pleasure, D.E., Mishler, K.C. and Engel, W.K. (1969) Science, N.Y., 166, 524-525.
4. Bird, M.T., Shuttleworth, E.Jr., Koester, A. and Reingloss, J. (1971) Acta Neuropath. Berl., 19, 39-50.
5. Bradley, W.G. and Williams, M.H. (1973) Brain, 96, 235-246.

6. Bradley, W.G. and Jaros, E. (1973) Brain, 96, 247-258.

7. Hebb, C. and Silver, A. (1961) Nature, Lond., 189, 123-125.

8. Lubinska, L. (1964) in Mechanism of Neural Regeneration Volume 13, Singer, M. and Schade, P. eds., Elsevier, Amsterdam, pp.1-71.

9. Lubinska, L. and Niemierko, S. (1971) Brain Res., 27, 329-341.

10. Ranish, N. and Ochs, S. (1972) J. Neurochem., 19, 2641-2649.

11. Fonnum, F., Frizell, M. and Sjöstrand, J. (1973) J. Neurochem., 21, 1109-1120.

12. Fonnum, F. (1975) J. Neurochem., 24, 407-409.

13. Ellman, G.L., Courtney, K.D., Andres, V.Jr., and Fleatherstone, R.M. (1961) Biochem. Pharmacol., 7, 88-95.

14. Morgan, J.L. and Seed, N.W. (1975) J. Cell Biol., 67, 136-145.

15. Komiya, Y. and Austin, L. (1974) Exp. Neurol., 43, 1-12.

16. Jablecki, C. and Brimijohn, S. (1974) Nature, Lond., 250, 151-154.

17. Brimijohn, S. and Jablecki, C. (1976) Exp. Neurol., 53, 454-464.

18. Fonnum, F., Frizell, M. and Sjöstrand, J. (1976) J. Neurochem., 26, 427-429.

19. Schmitt, F.O. (1969) Symp. Int. Soc. Cell Biol., 8, 95-111.

20. Wuerker, R.B. and Palay, S.L. (1969) Tissue and Cell, 1, 387-402.

21. Livett, B.G. (1976) Int. Rev. Physiol. Neurophysiol., II, 10, 37-124.

22. Weisenberg, R.C., Borisy, G.G. and Taylor, E.W. (1968) Biochemistry, Easton, 7, 4466-4478.

23. Dahlström, A. (1968) Eur. J. Pharmacol., 5, 111-113.

24. Karlsson, J-O. and Sjöstrand, J. (1969) Brain Res., 13, 617-619.

25. James, K.A.C., Bray, J.J., Morgan, I.G. and Austin, L. (1970) Biochem. J., 117, 769-777.

Supported by grants from the Muscular Dystrophy Association, the Muscular Dystrophy Group of Great Britain and NIH Grant No. AA03213-01

Peripheral Neuropathies
N. Canal and G. Pozza, eds.
© 1978 Elsevier/North-Holland Biomedical Press

EXPERIMENTAL INVESTIGATION OF ALCOHOLIC NEUROPATHY

E.P. BOSCH, M.D., R.W. PELHAM, Ph.D., C.G. RASOOL, Ph.D. and W.G. BRADLEY, M.A.,
B.Sc., D.M., F.R.C.P.
Department of Neurology, Tufts-New England Medical Center Hospital, Boston,
Massachusetts (U.S.A.)

ABSTRACT

An experimental model of chronic alcoholic neuropathy in the rat was produced by schedule-induced polydipsia. A mild distal axonal neuropathy in the
ventral caudal nerve was found after 16 weeks exposure to about 12g of absolute alcohol per Kg body weight per day. The rats appeared not to be deficient in thiamine, suggesting that the axonal degeneration was due to the
direct toxic effect of alcohol. Axonal transport studies indicated a significant increase in the amount of acetylcholinesterase transported in an orthograde direction in the sciatic nerves of alcoholic rats.

INTRODUCTION

For 150 years peripheral nerve damage has been recognized to be associated
with chronic alcoholism in man[1], but there are still conflicting opinions
about the nature of the pathological process and its pathogenesis. Most
recent studies of nerve biopsies have shown a significant reduction of fiber
density of both small and large myelinated fibers, with evidence of axonal
regeneration and some acute axonal degeneration[2-5]. However Denny-Brown
(1958)[6] stated that segmental demyelination was commonly seen in early acute
alcoholic neuropathy. In an electronmicroscopic study of 11 cases of alcoholic
neuropathy, Bischoff (1971)[7] found axonal degeneration in every case, though
4 had predominant segmental demyelination.

In man chronic alcoholic neuropathy is commonly associated with dietary
deficiencies[8]. Blood levels of thiamine and other group B vitamins are
significantly reduced in alcoholic patients with peripheral neuropathy[9]. The
absorption of thiamine is impaired in chronic alcoholics[10]. Experimental
thiamine deficiency in man[11], rats and other species[12-15] may produce a peripheral neuropathy. However Delaney et al. (1966)[16] could detect a thiamine
deficient state in only 37 per cent of chronic alcoholics and in only half of
their cases with neuropathy. Behse and Buchthal (1977)[5] found no evidence of
vitamin or other metabolic abnormalities in 37 chronic alcoholic patients with
peripheral neuropathy. They found a different histopathological picture from

that in alcoholic neuropathy in nutritional neuropathy following gastrectomy. They concluded that alcohol was directly toxic to the peripheral nervous system.

Because of the socioeconomic importance of chronic alcoholism, and because of the uncertainties concerning the pathology and pathogenesis of the human disease, experimental studies in animals are required to clarify the picture. Several different experimental models have been developed to induce a high alcohol intake in experimental animals, including the schedule-induced poly-dipsia model of Falk[17-20] and models in which animals are given alcohol in their drinking liquids[21].

The present report describes electrophysiological, morphological and bio-chemical studies of the peripheral nervous system of rats subjected to 16 weeks chronic alcohol intake in the schedule-induced polydipsia paradigm.

MATERIALS AND METHODS

Twenty-nine male Holtzmann rats were induced chronically to drink high doses of alcohol by the schedule-induced polydipsia technique[17-20]. The animals were individually housed in cages with food-pellet dispensers which released a single 45 mg pellet at 2 minute intervals for the first hour of every four hours around the clock. Before the rats were placed in the exper-imental cages, they were fasted to 80 per cent of their initial free-feeding weight. Experimental rats received 5% v/v ethanol in water containing 0.35% saccharin. Control rats received saccharin solution alone, plus daily supple-ments of standard laboratory pellets to keep their body weight equal to the experimental animals. Fluid intake[5] and body weights were measured twice weekly. The experiment was terminated after 16 weeks.

Electrophysiology. At the end of the study period the maximal motor nerve conduction velocity of the caudal nerve was measured by a technique similar to that of Miyoshi and Gotto (1975)[22]. Rats anesthetized with pentobarbital (25 mg/Kg i.p.) and a nitrous-oxide-oxygen-halothane mixture were studied in a heated foil-sheathed box (Figure 1).

Rectal temperature and skin temperature over the distal end of the rat tail were measured by thermistor-probes at the time of recording each conduction velocity. The skin temperature of the tail during the electrophysiologic studies was $36.7^\circ \pm 0.5$ c. Action potentials from a distal segmental tail muscle were recorded through surface ring electrodes placed around the distal tail. The caudal nerve was stimulated by ring electrodes at two proximal sites (rostral base of tail, and mid-tail). Stimulating and recording elec-trodes were connected to a Teca TE4 Electromyograph.

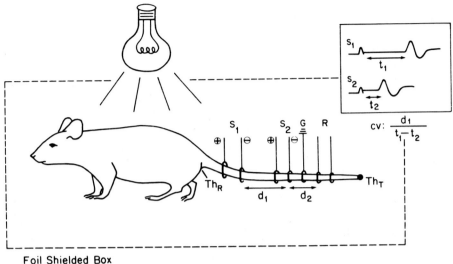

Foil Shielded Box

Figure 1: Diagram of experimental technique for measuring maximum conduction
velocity of the caudal nerves of the rat.

Axonal transport studies. Studies of axonal transport of acetylcholinesterase (AChE) and choline acetyltransferase (ChAT), and assays of specific
colchicine binding by neurotubulin were performed using methods described
elsewhere[23].

Morphologic studies. Following removal of the sciatic nerves for axonal
transport studies, the animals were heparinized through a cardiac puncture
and 3 ml of blood were taken for erythrocyte transketolase determinations
(Bio-Science Laboratories, Van Nuys, CA). The animals were then perfused
through the left ventricle with 2% paraformaldehyde in 0.1 M phosphate buffer
at pH 7.4, followed by 3.6% glutaraldehyde in the same buffer. Following perfusion, the posterior tibial nerve in the calf contralateral to the ligated
nerve and the ventral caudal nerve in the proximal and distal third of the
tail were removed. The techniques for further fixation embedding and sec-
tioning are described elsewhere[24]. Density of myelinated fibers per mm^2 of
fascicular area and myelinated fiber diameter histograms of caudal nerves at
proximal and distal levels were measured using photographs of whole nerves at
a magnification of X 1000, using a Zeiss TZG3 particle size analyzer in the
exponential mode. Portions of the caudal nerve 2 cm long from proximal and
distal levels were prepared for microdissection of single fibers as described
elsewhere[24]. Typing of single teased nerve fibers was performed according to

the descriptive categories of Dyck (1975)[25], using 50 single teased fibers at each level.

RESULTS

Ethanol consumption. During the study period the experimental (16) and control (13) animals gained weight and their mean weights at sacrifice were comparable (ethanol group 317.8 gm; controls 314.2 gm). The fluid intake remained constant throughout the study. The mean daily fluid intake was higher in control than ethanol exposed rats (ethanol group 306 ml/Kg/day; controls 350 ml/Kg/day). The experimental animals drank 12.1 ± 1.4 (SD) gm/Kg absolute ethanol per day, which provided 42 per cent of their total caloric intake.

Immediately following a feeding period the alcoholic rats were drowsy but returned to alertness before the next feeding cycle. At the end of the study there was no observable abnormality of motor behavior.

Electrophysiology. Maximal motor nerve conduction velocities and terminal latencies of the caudal nerve were determined for 8 alcoholic and 7 control rats. The mean conduction velocity (ethanol group 31.6 ± 6.4 m/sec; controls 32.3 ± 3.8 m/sec) and terminal latency (ethanol group 2.0 ± 0.7 msec; controls 2.3 ± 0.4 msec) were not significantly different between the control and alcoholic groups after 16 weeks.

Morphological findings. Sections for light and electronmicroscopy from the distal third of the ventral caudal nerve from 10 alcoholic and 7 control animals showed occasional fibers undergoing acute axonal degeneration in 4 ethanol and 2 control rats. In one of the alcoholic animals axonal degeneration was particularly conspicuous.

Morphometric data for the distal ventral caudal nerve are shown in Table 1. The mean densities was reduced by 16% in the ethanol group (one-tail t-test, $P<0.05$). The myelinated fiber diameter histograms indicated equal loss of small and large fibers (Figure 2).

One of the alcoholic rats had an abnormally high frequency of fibers undergoing degeneration into linear rows of myelin ovoids (condition E), but the difference between the mean frequencies of this pathologic change did not reach statistical significance. Rare fibers with paranodal segmental demyelination (condition C) were seen with equal frequency in both groups.

Sections for light and electronmicroscopy from the proximal level of the ventral caudal nerve from 10 alcoholic and 8 control rats showed occasional fibers undergoing axonal degeneration in both groups. Morphometric data for

Table 1: Morphometric data of single microdissected nerve fibers and myelinated nerve fiber densities of distal and proximal ventral caudal nerve.

DISTAL VENTRAL CAUDAL NERVE

FREQUENCY OF TEASED FIBER CONDITIONS								DENSITY OF MYELINATED FIBERS (No/mm^2)
A&B	C	D	E	F	G	H	I	
Controls (5)								
Mean: 93.6	4.4	0	1.6	0	0.4	0	0	13,556 ± 1505
Range: 88-100	0-8	0	0-8	0	0-2	0	0	11,916 - 15,671
Ethanol (5)								
Mean: 92	3.2	0	2.8	0.4	0.4	0	1.2	11,333 ± 2148 (P< 0.05)
Range: 80-98	0-10	0	0-14	0-2	0-2	0	0-4	8,734 - 13,525

PROXIMAL VENTRAL CAUDAL NERVE

FREQUENCY OF TEASED FIBER CONDITIONS								DENSITY OF MYELINATED FIBERS (No/mm^2)
A&B	C	D	E	F	G	H	I	
Controls (5)								
Mean: 99.2	0.8	0	0	0	0	0	0	10,974 ± 1769
Range: 98-100	0-2	0	0	0	0	0	0	8,540 - 12,761
Ethanol (5)								
Mean: 99	0.7	0	0	0.3	0	0	0	10,118 ± 2213
Range: 96-100	0-2	0	0	0-2	0	0	0	6,588 - 12,623

the proximal ventral caudal nerve are shown in Table 1. Mean densities, and myelinated fiber diameter histograms showed no difference between the control and the ethanol groups. Occasional, single, teased fibers with paranodal demyelination (condition C) were found in 2 animals of each group, and the mean frequencies of this condition were equal in ethanol and control rats. No single teased fiber undergoing axonal degeneration was found.

Sections from the posterior tibial nerve at the level of the calf revealed no light microscopic abnormalities in 5 alcoholic and 3 control animals.

Transketolase determinations. The erythrocyte transketolase levels of ethanol rats (0.51 ± 0.09 IU/g hemoglobin) did not differ significantly from the level in control rats (0.50 ± 0.03 IU/g hemoglobin).

Axonal transport studies. The parameters of axonal transport of AChE determined in sciatic nerves subjected to double ligature for 6 hours are shown in Table 2:

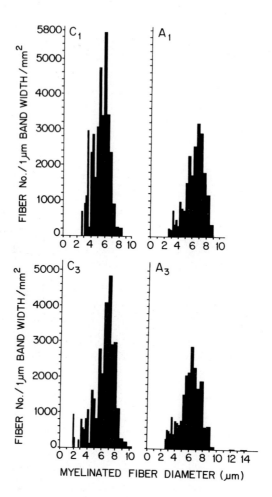

Figure 2: Representative fiber diameter histograms of distal ventral caudal nerves of 2 control (C) and 2 alcoholic (A) rats.

Table 2: Effect of alcohol on AChE transport in rat sciatic nerve.

Treatment	Apparent Transport Rate mm/24h	% of Enzyme Mobile	Absolute Transport Rate mm/24h	Amount of Enzyme Transported umol/24h
Control (4)	35.4 ± 6.9	12.4 ± 3.5	319.2 ± 150.9	0.84 ± 0.21
Ethanol (5)	39.8 ± 10.4	11.4 ± 2.1	347.6 ± 142.9	1.29 ± 0.25

The amount of AChE transported in the alcohol group was significantly increased (P<0.025) by 54 per cent. There was no change in the other parameters of transport of AChE, or in the transport of ChAT.

Colchicine binding to neurotubulin. Preliminary studies showed no major change in specific and nonspecifc colchicine binding of the sciatic nerves of the ethanol and control groups.

DISCUSSION

The schedule-induced polydipsia technique used in this experiment to produce a chronic high intake of alcohol in the rat has been shown to produce dependence as indicated by the consistent appearance of withdrawal seizures. In this model, the mean blood ethanol concentration one hour after feeding is 142.8 mg/100 ml[20]. The rats continue to grow, though at a slower rate than free-fed litter mates, and show no clinical evidence of dietary deprivation.

Rats consuming mean daily intake of absolute alcohol of 12.1 g/Kg for 16 weeks developed morphological evidence of a mild distal peripheral neuropathy in the caudal nerve. This is the first clear demonstration of the production of a neuropathy in animals chronically exposed to alcohol. The density and total number of myelinated fibers in the distal third of the ventral caudal nerve of alcoholic animals was significantly reduced by 16 per cent compared with controls. This loss of fibers was due to axonal degeneration, acute stages of which were seen to a greater extent in alcoholic than in control animals. The ultrastructural pattern of axonal degeneration was in no way different from Wallerian or other forms of axonal degeneration. There was no segmental demyelination, which was concordant with the absence of significant slowing of caudal nerve conduction velocity. More proximal parts of the ventral caudal nerve and of the posterior tibial nerve at the knee showed no abnormality compared with controls, indicating the distal nature of the neuropathy.

Transketolase is a thiamine dependent enzyme, and determinations of blood transketolase levels have proved to reflect the state of thiamine nutrition in patients with neurological damage from chronic alcoholism[26]. Our chronic alcoholic rats did not differ from controls in the erythrocyte transketolase level. Therefore this study supports the contention of Behse and Buchthal[5] that alcohol is directly toxic to the peripheral nervous system. However the 16 per cent loss of myelinated fibers in the distal ventral nerve of the ethanol rats in the present experiment was less than the 30 to 50 per cent reduction in fiber density occurring in sural nerves of chronic alcoholic patients[3,5]. The limited three month period of intoxication utilized in the current experiment may have been too short to produce a more severe neuropathy. It would be of value to study animals for a more prolonged period, and also to study the combined effect of chronic alcohol intoxication and vitamin B1 deficiency.

The present results may be compared with those of Juntunen et al. (1978)[27] who exposed rats for periods of up to $9\frac{1}{2}$ months to approximately half the dosage of alcohol used in the present experiment, utilizing alcohol administered in the drinking water. Nutritional deficiency occurred in these animals with a consequent 48 per cent reduction in body weight compared with controls. The blood thiamine levels of these animals were not determined. They found a statistically significant 12 per cent reduction in the conduction velocity of the largest myelinated fibers in the sciatic nerve. Despite intensive study, the morphologic evidence of a peripheral neuropathy is not very convincing. They reported a possible reduction in the density of myelinated fibers in two peroneal nerves of alcoholic rats; there was an increase in nonspecific cholinesterase staining of intramuscular nerve fibers and changes in Schwann cell cytoplasm in the sciatic nerve which are difficult to interpret.

Axonal transport of AChE and ChAT have been investigated in this experimental alcoholic neuropathy. The percentage of enzyme, which was mobile, determined by the double ligation technique[23], was used to calculate the absolute rate of transport of the enzymes. No significant change was seen in the rate of transport of AChE or ChAT, or in the proportion of the enzymes which was mobile within the nerve. However there was a significant increase of 54 per cent in the amount of AChE being transported in ethanol animals compared with controls. A further study has been performed on animals subject to a similar dose of alcohol administered in a liquid diet for 16 weeks[21]. The findings on axoplasmic transport studies were very similar. There was no change in the absolute transport rate of AChE and ChAT, and no change in the amount of ChAT transported. However the amount of AChE transported was increased by 49 per cent compared with control animals, though this just failed to reach statistical significance.

The implication of an increased amount of transport of AChE is not clear. We have not studied protein synthesis in the nerve cell body, nor protein turnover in the distal parts of the nerves to provide a complete picture of the protein metabolism within the neurons. One possible explanation of the increased amount of transport of AChE might be that it was related to attempted axonal regeneration. However, the amounts of AChE and ChAT being transported in a regenerating nerve above a distal lesion are decreased from 2 to 7 days after injury, and there is no evidence of increased amount of transport[28]. Increased fast axonal transport has been reported both in the cerebral cortex as demonstrated by studies of synaptosomal fractions and in the optic nerves and tracts of animals subject to alcohol intoxication[29,30]. However in neither study did the technique allow the determination of whether it was the rate or the amount of protein transported which was increased.

CONCLUSIONS

This study suggests that alcohol per se is toxic to the peripheral nervous system, though the extent of that toxicity in the present study appears to be small. Further studies of longer duration intoxication and combination with vitamin deficiency will enable the elucidation of the relative effects of the direct action and of vitamin deficiency in producing nerve degeneration in patients with alcoholic neuropathy.

REFERENCES

1. Jackson, J. (1822) N. Engl. J. Med. Surg., 11, 351-353.
2. Dyck, P.J., Gutrecht, J.A., Bastron, J.A., Karnes, W.E. and Dale, A.J.D. (1968) Mayo Clin. Proc., 43, 81-123.
3. Walsh, J.C. and McLeod, J.G. (1970) J. Neurol. Sci., 10, 457-469.
4. Tredici, G. and Minazzi, M. (1975) J. Neurol. Sci., 25, 333-346.
5. Behse, F. and Buchthal, F. (1977) Ann. Neurol., 2, 95-110.
6. Denny-Brown, D.E. (1958) Fed. Proc., 17, Suppl., 2, 35-39.
7. Bischoff, A. (1971) Dtsch. Med. Wochenschr., 96, 317-322.
8. Victor, M. and Adams, R.D. (1961) Am. J. Clin. Nutr., 9, 379-397.
9. Fenelly, J., Frank, O., Baker, H. and Leevy, C.M. (1964) Brit. Med. J., 2, 1290-1292.
10. Tomasulo, P.A., Kater, R.M.H. and Iber, F.L. (1968) Am. J. Clin. Nutr., 21, 1340-1344.
11. Williams, R.D., Mason, H.L., Power, M.H. and Wilder, R. (1943) Arch. Intern. Med., 71, 38-53.
12. Prickett, C.O., Salmon, W.D. and Schroeder, G.A. (1939) Am. J. Path., 15, 251-259.
13. North, J.D.K. and Sinclair, H.M. (1956) Arch. Path., 62, 341-356.
14. Collins, G.H., Webster, H.F. and Victor, M. (1964) Acta Neuropath., 3, 511-521.

15. Prineas, J. (1970) Arch. Neurol., 23, 541-548.
16. Delaney, R.L., Lankford, H.G. and Sullivan, J.F. (1966) Proc. Soc. Exp. Biol., 123, 675-679.
17. Falk, J.L. and Samson, H.H. (1972) Science, 177, 811-813.
18. Falk, J.L., Samson, H.H. and Tang, M. (1973) Adv. Exp. Med. Biol., 35, 197-211.
19. Falk, J.L. and Samson, H.H. (1976) Pharm. Rev., 27, 449-464.
20. Craig, J.R., Munsat, T.L. and Chuang, M. (1977) Ann. Neurol., 2, 311-314.
21. Freund, G. (1969) Arch. Neurol., 21, 315-320.
22. Miyoshi, T. and Goto, I. (1973) Electroencephalogr. Clin. Neurophysiol., 35, 125-131.
23. Rasool, C.G. and Bradley, W.G. (1978) in Peripheral Neuropathies, Canal, N. ed., Elsevier, Amsterdam, (In press)
24. Bradley, W.G. (1974) Disorders of Peripheral Nerves, Blackwell Scientific Publications, Oxford.
25. Dyck, P.J. (1975) in Peripheral Neuropathy, Volume I, Dyck, P.J., Thomas, P.K., and Lambert E.M. eds., W.B. Saunders Company, Philadelphia, pp. 296-336.
26. Embree, L.J. and Dreyfus, P.M. (1963) Trans. Am. Neurol. Assoc., 88, 36-42.
27. Juntunen, J., Teräväinen, H., Eriksson, K., Panula, P. and Larson, A. (1978) Acta Neuropath. (Berlin), 14, 131-137.
28. Frizell, M. and Sjöstrand, J. (1973) J. Neurochem., 22, 845-850.
29. Israel, M.A., Kuriyama, K. and Yoshikawa, K. (1975) Neuropharmacology, 14, 445-451.
30. Yamasaki, Y. and Kuriyama, K. (1974) Japan J. Pharmacol., 24, 285-290.

Supported by grants from the Muscular Dystrophy Association and the Muscular Dystrophy Group of Great Britain, and NIH Grant No. AA03213-01

Peripheral Neuropathies
N. Canal and G. Pozza, eds.
© 1978 Elsevier/North-Holland Biomedical Press

ON THE RELATION BETWEEN MICROTUBULE DENSITY AND AXOPLASMIC TRANSPORT IN
NERVES TREATED WITH MAYTANSINE IN VITRO

BERNARDINO GHETTI and SIDNEY OCHS
Departments of Pathology (Neuropathology) and Physiology, Indiana University
School of Medicine, 1100 West Michigan Street, Indianapolis, Indiana 46202

ABSTRACT

The effect of maytansine on the axoplasmic transport and on the density of
microtubules in myelinated and unmyelinated fibers of the sciatic nerve in vitro
was studied and a correlation between axoplasmic transport block and a reduction
of microtubule density in the large myelinated fibers was demonstrated.

INTRODUCTION

In recent years it has been proposed that microtubules play an important
role in axoplasmic transport[1,2]. Yet, their primary involvement in axoplasmic
transport remains a controversial issue[3,4].

The tubulin-binding agents, colchicine and vinblastine, have been among the
most useful tools available to clarify the relation between axoplasmic
transport[5,6,7] and microtubules. There is evidence that microtubules
depolymerize in cells when treated substoichiometrically with tubulin-binding
agents[8]. In vitro studies suggest that by inhibition of the polymerization
reaction[9], vinblastine depolymerizes microtubules which are in equilibrium with
tubulin in soluble pools.

Most investigations of the effects of colchicine and vinblastine on
axoplasmic transport indicate that these agents impair or block transport[5,6,10].
However, correlative morphological and physiological studies of the effects of
these agents are scant. In most investigations qualitative changes or an
approximate quantification of microtubules in unmyelinated fibers have been
given[4,7,11,12] without assurance that transport is being investigated in the
same type of fibers that are studied for microtubule quantification.

It has been shown that in motor and sensory nerves most of the labeled
material is likely carried by the myelinated fibers of large-diameter[13,14]; it
is, therefore, necessary to investigate whether a correlation exists between the
block of transport and the microtubule changes in myelinated fibers. This has
been undertaken in the present study using maytansine (MYT), a new potent
stathmokinetic agent[15,16]. Maytansine binds to tubulin[17,18], inhibits the

in vitro polymerization of tubulin[17], induces microtubule loss in vitro[19], and in vivo[20] and blocks axoplasmic transport[19]. The block of transport produced in vitro with this agent was assessed in the desheathed nerve preparation[19] and the microtubular density in both the large-diameter group of myelinated fibers and in the unmyelinated fibers was determined. It will be shown that a decrease in the microtubule density in the large-diameter group of myelinated fibers is correlated with the block of transport and that there is a much greater and earlier decrease in the microtubule density in the unmyelinated fibers.

MATERIALS AND METHODS

Cats were anesthetized and, following laminectomy, ^{3}H-leucine injected into the L_7 dorsal root ganglion for uptake by sensory cells. To determine the pattern of outflow of labelled activity in vitro in the desheathed peroneal nerve preparation[21], the animals were sacrificed two hours after injection of the precursor, the peroneal nerves desheathed over a length from 35 to 140 mm from the ganglion and these nerves then placed in flasks containing 0.05 to 72 µM of MYT in a lactate Ringer or in a Krebs-Ringer solution for 4 hours of in vitro downflow. In some cases shorter exposure times were studied. After the period of incubation, a 15-20 mm segment of peroneal nerve was removed from the distal end of the desheathed part of the nerve for ultrastructural studies. The distance of this segment was from 120 to 140 mm from L_7 ganglion taken as zero. The remainder of the desheathed peroneal branch and sheathed tibial branch were then sectioned into 5 mm pieces to determine the outflow of the labelled activity[13].

The segment of nerve taken for electron microscopy was fixed for two hours in 5% buffered glutaraldehyde at a pH of 7.3. After this time, a 5 mm segment was cut from the middle of the segment and further cut longitudinally into 4-5 specimens. These pieces were postfixed in Dalton's chrome osmium, dehydrated, and embedded in Epon 812. Ultrathin sections were stained with uranyl acetate and lead citrate.

Thirty-six peroneal nerves exposed to MYT were studied. As controls for ultrastructural studies, 17 desheathed peroneal nerves not exposed to MYT were used. While studies of the axoplasmic transport and of the morphological changes were carried out in all 36 experiments, the correlation between axoplasmic transport and microtubule density was done in 15 of these nerves exposed to concentrations of MYT ranging from 0.1 to 72 µM. For the analysis of microtubular density two Epon embedded blocks from each experimental and

control nerve were cut in cross section. The peroneal is a mixed nerve and
the myelinated axons randomly selected for microtubule counting were not
necessarily sensory axons in which transport was evaluated. To quantify the
microtubules, electron micrographs of 5 large myelinated axons, 9-14 μm in
diameter, and 15-25 unmyelinated axons were taken from sections obtained from
each Epon-embedded block. From each control nerve, 5 myelinated fibers and
30-50 unmyelinated fibers were used. Electron micrographs of the nerve cross
sections were randomly taken at a constant magnification of 5400 and printed
at a magnification of three times, the final magnification of the prints being
16,200. The cross sectional areas of the individual myelinated axons were
determined as follows: the axonal perimeter was measured on the prints, and
then divided by the magnification factor. When the true axonal perimeter was
determined, then the area of an ideal circle having a circumference equal to
the axonal perimeter was calculated. The microtubules were counted from the
prints using a 5X magnifying lens. Counts were reproducible to within $\pm 5\%$.
To determine microtubule density, 15 experimental groups each composed of
10 myelinated fibers and 15 groups each composed of 30-60 unmyelinated fibers
were used. As controls, 40 myelinated and 326 unmyelinated fibers were taken
from 8 nerves. The microtubule density was determined for each axon, and the
mean densities were calculated for the controls and for each of the
experimental groups of myelinated or unmyelinated fibers. The fibers were
also pooled into 3 groups of myelinated and 3 groups of unmyelinated on the
basis of the following 3 ranges of MYT concentration: 0.1-3, 4-10, and 17-72 μM.
The mean densities of these groups were obtained. The Student T-test was
used to test for significant differences between means of each group. The
F-test was used to test significant differences between variances.

For studies of time changes of microtubular density, 15-20 mm segments taken
from desheathed peroneal nerves were ligated at both ends and exposed to 5 μM
MYT for 0.33, 0.67, 1,2,3,4,5 hours. The experimental specimens and
controls were then fixed in glutaraldehyde. For microtubule counting the
procedure already described was followed.

RESULTS

Block of axoplasmic transport with maytansine

The downflow of labelled components in the sheathed tibial branch of the
sciatic nerve showed little effect of MYT at concentrations as high as 72 μM.
In the desheathed peroneal branch, a block of axoplasmic transport was seen at
concentrations between 5 and 72 μM. Evidence of block was seen within 1 to 3.2

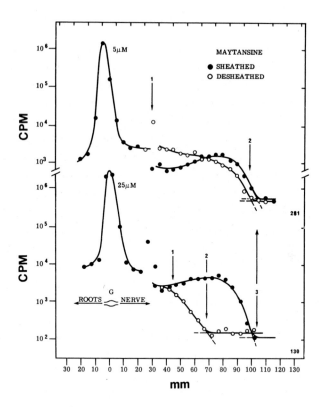

Fig. 1. Distribution of radioactivity in the dorsal root ganglia and sheathed tibial branches (●) and desheathed peroneal branches (o) of two cat sciatic nerves. Two hours after downflow of incorporated ^{3}H-leucine in the animal, nerves were exposed (arrow 1) to 5 and 25 μM MYT for 4 hours in vitro. The activity present in 5 mm segments of roots, ganglia, and nerves are given on the ordinate in logarithmic divisions. Abscissa is in millimeters, taking the distance from the center ganglion as zero. Arrow 3 indicates the position to which the fronts of the crests are calculated to have moved at the usual rate of 410 mm per day. With 5 μM MYT the front of the crest of the desheathed branch (arrow 2) is only a little behind the front of the sheathed branch. With 25 μM MYT present in vitro, the front of the desheathed branch has advanced only a little before block occurs (arrow 2).

hours after the nerve was placed in the incubating medium containing MYT in concentrations of 72 to 5 μM. A full block of transport was seen at successively earlier times as the concentration of MYT was increased. A comparison of the block seen with 5 μM and with 25 μM of MYT shows the difference in these two cases (Fig. 1). The block time in this example at a concentration of 5 µM occurred 3.2 hours after placing the nerve in the flasks for incubation, and with 25 µM, 1.5 hours after incubation. Notice that in each case transport in the sheathed nerve appears not to be affected and the front of the crest moved down to a distance close to that expected after a total 6 hours of downflow (2 in vivo + 4 in the incubation media). Much higher concentrations are required for MYT to pass through the perineurial sheath in effective amounts. At concentrations below 3 µM little effect was evident in the desheathed nerves on axoplasmic transport.

Microtubules in myelinated fibers

Myelinated fibers with axonal diameter measuring 9-14 µm were taken to represent the group of large myelinated fibers. Clusters of microtubules were readily observed in control large myelinated fibers (Fig. 2A). In the fibers exposed to MYT concentrations ranging from 4 µM to 72 µM, the microtubules although reduced in number as compared with control fibers, were always relatively easy to find and were scattered throughout the axoplasm; however, clusters were rarely seen (Fig. 2B). At concentrations of 4-5 µM MYT the reduction of microtubules was not readily detectable. Neurofilaments appeared to be more numerous at concentrations of MYT between 5 and 72 µM. No other organelles were affected. No paracrystalline structures were observed in the fibers at any of the maytansine concentrations studied. At concentrations of 3 µM MYT and below, the number of microtubules were comparable with those of the controls.

The mean microtubules density of each of 8 control groups of large myelinated fibers ranged from 4.21 to 6.97 microtubules/µm^2, the mean microtubule density of the total population was 5.65/µm^2. In the fibers exposed to MYT concentrations ranging from 17 to 72 µM, the mean microtubule density was 23.5% of the pooled control fibers. In fibers exposed to concentrations of 5 µM the mean microtubule density was 52.2% of the controls. At 2 and 1 µM concentrations, the microtubule density was 81.9 and 83.7 per cent respectively of the pooled control. At lower concentrations of the agent no change in microtubular density could be detected.

Microtubules in unmyelinated fibers

The microtubule changes observed in unmyelinated fibers of nerves exposed to concentrations of MYT between 25 and 72 µM were more dramatic; all the axons in this concentration range were severely depleted of microtubules. In nerves exposed to concentrations of MYT between 4 and 25 µM, the microtubules,

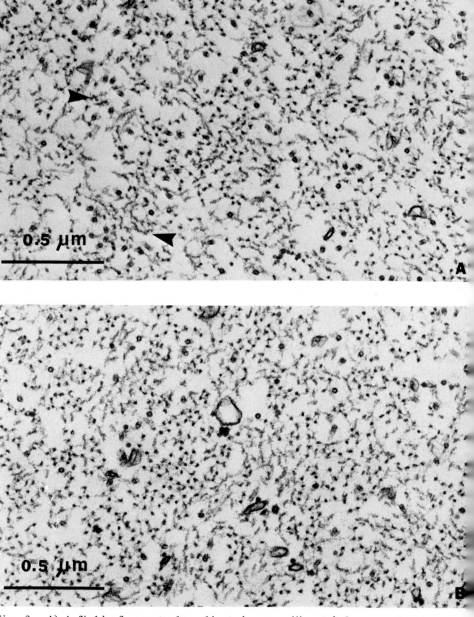

Fig. 2. A) A field of a control myelinated axon. Microtubules are clearly
evident, often in clusters (arrows). B) Myelinated axon from a nerve exposed to
10 μM MYT. The microtubules are fewer in number than in controls and do not
form clusters.

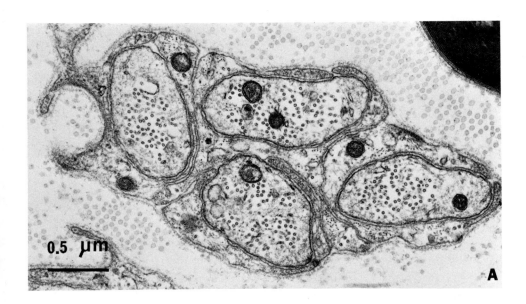

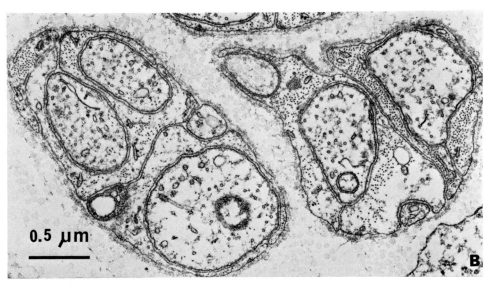

Fig. 3. A) Unmyelinated axons from a control nerve. Microtubules are clearly seen. B) Unmyelinated axons from a nerve exposed to 1 μM MYT. Note that the microtubules are markedly reduced in number.

although present, were markedly reduced in number in comparison with control
(Fig. 3A) unmyelinated axons. At concentrations below 4 μM the depletion of
microtubules was still readily recognizable (Fig. 3B). It was much less severe
in nerves exposed to concentrations of MYT below 1 μM, and at 0.05 μM MYT, the
microtubule loss was not appreciable. An increase in the number of neurofilaments and the presence of an amorphous floccular material was observed in fibers
exposed to MYT concentrations ranging from 3 to 72 μM. No paracrystalline
structures were observed in the unmyelinated fibers at any of the MYT concentrations studied. The mean microtubule density of each of the control groups
ranged from 61.5 to 86.5 microtubules/μm^2. The mean microtubule density of the
total control population of unmyelinated fibers was 78.13 microtubules/μm^2. In
fibers exposed to concentrations of MYT in the range from 17 to 72 μM, the mean
density was 6.3% of the controls. In fibers exposed to concentrations of 5 μM
the mean microtubule density was 8.85% of the controls. At 1 μM and 0.1 μM
concentrations of MYT the microtubule densities were respectively 35.3% and
73.8% of control unmyelinated axons.

Temporal changes

Preliminary studies on the time sequence of the changes in microtubule
density indicated that in vitro the microtubule density in control myelinated
fibers showed only a small decrease during an incubation time lasting 5 hours.
In the myelinated fibers exposed to MYT, the microtubule density after a 2-hour
exposure was only slightly lower than the controls with a marked fall occurring
between 3 and 4 hours. In the unmyelinated fibers on the contrary, a dramatic
microtubule loss developed between 20 and 60 minutes and the same low number of
microtubules (8% of controls) then remained over the next 4 hours.

DISCUSSION

The aim of our investigation was to correlate changes in microtubule density
with alterations in axoplasmic transport in the cat peroneal desheathed nerve
preparation in vitro as affected by different concentrations of MYT. It was
shown that a concentration of 5 μM MYT blocked transport after approximately
3.2 hours of exposure in vitro. At the end of the incubation, after 4 hours
of in vitro exposure the microtubules were reduced by 50%.

The lack of effect of MYT over the whole range of concentrations up to
72 μM on transport in the sheathed tibial branch shows that the perineurial
sheath is an effective permeability barrier to the agent in this range and it
has been reported that a block occurs in the sheathed vagus nerve in vitro[23]
when 100 μM MYT are used.

Autoradiographic studies, carried out in a nerve preparation similar to that used for this study[13] indicated that the bulk of material transported along the axon is carried by the myelinated fibers of larger diameter. The total cross-sectional area of the unmyelinated fibers is estimated to be only a small per cent of the total axonal cross-sectional area and these axons contribute little to the total radioactive downflow in this system[13,22]. Thus, after a 4-hour incubation time with 5 μM MYT we can correlate the approximately 50% reduction of the microtubules in the large myelinated fibers with block of transport. The much more severe and early losses of microtubules in unmyelinated fibers is not causally related. Calculation of microtubular disassembly in the unmyelinated fibers could, on this account, be misleading if it is not compared directly with transport in unmyelinated fibers.

If we assume a direct relationship between the microtubules and axoplasmic transport, it is of interest to observe that transport is blocked only when a 50% loss is reached after 3 to 4 hours. Prior to that, microtubular losses do occur, but transport is not blocked. The approximately 50% loss of microtubules we found at the time of the block of transport is a figure comparable with some recently published data showing that a block of transport of mitochondria was associated with a loss of more than 50% of microtubules[24].

Considering that a block of transport occurred when approximately 50% of the microtubules were lost raises a question as to the role of the remaining microtubules. Are they functionally altered, or if they are normal and functional, is the block due to the numerical insufficiency of the remaining microtubules? Further knowledge of the mechanism of disruption of the microtubules induced by MYT and other tubulin-binding agents in vivo and in vitro should allow additional insight into a differentiation between these alternatives.

SUMMARY

The present studies have shown that maytansine, a new antimitotic agent that binds to tubulin, blocks the axoplasmic transport at concentrations of 5 μM and above. At the time of block the microtubule density in the large myelinated fibers was approximately 50% of the controls, while the density in the unmyelinated was 8.85% of the controls. Considering that most of the material moving down along the nerve fibers is carried by the large myelinated fibers, our data show a correlation between axoplasmic transport and microtubules.

ACKNOWLEDGMENTS

We thank Dr. A. T. Sneden for supplying maytansine and Constance J. Alyea,

Anna M. Mullen, Shew-Yin Chan and Jennifer A. Gallagher for their help. This work was supported by the following grants: PHS grant S01 RR 5331, American Cancer Society IN-46R, NIH PHS R01 NS 8706-09, and NSF 77-24176.

REFERENCES

1. Porter, K.R. (1966) in Principles of Biomolecular Organization, Wolstenholme, G.E.W. and O'Connor, M. eds., Little, Brown and Company, Boston, pp. 308-356.

2. Schmitt, F.O. (1968) Proc. nat. Acad. Sci., 60, 1092-1101.

3. Fernandez, H.L., Huneeus, F.C. and Davison, P.F. (1970) J. Neurobiol., 1, 395-409.

4. Byers, M.R. (1974) Brain Research, 75, 97-113.

5. Kreutzberg, G.W. (1969) Proc. nat. Acad. Sci., 62, 722-728.

6. Karlsson, J. and Sjöstrand, J. (1969) Brain Research, 13, 617-619.

7. Bunt, A.H. (1973) Invest. Ophthal., 12, 579-590.

8. Margolis, R.L. and Wilson, L. (1977) Proc. nat. Acad. Sci., 74, 3466-3470.

9. Wilson, L., Anderson, K. and Chin, D. (1976) in Cell Motility (Cold Spring Harbor Conferences on Cell Proliferation, Cold Spring Harbor, N.Y.), Goldman, R., Pollard, T., Rosenbaum, J. eds, Cold Spring Harbor Laboratory, 3, 1051-1064.

10. Edström, A., and Mattsson, H. (1972) J. Neurochem. 19, 205-221.

11. Green, L.S., Donoso, J.A., Heller-Bettinger, I.E. and Samson, E. (1977) Ann. Neurol., 1, 255-262.

12. Donoso, J.A., Green, L.S., Heller-Bettinger, I.E. and Samson, F.E. (1977) Cancer Research, 37, 1401-1407.

13. Ochs, S. (1972) J. Physiol., 227, 627-645.

14. Ochs, S. and Jersild, R.A. (1974) J. Neurobiol., 5, 373-377.

15. Kupchan, S.M., Komoda, Y., Court, W.A., Thomas, G.J., Smith, R.M., Karim, A., Gilmore, C.J., Haltiwanger, R.C., and Bryan, R.F. (1972) J. Am. Chem. Soc., 94, 1354-1356.

16. Wolpert-DeFilippes, M.K., Bono, V.H., Dion, R.L. and Johns, D.G. (1975) Biochem. Pharmacol., 24, 1735-1738.

17. Remillard, S., Rebhun, L.I., Howie, G.A. and Kupchan, S.M. (1975) Science 189, 1002-1005.

18. Mandelbaum-Shavit, F., Wolpert-DeFilippes, M.K. and Johns, D.G. (1976) Biochem. Biophys. Res. Comm., 72, 47-54.

19. Ghetti, B. and Ochs, S. (1977) Abstracts, Soc. Neuroscience, III, 30.

20. Ghetti, B. (1978) Brain Research (in press).

21. Ochs, S., Worth, R.M. and Chan, S. (1977) Nature 270, 748-750.

22. Ochs, S., Erdman, J., Jersild, R.A. and McAdoo, V. (in preparation).

23. Donoso, J.A., Watson, D.F., Heller-Bettinger, I.E. and Samson, F.E. (1978) Cancer Research, 38, 1633-1637.

24. Friede, R.L. and Ho, K. (1977) J. Physiol., 265, 507-519.

Peripheral Neuropathies
N. Canal and G. Pozza, eds.
© 1978 Elsevier/North-Holland Biomedical Press

CONDUCTANCES OF RAT SKELETAL MUSCLE FIBERS DURING RECOVERY FROM CHRONIC
APPLICATION OF VINCRISTINE TO THE MOTOR NERVE

D. CONTE-CAMERINO, S.H. BRYANT and F. DE FILIPPIS

D.C.C. and F.D.F.: Istituto di Farmacologia, Facoltà di Medicina, Bari, Italia

S.H.B.: Department of Pharmacology and Cell Biophysics, University of Cincinnati, Cincinnati (OHIO) U.S.A.

ABSTRACT

Membrane potassium and chloride conductances were measured in rat extensor digitorum longus fibers at 1 to 8 months after removal of a silicone cuff containing vincristine (0.05% and 0.1%) from the nerve. Potassium conductance remained high and did not return to normal, whereas chloride conductance overshoots the normal value by about 30%.

INTRODUCTION

In mammalian skeletal muscle chloride conductance G_{Cl} is about 80% of the total surface and tubular membrane conductance G_m; the remainder is largely potassium conductance G_K, the sodium and other ionic conductances are negligible[1,2,3]. G_{Cl} and G_K must be maintained at appropriate levels for normal excitability of the mammalian muscle fiber. An abnormally low G_{Cl} has been shown to be the basis for the repetitive firing seen in some forms of hereditary myotonia and is the mechanism of myotonia produced by certain drugs[4,5,6,7,8].

Denervation of mammalian skeletal muscle has recently been shown to lead to a delayed fall of G_{Cl} and rise of G_K[9,10,11]. Thus, the motor nerve exerts control over the resting conductances, but it is not yet certain through what mechanism this is accomplished. In previous studies we have attempted to evaluate the importance of factors brought by axoplasmic transport to the muscle fiber by the use of agents such as colchicine, vinblastine and vincristine, which when applied to the motor nerve can interfere with axoplasmic transport without blocking impulse transmission[10,12,13,14,15].

We have concluded from these studies that factors transported by the microtubular or microfilament systems of the axon are necessary for maintenance of a high G_{Cl} and for suppressing G_K.

In the course of the vincristine study the question arose as to whether the nerve is capable of normal functioning after we remove the vincristine-containing silicone cuff from the nerve following chronic application of the drug for one month. We report here that G_K remained high and never returned to normal during a 1 to 8 months period, but G_{Cl} increased to values about 30% higher than normal. This study further supports the existence of separate factors for controlling G_K and G_{Cl}.

MATERIALS AND METHODS

The right peroneal nerve of 25 adult (250-300 g) Wistar rats was exposed under surgical anesthesia and a silastic cuff containing vincristine Vc or a blank was placed around the nerve approximately 10 mm from the extensor digitorum longus (EDL) muscle. The rats were in three groups which contained the following treatments: in 13 the cuff contained 0.1% Vc, in 10 the cuff contained 0.05% Vc, and in 2 control animals the cuff was prepared blank. Of the operated animals 5 (20%) were rejected for the study because they showed some paralysis, the remainder appeared to have normal function of the EDL muscle. The preparation of the silicone-rubber nerve-cuffs was as described previously[13].

A second operation was performed to remove the cuffs from the nerve in order to observe recovery. The 0.1% Vc cuffs were removed at 15 days along with one blank, and the 0.05% Vc cuffs were removed at 30 days again with one blank. Following the second surgery 3 more animals were rejected because of partial paralysis from the procedure.

Electrophysiological measurements were made on the EDL muscles in vitro at 25°C with microelectrodes at different times (32 to 240 days) from the removal of the cuff. Two microelectrodes inserted into the same fiber were used, one for passing current and the other for recording membrane potentials. Excitability was measured by observing the response of the membrane to stimulating pulses in presence and absence of tetrodotoxin (TTX) at 10^{-6} M. Cable parameters of the fibers were measured from the subthreshold electrotonic potentials in response to hyperpolarizing constant current pulses passed into the fiber at two spacings of the voltage and current electrodes. A close spacing of 0.05 mm and one about 1 space constant were used. Membrane time constant was estimated from the time of rise of the electrotonic potential to 84% of steady state value when the electrodes were spaced at 0.05 mm.

Membrane resistance (R_m), membrane capacitance (C_m) and a fiber diameter (d_{calc}) were calculated and tabulated for each fiber from estimates of the input resistance and space constant, and by assuming a value of 125 ohm·cm for myoplasmic resistivity. The cable measurements were made from random surface fibers in a chloride-containing and a chloride-free physiological solution. Component conductances were estimated from the mean reciprocals of R_m in chloride-containing (G_m) and chloride-free (G_K) solutions. It is assumed that membrane conductance G_m when chloride is present is the sum of G_K and G_{Cl}. It is further assumed that in the absence of chloride in the solution the membrane conductance is G_K, thus G_{Cl} may be calculated as G_m minus G_K. All of these electrophysiological methods have been described in detail earlier[1,8].

The normal chloride-containing physiological solution had the following composition (mM): NaCl 160; KCl 4.5; $CaCl_2$ 2.0; $MgCl_2$ 1.0; NaH_2PO_4 0.44; $NaHCO_3$ 12.0; and glucose 5.5.

The chloride-free solution contained equimolar amounts of sodium and potassium methylsulfates in place of NaCl and KCl, and $Ca(NO_3)_2$ and $Mg(NO_3)_2$ in place of $CaCl_2$ and $MgCl_2$. The physiological solutions were gassed with a 5% CO_2/95% O_2 mixture.

Vincristine was obtained from Lilly S.p.A., Italy and the tetrodotoxin from Sankyo Ltd., Tokyo. TTX was stored as 10^{-4} g/ml stock solution and added to the bath to produce a final concentration of 10^{-6} M.

RESULTS

The cable parameters in the recovery period following removal of the Vc-cuff are summarized in Table 1. Here the data from the 0.05% and 0.1% Vc-cuffs are compared with the mean of 7 control preparations. The control preparations included 2 in which the cuff contained no drug, 4 contralateral muscles from cuffed animals, and 1 muscle from an unoperated animal. Because there were no differences between the individual control preparations the values were averaged.

Both the treated preparations and the controls gave no signs of fibrillation, no anode-break stimulation after TTX, and no TTX-resistant action potentials. Some anode-break excitation was observed in control and experimental preparations prior to adding TTX.

TABLE 1 — Cable Parameters of Rat EDL fibers during the recovery from chronic Vincristine treatment.

				Normal Physiol. Solution				Chloride-free Physiol. Solution		
Preparation	Drug Concentration	Days	N	d_{calc} (μm)	R_m ($\Omega \cdot$ cm^2)	C_m (μF/cm^2)	N	d_{calc} (μm)	R_m ($\Omega \cdot$ cm^2)	C_m (μF/cm
Mean of 7 Controls:			44	42.9±1	324±14	3.9±0.3	31	54.3±2	7576±744	3.6±0.3
Mean of 3 Vincristine Treated:	0.05%	32-240	29	51.3±1*	239±9*	2.5±0.2*	25	60.7±3	6175±937	3.7±0.7
Mean of 5 Vincristine Treated:	0.1%	36-62	53	48.9±1*	261±12*	2.8±0.2*	35	55.6±3	4056±587*	3.9±0.3

* Significantly different from mean of control group (p < 0.001)
The columns from left to right are as follows: Preparation, each from a different rat; Drug concentration during the treatment; days from removal of the cuff; N, number of fibers; d_{calc}, R_m and C_m, are the cable parameters in normal physiological solution; the remaining columns are the same parameters in chloride-free medium.

The mean resting potentials in normal solution of control and experimental groups were somewhat depolarized compared to previous studies. In the chloride--free solution however all of the preparations hyperpolarized by a mean of from 4 to 16 mV to give mean potentials of 60.0±1.8 mV for control and 60.8±0.9 mV and 64.0±1.8 mV for the low and high concentrations of Vc, respectively.

The mean R_m fell significantly for both Vc concentrations from a control of 324±14 ohm·cm^2 to 239±9 and 261±12 ohm·cm^2 for 0.05% and 0.1%, respectively. In chloride-free solution R_m at both Vc concentrations was lower than control (7576±744 ohm·cm^2),but only the value at the 0.1% Vc concentration (4056±587 ohm·cm^2) was significant. In normal solution some small changes were also observed in the calculated diameter and in fiber capacitance, but these did not occur in chloride-free solution.

The resting component conductances are given in Table 2. As with the cable parameters of Table 1 the data from the control preparations and from the different periods during recovery at each concentration of Vc were combined. The total conductance G_m was increased significantly from a control of 3359 ± 161 μmhos/cm^2 to 4327 ± 151 and 4302 ± 194 μmhos/cm^2 for Vc concentrations of 0.05% and 0.1%, respectively. The increases in G_m can be seen to be reflected in parallel increases in both G_K and G_{Cl}. The increase in G_K from a control value of 185 ± 22 μmhos/cm^2 to 363 ± 30 μmhos/cm^2 at 0.1% Vc is significant, but the increase at the lower concentration of Vc (0.05%) to 240 ± 31 μmhos/cm^2 is only of borderline significance; G_{Cl}, on the other hand, significantly increased from the control of 3174 ± 125 μmhos/cm^2 to 4087 ± 112 μmhos/cm^2 and 3939 ± 151 μmhos/cm^2 at 0.05% and 0.1%, respectively.

TABLE 2   Component Resting Conductances of Rat EDL Fibers during the recovery from chronic Vincristine treatment.

Preparation	Drug Concentration	Days	N	G_m (μmhos/cm^2)	N	G_K (μmhos/cm^2)	G_{Cl} (μmhos/cm^2)
Mean of 7 Controls:			44	3359·161	31	185·22	3174·125
Mean of 3 Vincristine Treated:	0.05%	32–240	29	4327·151*	25	240·31	4087·112*
Mean of 5 Vincristine Treated:	0.1%	36–62	53	4302·194*	35	363·30*	3939·151*

* Significantly different from mean of control group (p < 0.001)

The columns from left to right are as follows: Preparation, each from a different rat; Drug concentration during the treatment; Days from the removal of the cuff; N, number of fibers for G_m and G_K respectively; G_m, total membrane conductance; G_K and G_{Cl} are the component conductances.

DISCUSSION

In a previous study[14] vincristine was applied in two concentrations (0.05% and 0.1%) in cuffs to the peroneal nerve for periods from 11 to 23 days in the same way as we have done in the present study. It was found that G_K increased significantly by factors of 2.8 and 2.1 times for the low and high concentrations, respectively. G_{Cl} in that study decreased significantly to half of control but only at the high concentration.

In a report from another laboratory[17] it is claimed that denervation occurs regularly with use of the silicone nerve cuff technique. We did not experience this difficulty as indicated from the few animals that we had to reject, and that the preparations which were used showed no evidence of fibrillation.

In the present study Vc was applied in the same concentrations for about the same periods of time (30 days, 0.05% and 15 days, 0.1%), and it is assumed that the drug produced similar levels of effects on the conductances at the time that the cuffs were removed. A comparison of effects during exposure and after recovery from Vc is shown in Fig. 1. During exposure G_K increases and G_{Cl} decreases similar to the effects of denervation. For several months after removal of the cuff G_K tends to remain high and does not return to normal, whereas G_{Cl} returns to supernormal values, overshooting by 24-29%. Previously it also was not clear whether there would be any recovery from vincristine since disaggregation or reconstitution of the microtubules would be necessary for this to occur. The present results suggest that recovery occurs most quickly for G_{Cl}.

Our earlier results with colchicine[9] do not fit the pattern seen with the vinca alkaloids since the former agent caused a decrease in G_K, however in those experiments colchicine was given in high concentrations by epineural injection. Recently, the colchicine experiments were repeated using the less traumatic "soaking" technique[16] to apply the colchicine and it was found that G_K was not significantly affected although G_{Cl} decreased as before.

The fact that G_K and G_{Cl} act differently toward recovery again suggests that there may be separate controlling systems for these conductances. The G_K suppressing factor appears to be more sensitive to blockade by vincristine and vinblastine, and it is resistant to recovery from vincristine in the present experiments.

A useful hypothesis to come out of our vincristine studies is that there are at least two factors, possibly two axoplasmic transport pathways, that separately control G_K and G_{Cl}. The factors controlling G_K are affected at lower drug concentrations and recover slowly; the factors controlling G_{Cl} need higher concentrations but recover more quickly.

ACKNOWLEDGEMENTS

This work was supported by a grant from the Italian National Research Council (C.N.R. No. CT 77.01272.04).

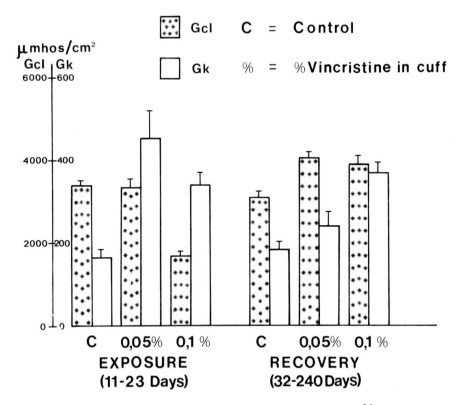

Fig. 1. Comparison of membrane conductances upon exposure to ^{14}, and after recovery from application of vincristine to the motor nerve.

REFERENCES

1. Bryant, S.H. and Morales-Aguilera, A. (1971) J. Physiol., 219, 367-383.

2. Palade, P.T. and Barchi, R.L. (1977) J. Gen. Physiol., 69, 879-896.

3. Bryant, S.H. (1976) in Membranes and Disease, Bolis, L., Hoffman, J.F., and Leaf, A. eds., Raven, New York, pp. 197-205.

4. Adrian, R.H. and Bryant, S.H. (1974) J. Physiol.,240, 505-515.

5. Adrian, R.H. and Marshall, M.W. (1976) J. Physiol., 258, 125-143.

6. Rudel, R. (1976) in Membranes and Disease, Bolis, L., Hoffman, J.F. and Leaf, A. eds., Raven, New York, pp. 207-213.

7. Lipicky, R.J., Bryant, S.H. and Salmon, J.H. (1971) J. Clin. Invest., 50, 2091-2103.

8. Bryant, S.H. (1969) J. Physiol., 204, 539-550.

9. Bryant, S.H. and Camerino, D. (1976) J. Neurobiology, 7, 229-240.

10. Camerino, D. and Bryant, S.H. (1976) J. Neurobiology, 7, 221-228.

11. Lorcovic, H. and Tomanek, R.J. (1977) Am. J. Physiol., 232, C109-C114.

12. Conte-Camerino, D. and Bryant, S.H. (1976) in Membranes and Disease, Bolis, L., Hoffman, J.F. and Leaf, A. eds., pp. 215-218.

13. Conte-Camerino, D. and Bryant, S.H. (1977) Pharm. Res. Comm., 9, 223-233.

14. Conte-Camerino, D. (1978) Pharm. Res. Comm., In Press.

15. Samson, F. (1976) Ann. Rev. of Pharmacol. and Toxicol., 16, 143-159.

16. DeCoursey, T., Younkin, S. and Bryant, S.H. (1978) J. Exp. Neurol., In Press.

17. Cangiano, A. and Fried, J.A. (1977) J. Physiol., 265, 63-84.

NEUROPATHIES IN
CHRONIC RENAL FAILURE

Peripheral Neuropathies
N. Canal and G. Pozza, eds.
© 1978 Elsevier/North-Holland Biomedical Press

PATHOPHYSIOLOGICAL ASPECTS OF URAEMIC NEUROPATHY

VIGGO KAMP NIELSEN

Laboratory of Clinical Neurophysiology, University Hospital,
(Rigshospitalet), Blegdamsvej 9, 2loo Copenhagen (Denmark)

ABSTRACT

Clinical and electrophysiological findings in uraemic neuropathy
and the effect of dialysis treatment and renal transplantation are
reviewed. Pathophysiologically, the neuropathy can be characterized by a readily reversible peripheral nerve dysfunction, which appears to be generalized in nature, e.g. as judged from a widespread
slowing of the nerve conduction. The pathogenesis is probably multifactorial. As the only factor, histopathological findings (distal
axonal degeneration with segmental demyelination) seem inconsistent
with the variety and extent of electrophysical disturbances and do
not fit in with the rapid remission of the neuropathy immediately
after renal transplantation. According to current concepts, the
uraemic intoxication is basically caused by an accumulation of enzymatic inhibitors in body fluids, a.o. impairing the Na-K transport across cell membranes. This concept has wide applications to
pathophysiological observations in uraemic neuropathy, and the hypothesis is advanced that a reversible reduction of the resting potential difference of the nerve axon membrane is a dominant factor
in the pathogenesis.

INTRODUCTION

Uraemic neuropathy has only been fully recognized for the last
15 years[1], although the clinical picture was described about loo
years ago[2,3]. The rediscovery coincided with the introduction of
regular dialysis treatment, by which the lifetime of patients with
terminal uraemia was considerably prolonged. An increasing number
of reports soon placed the neuropathy among the most feared complications to the treatment, but with more comprehensive studies it
was realized that the neuropathy should rather be considered as an
integral part of the uraemic syndrome. During the present decade
most nephrological centers have witnessed a remarkable decline in
the frequency of clinical neuropathy[4], a.o. resulting from an ear-

lier institution of regular dialysis. Similarly the number of severe neuropathies has decreased due to the access to renal transplantation, for which patients with impending sensory-motor neuropathies are usually given priority. Detailed descriptions of the
uraemic neuropathy have been published elsewhere[5,6,7]. This review
primarily focus on the pathophysiology of the neuropathy. Besides,
recent studies on the uraemic intoxication may elucidate the pathogenesis of the neurological findings.

CLINICAL NEUROPATHY

   Uraemic neuropathy is predominantly a sensory neuropathy without any destinctive features. Late in the course of chronic renal
failure patients may present with mild, often intermittent sensory
symptoms confined to the distal part of the extremities. Clinical
examination is often negative or may show weak or absent achilles
reflexes and impaired vibratory perception as the only abnormality.
In the majority of patients the neuropathy never progress any further. A small group of patients, however, may suddenly develop a
progressive, ascending, mixed sensory-motor neuropathy, where
muscle weakness and wasting soon becomes the dominant feature. It
is still unknown what elicits this often invalidating course. The
onset may be preceded by a period of severe catabolism due to severe dyspepsia, surgical trauma, gastro-intestinal bleeding or infections with prolonged bed-rest. Apart from dialysis or transplantation there is no effective treatment. Thus, the aim of conservative management in uraemia has rather been the prevention of clinical neuropathy, e.g. by dietary restrictions[8].

ELECTROPHYSIOLOGICAL FINDINGS

   The frequency of electrophysiological indices of impaired peripheral nerve function is considerably higher than that of clinical
symptoms and signs. Moreover, electrophysiological abnormalities
are present at an earlier stage of chronic renal failure and have
a wider distribution than clinical findings. This led to the early
recognition of the so-called subclinical neuropathy in uraemia[9].
However, this distinction is obviously arbitrary and may be one of
the main reasons for the considerable variation in the reported
incidence of uraemic neuropathy.

Conduction velocity

The motor and sensory conduction velocity is the most extensively studied single parameter. The reported findings are rather concordant: Slowing of the conduction has been demonstrated in almost all nerves examined and often to about the same degree. This applies to nerves in lower and upper extremities, to motor and sensory fibres, and to fast and slowly conducting fibres[10]. Although nerves in the legs are usually more severely affected, this is not a rule without exceptions. Therefore, the average value of the conduction velocity in the median, ulnar, common peroneal, and posterior tibial nerves has been suggested as a more reliable indicator of the peripheral nerve function[11]. Although differences between mean velocities in uraemics and normal controls are statistically significant, the average decrease in patients only amounts to about 15-2o% of the normal mean value, and the distribution of data shows considerable overlapping. Thus, velocities below 4o m/s in the median nerve and 3o m/s in the common peroneal nerve are exceptional. This would seem consistent with a selective loss of a large diameter fibres, as demonstrated in fibre diameter histograms of sural nerve biopsies[12]. However, in the median nerve with a similar degree of slowing of the conduction, there was no electrophysiological evidence in favour of a reduction in the number of fibres. The reduction of the sensory potential amplitude showed a perfect correlation with the concomitant increase of the temporal dispersion, i.e. within the limits obtained in normal nerves[10].

The conduction velocity is closely correlated with the kidney function as expressed by the endogenous creatinine clearance, while there is no direct relationship with the degree of azotaemia, i.e. the serum levels of urea and creatinine. Accordingly, a neurotoxic effect of these substances per se cannot be demonstrated[13]. A similar multiple correlation should be taken into consideration before postulating a neurotoxic effect of any other substance accumulating in uraemic serum. A significant slowing of the conduction in the common peroneal nerve was seen in about 5o% of patients, when the creatinine clearance was reduced to lo% of normal. With further progression in renal failure the velocities invariably showed a down-hill course and in end-stage ureamia a

slowing in one or more nerve segments was present in nearly all patients. As distinct from clinical findings, this course was the
same in upper and lower extremities, and in distal and proximal
nerve segments. Neither was the degree of slowing well correlated
to the presense or absense of clinical findings, as the difference
between mean conduction velocities could be accounted for by a concomitant difference in kidney function. Finally, there was no critical conduction level for the appearence of clinical neuropathy[13].

Distal vs. proximal nerve segments. A phenomenon of considerable pathophysiological interest is the fact that the nerve conduction in uraemic patients is slowed in both distal and proximal segments of the same nerve. Thus, with simultaneous recording of sensory action potentials in the median nerve at wrist, elbow, and
axilla following stimulation of digit I or III, a significant reduction of the conduction velocity could be demonstrated in all
three segments. Moreover, the distal segment was not the most affected[14]. When pooling all measurements of distal and proximal
conduction velocities in my final material, a regression analysis
showed that a reduction in the digit-wrist segment of 1 m/s was in
average accompanied by a reduction of 2 m/s in the wrist-elbow
segment[15]. The same tendency was demonstrable in motor fibres of
the median nerve in that the distal motor latency was normal in 58
out of 65 nerves with reduced motor conduction velocity in the elbow-wrist segment.

Impaired nerve conduction in proximal nerve segments has recently been demonstrated by other groups using different techniques.
Guiheneuc and Bathien studied the H-reflex of the soleus muscle in
79 uraemic patients[16]. The latency was increased in nearly all patients, whereas the reflex response had a normal amplitude. The
conduction velocity of the H-reflex showed a linear relationship
with the distal motor conduction in the lateral peroneal nerve.
These findings were confirmed in 64 patients studied by Knoll[17].
He considered the latency of the H-reflex to be a more sensitive
parameter than the motor conduction in distal segments, as the reflex response latency was prolonged earlier in the course of uraemia and in patients with normal motor conduction velocities in distal nerve segments. Panayiotopoulos and Scarpalezos[18], studying
the F-response in uraemic patients, found that the conduction ve-

locity in the proximal segment (ant. horn cell-knee) was reduced to the same degree as the motor conduction in the distal (knee-ankle) segment of the deep peroneal nerve.

These findings reinforce the previously advanced statement that a generalized slowing of the nerve conduction is an integral part of the uraemic syndrome[5].

Excitability of nerves

Tackmann et al.[19] found that the absolute and the relative refractory period in sensory action potentials was increased in uraemic patients. With stimulus intervals shorter than 3 ms the test response showed a greater reduction in amplitude than seen in normal controls and also a greater increase in latency relative to the conditioning response. Similar results were obtained in alcoholic and diabetic neuropathy and the interesting suggestion is made that these findings may implicate changed membrane properties with a lower safety factor. However, the observation awaits further confirmation, as Delbeke et al.[20] were unable to demonstrate increased refractoriness in motor fibres of the median nerve in four uraemic patients.

Resistance to ischaemia

In patients with certain metabolic disorders peripheral nerves sustain limb ischaemia much longer than normal nerves. This was originally demonstrated in diabetics[21,22], but has also been demonstrated in hypercalcaemia[23] and in chronic hepatic failure[24,25,26]. In uraemic patients the phenomenon was first described by Christensen and Ørskov[27] who showed that vibratory perception was retained during 3o min of ischaemia in 16 of their 19 patients. This was not related to abnormalities in the glucose tolerance. Meilvang[28] was only able to reproduce this observation in two of his 23 patients, but most of his patients had a mild to moderate renal failure. We defined the ischaemic perception time (IPT) as the duration of ischaemia (min) in which vibrations with the maximally available stimulus strength could be perceived[25]. In 16 of my patients on regular haemodialysis, IPT (25.8 ± 1.1 min) was significantly longer than in 16 normal controls (17.9 ± 0.5 min), $P < 0.001$. Four patients retained vibratory perception for more than 3o min

202

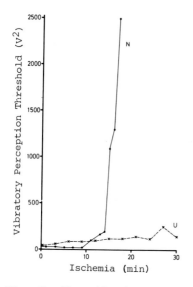

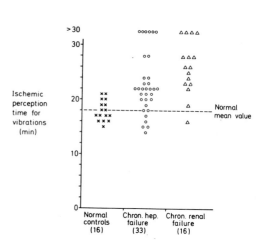

Fig. 1. The vibratory perception threshold (pulp, dig.II)
during ischaemia of the arm
in a normal person (N) and a
uraemic patient (U).

Fig. 2. Ischaemic perception time
(see text) in normal controls and
chronic hepatic failure (Kardel &
Nielsen, 1974), and in dialysis
patients (Nielsen, 1973, unpubl.)

(figs. 1,2). In normal nerves subjected to ischaemia the amplitude
of the sensory action potential decreases at a faster rate proximally than distally, and the sensory conduction velocity is slowed
more rapidly in proximal than in distal segments[29,30]. The increase in sensory threshold coincides with the extinction of the action potential proximally, just below the occluding cuff, while
potentials can be recorded more distally also after sensory perception is abolished[30]. We studied these parameters in hepatic patients with prolonged resistance to ischaemia[26]. Two aberrations
from the normal response were observed: (1) Axon membrane polari-
zation along the nerve was maintained for a longer period of time,
as evidenced by the slow decrease of the potential amplitude at
the proximal site of recording. At a more distal level, Castaigne
et al. made the same observation in uraemic patients[31]. (2) The
decrease in amplitude and sensory conduction velocity was considerably slower, and the slope of the decrease was nearly the same in
distal and proximal segments and sites of recording. The ischaemia
resistance phenomenon following dialysis is further discussed below.

Electromyography

Surprisingly few reports have appeared on electromyographic findings in chronic renal failure. These have shown EMG changes consistent with a neurogenic atrophy with moderate to severe loss of motor units and fibrillation activity[32,33]. Abnormal findings are usually confined to distal muscles and appear later in the course of renal failure than slowing of the motor conduction[34]. Single fibre EMG in the extensor dig. comm. muscle has shown a normal fibre density and a normal jitter, suggesting absence of reinnervation and a normal neuromuscular transmission. These patients had a significant slowing of the motor conduction velocity[35]. Floyd et al.[36] found clinical and electromyographic evidence of a proximal myopathy in a group of uraemic patients without signs of neuropathy. This has not been confirmed by later reports.

REGULAR DIALYSIS TREATMENT

It is generally agreed that regular dialysis may prevent the progression and in quite a number of patients induce an improvement of clinical neuropathy. On the other hand, a low conduction velocity at best remains stationary, at least within the first year. The latter observation characterizes the limitations of dialysis as a treatment, especially when compared with the dramatic effect of a succesful renal transplantation. Even the well dialysed patient remains a "uraemic". Hence the conduction velocity is regarded as unsuited for the running control of the effect of the treatment. The vibratory perception threshold is maybe a more sensitive indicator of the clinical course[37]. In spite of a notable intraindividual variation within the pathological range, the method has proved to be useful as a supplement to clinical bed-side examination. In keeping with our findings, other groups have confirmed that effective dialysis causes an improvement of the vibratory perception, which parallels or precedes the remission of other clinical symptoms and signs of neuropathy[38,39].

Effect of single dialyses. It is well documented that there is no systematic change in the conduction velocity of nerves following single dialyses[31,40,41]. However, a temporal and significant drop of the vibratory perception threshold has been shown within the first 36 hours after a dialysis followed by a new rise up to the next dialysis[42,38]. Another group recorded a significant increase of the amplitudes of muscle and mixed nerve action potentials immediately after dialysis. The same tendency was seen for amplitudes of sensory action potentials, but probably due to the low number of observations the difference was not statistically significant[41].

Castaigne et al.[31] studied changes in the resistance to ischaemia effected by single dialyses. They observed that the ischaemic resistance was further increased the day after a dialysis with induced hypovolaemia. However, when the hypovolaemia was corrected by infusion of macromolecular plasma expander (Rheomacrodex[R]) the ischaemic perception time was significantly shortened approaching normal values. These findings have gained particular interest in the light of new observations in experimental diabetes[43]. Some years ago, Seneviratne and Weerasuriya[44] advanced the hypothesis that the increased resistance to ischaemia might be due to inability to built up a sufficiently high potassium concentration in the endoneurial space, hence delaying the depolarization of the axon membrane. As the morphological basis they suggested that there was an increased permeability of the cation binding barrier substance in the nodal gab, previously described by Landon and Langley[45]. Their histopathological studies in diabetic rats appeared compatible with this hypothesis, but their findings could not be confirmed by Sharma and Thomas[46]. Recently, Jakobsen[43] has re-advanced the hypothesis, but as a morphological basis he suggests an expansion of the endoneurial space ("endoneurial oedema"), which he was able to demonstrate in streptozotocin diabetic rats by morphometric measurements. The above mentioned changes in the ischaemic resistance produced by dialysis with hypovolaemia and subsequent infusion of plasma expanders could be explained on the basis of hydration and dehydration of the endoneurial space, but other factors should be considered such as the clearance of neurotoxic enzyme inhibitors.

KIDNEY TRANSPLANTATION

It is an impressive experience to observe how even severe sensory-motor disturbances may vanish within a few days or weeks after a succesful kidney transplantation. This was already recognized in

the early days of transplantation[47,48]. The remission of clinical
and electrophysiological signs of neuropathy follows a two-phasic
course with a short lasting rapid recovery phase followed by a
more protracted phase with slow improvement which may go on for
more than a year before full recovery is established[49,50,51,52].
Typically, the remission of clinical symptoms and signs is completed long before the nerve conduction reaches normal values. The
recovery of electrophysiological parameters exhibits the following
characteristics: An abrupt increase in the conduction velocity is
seen early after the transplantation. This has been demonstrated
already during the first few days[53,54], whereas Bolton[55] was less
impressed, although his data also showed the greatest improvement
early after transplantation. The course is nearly the same in different nerves and nerve segments and in mildly and severely affected nerves. Even conduction velocities in the lower normal range
may improve significantly, i.e. more than expected from the intraindividual variation[52]. During the second phase the nerve conduction shows a continuous but slow improvement, which may last for
many months and which does not always reach normal levels. The amplitude of nerve and muscle action potentials recovers with the
same two-phasic course and is usually fully restored before normalization of the conduction velocity. Late sequelae after uraemic
neuropathy are few and clinically unimportant, and only seen in
patients with very severe and longstanding neuropathy. Apart from
a subnormal conduction velocity, permanent sequelae may comprise
atrophy of isolated distal muscles, absent achilles reflexes, absent vibration sense on the big toe, and slight dysaesthesia of
the feet[51].

It was previously assumed that a normal excretory function of
the kidney graft (high endogenous creatinine clearance) was a pre-
condition for the recovery of uraemic neuropathy. However, there
are some casuistic reports on patients in whom a dramatic recovery
was observed even before the graft started functioning or functio-
ned subnormally[56,57]. This remarkable situation might indicate that
an endogenous degradation of neurotoxic substances may take place
in the normal kidney tissue of the graft, even when the graft is
in a state of acute renale failure with reduced excretory function.
This could be a key to the peculiar fact that patients with acute

renal failure ("shock kidney") despite severe azotaemia rarely if ever exhibit signs of uraemic neuropathy.

PATHOGENESIS

The electrophysiological findings described above, not least the recovery pattern after transplantation, cannot alone be explained by the reported histopathological abnormalities in uraemic nerves. These comprise random axonal degeneration with secondary demyelination[12] mainly confined to the distal segments of the nerves[58], suggesting a "dying back neuropathy". The multiple and widespread electrophysiological changes rather implicate that a more generalized and reversible impairment of the axon membrane function is a basic feature in the pathogenesis of uraemic neuropathy. This hypothesis is compatible with the current concept of the pathogenesis of the uraemic intoxication, which is "generally regarded as a consequence of accumulation of enzymatic inhibitors in the body fluids" (Giovannetti and Barsotti[59]).

In previous reports[5,10] I reviewed biophysical data showing that dialysable substances in uraemic serum reversibly inhibit the ouabain-sensitive Na-K-activated ATPase of cellular membranes resulting in a reduced Na efflux, an increased intracellular Na concentration, and accompanied by a decrease in the transmembrane potential difference. A reduction of the muscle membrane potential difference was in fact observed in vivo in uraemic patients[60,61]. In recent years several pieces of evidence have been added in support of this pattern of events. The original and many subsequent Na transport studies were performed on erythrocyte membranes[62,63,64,65], but similar studies have come out with concordant results also in other cellular systems such as crab muscle fibres[66], toad oocytes[67], and frog skin[68] incubated with uraemic serum, brain cells in uraemic rats[69], and leucocytes from uraemic patients[70]. Thus, there is abundant evidence in favour of the concept that inhibition of the Na transport over cell membranes is a generalized phenomenon in chronic renal failure.

It seems justified to assume that the same defect may result in a reduction of the potential difference in nerve axon membranes. The immediate effect would a.o. be a generalized slowing of the nerve conduction, in keeping with observations. Recently, Cole et

al.[71,72] have demonstrated a rapid increase of the ouabain-sensitive Na-K-ATPase activity after renal transplantation even to
supernormal levels with a concomitant reduction of the intracellular Na concentration to below normal values. The high ATPase activity level showed no tendency to normalize even several months
after the transplantation. This observation correlates well with
the initial rapid increase in the nerve conduction velocity after
transplantation, while it appears more difficult to account for
the second recovery phase with a slow and sometimes incomplete
normalization of the nerve conduction.

As to the more pronounced slowing of the nerve conduction in
proximal than in distal nerve segments, we were able to reproduce
this pattern in normal nerves subjected to short-lasting ischaemia
where the axon membrane function is temporarily impaired due to
hypoxia[30]. With this model, morphological changes in the nerve
fibres can be disregarded as evidenced by the fast normalization
of the nerve conduction parameters within minutes after restoration
of the blood circulation. However, while a reduction of the resting
membrane potential can explain the slowing of nerve conduction, it
does not readily explain why the conduction velocity along the sensory nerves showed a progressive decrease with the distance from
the point of stimulation. Our preliminary assumption that this
might indicate decremental conduction under these circumstances
(uraemia, hypoxia) seems to be ruled out by recent results from
studies of the orthodromic and antidromic sensory nerve conduction
over two adjacent nerve segments during ischaemia. These showed
that the proximal nerve segment was more sensitive to ischaemia
than the distal, irrespective of the direction of the conduction
and hence independent of the conduction distance from the point
of stimulation[73]. A possible explanation for the different degree
of slowing could be that the internodal length is greater in the
proximal than in the distal, or more precisely, in the terminal
nerve segment[74]. It is conceivable that a reduction of the resting
axon membrane potential, reducing the current density at the nodes
of Ranvier, may delay the depolarization of the membrane potential
at the adjacent nodes, and hence the rate of impulse propagation,
and that this effect may be more pronounced, the longer the internodal length. This could result in the relatively greater slowing

of conduction and the earlier conduction block during ischaemia in proximal nerve segments with long internodes.

The pathogenesis of uraemic neuropathy is in all probability multifactorial, and it is still premature to formulate a general concept. There is a reciprocal relation between the studies of the pathophysiology of uraemic nerves and of the biophysics of uraemic cells. A joint approach may be rewarding for a better understanding of the neuropathy.

REFERENCES

1. Asbury, A.K., Victor, M. and Adams, R.D. (1963) Arch. Neurol. (Chic.) 8,413.
2. Kussmaul, A. (1864) Würzburger med. Zschr. 4, 55.
3. Lanceraux, E. (1887) Troubles nerveux de l'urémie. Union médicale.
4. Thomas, P.K. (1976) Proc. Europ. Dial. Transpl. Ass., 13, 1o9.
5. Nielsen, V.K. (1974) Acta med. scand. Suppl. 573, pp. 1-32.
6. Asbury, A.K. (1975) in Peripheral Neuropathies, Dyck, P.J., Thomas, P.K. and Lambert, E.H. eds., W.B. Saunders, Philadelphia, London, Toronto, pp. 982-992.
7. Raskin, N.H. and Fishman, R.A. (1976) New Engl. J. Med., 294, 2o4.
8. Bergström, J., Lindblom, U. and Norée, L.-O. (1975) Acta neurol. scand. 51, 99.
9. Preswick, G. and Jeremy, D. (1964) Lancet 2, 731.
1o. Nielsen, V.K. (1973) Acta med. scand. 194, 445.
11. Jepsen, R.H. and Tenckhoff, H.A. (1969) Arch. phys. Med. 5o, 124.
12. Thomas, P.K., Hollinrake, K., Lascelles, R.G., O'Sullivan, D.J., Baillod, R.A., Moorhead, J.F. and Mackenzie, J.C. (1971) Brain 94, 761.
13. Nielsen, V.K. (1973) Acta med. scand. 194, 455.
14. Nielsen, V.K. (1967) Proc. Europ. Dial. Transpl. Ass., 4, 279.
15. Nielsen, V.K. (1974) Acta med. scand. 196, 83.
16. Guiheneuc, P. and Bathien, N. (1976) J. neurol. Sci., 3o, 83.
17. Knoll, O. (1977) Electroenceph. clin. Neurophysiol. 43, 593.
18. Panayiotopoulos, C.P. and Scarpalezos, S. (1977) J. neurol. Sci., 31, 331.
19. Tackmann, W., Ullerich, D., Cremer, W. and Lehmann, H.J. (1974) Europ. Neurol. 12, 331.
2o. Delbeke, J., Kopec, J. and McComas, A.J. (1978) J. Neurol. Neurosurg. Psychiat. 41, 65.
21. Steiness, I. (1959) Acta med. scand. 163, 195.
22. Gregersen, G. (1968) J. Neurol. Neurosurg. Psychiat. 31, 175.
23. Gregersen, G. and Pilgaard, S. (1971) Acta neurol. scand. 47, 71.
24. Seneviratne, K.N. and Peiris, O.A. (1970) J. Neurol. Neurosurg. Psychiat. 33, 6o9.

25. Kardel, T. and Nielsen, V.K. (1974) Acta neurol. scand. 5o, 513.

26. Nielsen, V.K. and Kardel, T. (1975) J. Neurol. Neurosurg. Psychiat.38, 966.

27. Christensen, N.J. and Ørskov, H. (1969) J. Neurol. Neurosurg. Psychiat. 32, 519.

28. Meilvang, S. (1974) Ugeskr. Læg. 136, 1386.

29. Caruso, G., Labianca, O. and Ferrannini, E. (1973) J. Neurol. Neurosurg. Psychiat. 36, 455.

3o. Nielsen, V. K. and Kardel, T. (1974) Acta physiol. scand. 92, 249.

31. Castaigne, P., Cathala, H.-P., Beaussart-Boulengé, L. and Petrover, M. (1972) J. Neurol. Neurosurg. Psychiat. 35, 631.

32. Sodi, A., Campanella, G., Rizzo, M. and Durval, A. (1967) Minerva Nefrol. 14, 174.

33. Isaacs, H. (1969) S.A. Med. J. 43, 683.

34. Liberson, W.T., Gratzer, M. and Zalis, A.W. (1969) Electroenceph. clin. Neurophysiol. 27, 724.

35. Thiele,B. and Stålberg, E. (1975) J. Neurol. Neurosurg. Psychiat.38, 881.

36. Floyd, M., Ayyar, D.R., Hudgson, P. and Kerr, D.N.S. (1969) Proc. Europ. Dial. Transpl. Ass., 6, 2o3.

37. Nielsen, V.K. (1974) Acta med. scand. 195, 155.

38. Edwards, A.E., Kopple, J.D. and Kornfeld, C.M. (1973) Arch. int. Med. 132, 7o6.

39. Daniel, C.R., Bower, J.D., Pearson, J.E. and Holbert, R.D. (1977) Southern Med. J. 7o, 1311.

4o. Jepsen, R.H., Tenckhoff, H.A. and Honet, J.C. (1967) New Engl. J. Med. 277, 327.

41. Stanley, E., Brown, J.C. and Pryor, J.S. (1977) J. Neurol. Neurosurg. Psychiat. 4o, 39.

42. Kopple, J.D., Kornfeld, C.M. and Edwards, A.E. (1973) Clin Res. 19, 151.

43. Jakobsen, J. (1978) Diabetologica 14, 113.

44. Seneviratne, K.N. and Weerasuriya, A. (1974) J. Neurol. Neurosurg. Psychiat. 37, 5o2.

45. Landon, D.N. and Langley, O.K. (1969) J. Anat. (Lond.) 1o5, 196.

46. Sharma, A.K. and Thomas, P.K. (1974) J. neurol. Sci. 23, 1.

47. Funck-Brentano, J.L., Chaumont, P., Mery, J.Ph., Vantelon, J. and Zingraff-Kok, J. (1964) Proc. Europ. Dial. Transpl. Ass. 1, 23.

48. Tyler, H.R. and Gottlieb, A.A. (1965) Proc. 8th Int. Congr. Neurol. Excerpta Medica, 2, 129.

49. Dobbelstein, H., Altmeyer, B., Edel, H., Gurland, H.J., Müller, R., Picklmaier, H. and Jabour, A. (1968) Med. Klin. 63, 616.

5o. Nielsen, V.K. (197o) Acta neurol. scand. Suppl. 46, 2o7.

51. Nielsen, V.K. (1974) Acta med. scand. 195, 163.

52. Nielsen, V.K. (1974) Acta med. scand. 195, 171.

53. Ibrahim, M.M., Crosland, J.M., Honigsberger, L., Barnes, A.D., Dawson-Edwards, P., Newman, C.E. and Robinson, B.H.B. (1974) Lancet 2, 739.

54. Oh, S.J., Clements, R.S., Lee, Y.W. and Diethelm, A.G. (1977) Electroenceph. clin. Neurophysiol. 43, 592.

55. Bolton, C.F. (1976) Neurology, 26, 152.

56. Barnes, A.D., Dukes, D.C., Robinson, B.H.B. and Blainey, J.D. (1971) Lancet 2, 610.

57. Nielsen, V.K., Ølgaard, K. and Ladefoged, J. (1974) Lancet 2, 1326.

58. Dyck, P.J., Johnson, W.J., Lambert, E.H. and O'Brien, P.C. (1971) Mayo Clin. Proc. 46, 400.

59. Giovannetti, S. and Barsotti, G. (1975) Nephron 14, 123.

60. Bolte, H.D., Riecker, G. and Röhl, D. (1963) 2nd Intern. Congr. Nephrol. 78, 114.

61. Cunningham, J.N., Carter, N.W., Rector, F.C. and Seldin, D.W. (1971) J. clin. Invest. 50, 49.

62. Welt, L.G., Sachs, J.R. and McManus, T.J. (1964) Trans. Ass. Amer. Phycns. 77, 169.

63. Welt, L.G. (1970) Proc. 4th Congr. Nephrol. Karger, Basel, München, New York, vol. 2, p. 263.

64. Cole, C.H. (1973) Clin. Sci. molec. Med. 45, 775.

65. Kramer, H.J., Gospodinov, D. and Krück, F. (1976) Nephron 16, 344.

66. Bittar, E.E. (1967) Nature (Lond.) 214, 310.

67. Bittar, E.E. (1970) Proc. 4th Congr. Nephrol. Karger, Basel, München, New York, vol. 2, p. 267.

68. Bourgoignie, J., Klahr, S. and Bricker, N.S. (1971) J. clin. Invest. 50, 303.

69. Minkoff, L., Gaertner, G., Darab, M., Mercier, C. and Levin, M.L. (1972) J. lab. clin. Med. 80, 71.

70. Edmondson, R.P.S., Hilton, P.J., Jones, N.F., Patrick, J. and Thomas, R.D. (1975) Clin. Sci. molec. Med. 49, 213.

71. Cole, C.H. and Maletz, R. (1975) Clin. Sci. molec. Med. 48, 239.

72. Cole, C.H., Steinberg, R. and Guttmann, R. (1978) Nephron 20, 248.

73. Nielsen, V.K. In prep.

74. Ludin, H.P. (1978) Pers. comm.

Peripheral Neuropathies
N. Canal and G. Pozza, eds.
© 1978 Elsevier/North-Holland Biomedical Press

MOTOR NERVE CONDUCTION VELOCITIES AS AN INDEX OF THE EFFICIENCY OF
MAINTENANCE DIALYSIS IN PATIENTS WITH END-STAGE RENAL FAILURE.
(A long-term follow-up study).

J. CADILHAC, Ch. MION, H. DUDAY, G. DAPRES and M. GEORGESCO
Service d'Explorations Fonctionnelles Neuro-Musculaires, C.H.U.,
Centre Gui de Chauliac, 34000 Montpellier (France)

in collaboration with Dr R. ISSAUTIER (AIDER), Dr Ch. POLITO (STIR)
and Dr P. FLORENCE (C.H.L.) medical directors of different hemodia-
lysis centres of the Montpellier area.

Uraemic neuropathy, first described by Charcot in 1873, was for a
long time regarded a terminal manifestation of chronic renal failure[1,2]. With the advent of maintenance dialysis, this neuropathy
has now been supplemented by EMG studies which have shown, among
other things, marked slowing of motor nerve conduction velocities
(N.C.V.). This phenomenon often precedes clinical signs of neuropathy, corresponds to the severity of renal failure (particularly the
serum creatinine level), and is widely accepted as an indication
for starting dialysis treatment[3-6]. Many also use repeated motor
NCV measurements during dialysis as a guide to adequacy of treatment[7-10].

Nevertheless, the value of single motor NCV studies in end stage
renal failure has been criticised[11], and other neurophysiological
indices have been recommended i.e.: the mean motor NCV of median,
ulnar, peroneal and tibialis posterior nerves[12], measurement of NCV
in the faster and slower nerve fibres[13], sensory NCV[14], latency of
the H reflex[15], and unitary EMG[16].

In summary,despite minor discrepencies, these neurophysiological
studies all produced valuable information about the main characteristics of uraemic neuropathy : functional changes are seen in both
motor and sensory peripheral nerves, in fast and slow fibres, in
the nerve trunk [13] and in its terminals[14]. There are, at the same
time, signs of axonal degeneration (loss of motor units) and of
segmental demyelination (slowing of NCV). A single dialysis session
has minor effects on these changes[12-17], but they are completely
reversible after renal transplant.

Nevertheless the significance of NCV in the follow-up of hemodialised patients is still controversial. Initial studies, especially those of the Seattle group[12], suggested that motor NCV were a very reliable index of the efficiency of maintenance dialysis. During the last ten years however, the dialysis treatment in end-stage renal failure has become available to a greater number of patients ; dialysis is started earlier, and the dialyzers heve become more effective. A reappraisal of the usefulness of NCV measurements seems timely, as many authors have questioned its significance : NCV failed to improve during several months of "adequate" dialysis control of uraemia[18] ; NCV can show enormous daily variations[19] and is an "unreliable tool when major therapeutic decisions are to be taken"[20] ; there is no relationships between impaired neurophysiological parametres and the improving clinical signs of neuropathy[21]. Thus, NCV could not be a reliable means of demonstrating the efficacy of maintenance dialysis[22]. Although these studies appear to cast doubt on the value of NCV as an index of adequate dialysis, most of the data were concerned with patients followed up for relatively short periods of time and in whom NCV was measured in only one or two nerves.

Our experience with serial mean motor NCV measured in four nerves over a much longer time fails to uphold these doubts and supports our previous statement[10].We report here further data on sum of motor NCV monitoring in a larger group of dialysed patients, analyzed by more sophisticated techniques.

MATERIALS AND METHODS

552 out of 800 patients with chronic renal failure were treated by maintenance dialysis and submitted to EMG examinations with motor NCV systematically measured in the median, ulnar, peroneal and tibialis posterior nerves. Only 213 patients (116 males, 87 females) followed-up for more than 3 years (mean : 5,07 $\pm$ 2,06 SD) were retained for this study. Their ages at the time of the first examination ranged from 4 to 71 years (mean age 40,52 $\pm$ 14,02 SD). The delay of survey was more than 5 years in 108 patients and more than 9 years in 25.

Nerve stimulation and EMG recording was carried out using the technique previously described[10].

RESULTS

I - Incidence of signs of neuropathy (table I)

TABLE 1

FREQUENCY OF SIGNS OF NEUROPATHY IN 213 PATIENTS

	Median	Ulnar	Peroneal	Tib. Post.
EMG anomalies[a]	79(37,1)	65(30,5)	172(80,8)	184(86,4)
MCV reduced	71(33,3)	65(30,5)	142(66,7)	153(71,8)
Nerve inexcitable	8(3,8)	0	30(14,1)	31(14,6)
Clinical manifestations in patients with EMG anomalies[b]				
Objective	12(15,2)	5(7,7)	35(20,3)	48(26,1)
Only subjective	20(25,3)	11(16,9)	42(24,5)	41(22,3)
No signs	39(49,3)	40(61,6)	80(46,5)	81(44)
Unknown	8(10,2)	9(13,8)	15(8,7)	14 7,6)

[a] in brackets, percentage of the 213 patients
[b] in brackets, percentage of the number of patients with EMG anomalies

Slowing of motor NCV was demonstrated in the vast majority of patients at one time or another and the lower limbs were more often affected than the upper. In 67 patients (31,4 %) there was a global involvment of the 4 nerves in upper and lower limbs and for each nerve, the distal motor latency increase was statistically less than the reduction in motor NCV.

The manner in wich the slowing of motor NCV presented was inconstant. In two-thirds of the patients (144 cases) slowing was detected at the first examination, before dialysis was begun, but in the remaining third, functionnal abnormalities of peripheral nerves were seen later, during the course of treatment.

Clinical manifestations of neuropathy were not always detectable and, in many cases, EMG signs only were present. Marked clinical evidence of neuropathy, in the form of motor disturbances (amyotrophy, areflexia, paresis) or objective sensory loss, was only seen in cases of very slow NCV or of inexcitable nerves. Subjective sensory symptoms, such as paresthesiae, cramps, burning feet, were more frequently but nevertheless not consistently correlated with reduction of motor NCV. They sometimes diminished or disappeared even when motor NCV remained extremelly slow. Furthermore, simultaneous measures of motor and sensory NCV in the median nerve in 50 patients show no significant difference. On this basis, it seems that motor NCV is a very sensitive test for detecting the presence and the degree of neuropathy.

The distribution of affected nerves is variable. Frequently, when several nerves were involved, their disturbances did not appear at the same time. In the lower limbs, the posterior tibial nerve was generaly involved earlier and more severely than the peroneal. In the upper limbs, involvment of the median and ulnar nerves was sometimes dissociated. Slowing of motor NCV could appear in only one nerve, although motor NCV in the lower limbs remain unchanged. We have carefully documented these rather unexpected findings : the role of the arterio-veinous fistula was, in some cases preeminent.

In order to avoid the dissociated timing of reduce NCV in the various nerves of a given patient, we used the sum of NCV in the upper and lower limbs and, as far as possible, we measured the motor NCV in the upper limb, on the side opposite to the fistula.

II - Time course of motor NCV

The long-term variations of motor NCV in individual produce a chronological pattern of events (time series) similar to these studied in statistical geography[24]. Von Neuman's test was applied to determine whether the fluctuations in the curve were organised or simply random.

$$\delta^2 = \frac{1}{n-1} \sum_{i=1}^{n} (y_{ti+1} - y_{ti})^2$$

$$\sigma^2 = \frac{1}{n-1} \sum_{i=t}^{n} (y_{ti} - \bar{y})^2$$

(σ is the standard deviation of the complète set of values)
If δ^2/σ^2 approaches 2, the fluctuations are random
If δ^2/σ^2 is significantly different from 2, the fluctuations are organised and meaninful.

Owing the large number of similar consecutive values, Spearman's ranking test was not appropriate to analysis trends in the NCV time series. Instead we first adjusted each series by application of the method of moving means[25], so that only fluctuations which

affected successive examinations remained. The significance of
trends in the adjusted curves was then tested by calculating r,
the correlation coefficient between the ranck of NCV and its value
in m/s*.

The different types of response pattern in NCV were identified
from combining the values of r and δ^2/σ^2 (table 2 anf Fig. 1).

TABLE 2

	$\delta^2/\sigma^2 \neq 2$		
	NS	S	HS
r > 0 trend to increase		random	non random
r $\neq$ 0 stable trend	random		non random
r < 0 trend to decrease		random	non random
	fluctuations		

The above statistical tests were applied both to the sum of the
motor NCV's of the two nerves in upper and lower limb and to the
NCV's of the four nerves. In many cases the curve relating to the
sum of NCV's showed major deflections of short duration affecting
nerves of upper and lower limbs alike. These fluctuations although
greater than 2 SD from the mean, reflected periods of transient
deterioration and, on statistical testing, were shown to be random. The data relating to inexcitable nerves will be considered
separately.

The data from 35 patients undergoing maintenance dialysis for more than six years was submitted to the statistical analysis described above.

A) - Transient (random) deteriorations of sufficiently short duration to be "smoothed out" during adjustement of the time series
curve were observed 7 times in only 4 patients. Local lesions due
for example to posture or shunt, could easily be excluded as a

* The results were identical wether rank or timing of the examination were used, since NCV measurements were made at fairly regular
intervals (every 3-5 months)

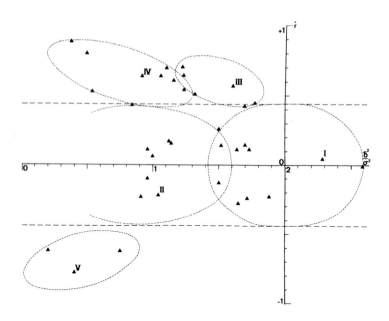

Fig. 1. Distribution of patients in function of Von Neuman's coefficient ($\delta 2/\sigma 2$) and of correlation coefficient (r). Five groups may be identified. The roman figures indicate a representative patient of each category.

cause because they would only affect one nerve. Transient deterioration could result from several factors. Frequently it was seen after a haemodialysis session which may have been inadequate due to poor functioning of the shunt, inappropriate composition of the dialysate or too long an interval between dialysis sessions due to vacation. It could also result from various complications such as infections, hepatitis, or other disorders independent of the primary disease.

Two such transient fluctuations are shown in fig. 3. The first occurred in 1968 as a result of infection during peritoneal dialysis and the second, a year later, as a result of anoxic coma following anaesthesia for the creation of an A-V fistula. The latter event was followed by a total inexcitability of the peroneal nerve which nevertheless recovered rapidly.

B) - <u>Long-term (non random) fluctuations</u>, spanning several months, were seen in 19 patients, and were clearly defined on the adjusted

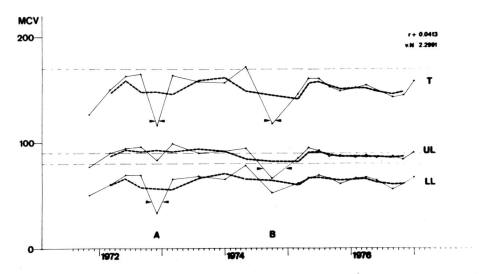

Fig. 2. Time course of motor NCV's in patient I (cf. Fig.1.). Continuous lines : sums of values of NCV in the lower limb (LL), the
upper limb (UL) and the four nerves (T). Haevy broken lines : adjusted values by application of the method of·moving means. Hori-
zontal thin broken lines : inferior normal values of the sum of
NCV (80 m/sec for LL, 90 m/sec for UL, 170 m/sec for T). Between
arrows , transient deflections of short duration (m - 2 σ). r :
correlation coefficient. v.N. : Van Neuman's coefficient for T.
A : too long an interval between dialysis sessions during vacation. B : hepatitis. Trend to stability.

curves. In four patients the fluctuations in NCV recurred in a si-
nusoidal pattern, but in the other patients they were isolated
events. These fluctuations frequently corresponded to other clinical and/or biological signs of deterioration (increased dry weight
or mean monthly serum creatinine level before dialysis). Furthermore, they were always a function of the individual quality of dialysis with sex, weight , residual renal function and nitrogen balance, of the dialysis system it-self (i.e. blood flow, dialysis
time, type of dializer and its own clearence) and finally of the
"unphysiology" of dialysis treatment. On the majority of occasions,
we could link these fluctuations to one or several such factors.
For instance, Fig. 4 shows the deterioration and subsequent recovery resulting from use of the wrong dialysis treatment. A tendancy to slowing of the NCV's is a certain sign inadequate dialysis
while improvement indicates satisfactory treatment once again.

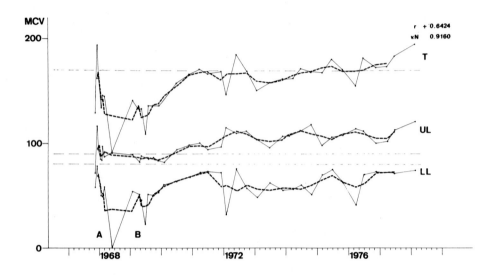

Fig. 3. Time course of motor NCV's in patient IV. Same legend as Fig. 2. A : infection after peritoneal dialysis. B : anoxic coma after anaesthesia. Transient deterioration. Trend to improvement

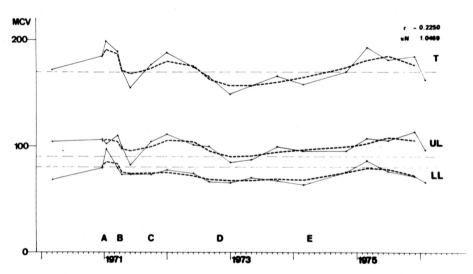

Fig. 4. Time course of motor NCV's in patient II. A : first dialysis. B : 3 x 12 h a week. C : 3 x 12 h a week, by night, at home. D : change of dialyzer . E : reduction of dialysis time to 3 x 9 h a week. Long term fluctuations. Trend to stability.

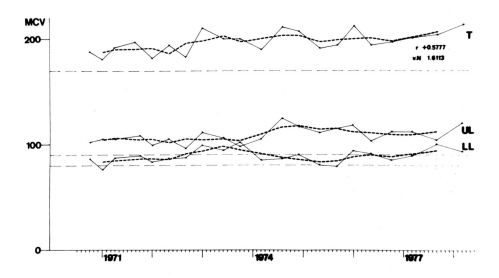

Fig. 5. Time course of motor NCV's in patient III. Long term random fluctuations in the normal values range. Trend to stability.

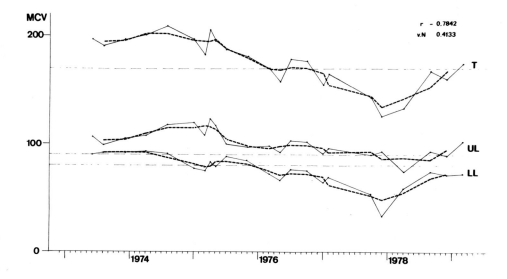

Fig. 6. Time course of motor NCV's in patient V. Trend to deterioration.

C) - Long term trends

- stability of the motor NCV during treatment was noted in 18/35 (51 %) of cases. In 10 patients, the mean motor NCV always remained at the level of normal values (above 45 m/sec in the upper limb. 40 m/sec in the lower limb). In 8 patients, it remains below these limites despite maintenance of good clinical state. We can only speculate that, in the latter cases, the dialysis was suboptimal.

- slow imrovement occured over a period of several years in 14 patients. In 3 cases there was complete recovery of the mean NCV, indicating that adequate dialysis can reverse even established neuropathies (commonly considered as irreversible).

- slow deterioration , on the other hand, was seen in only 3 cases : in two of them, however, recent intensification of the dialysis programme has led to some improvement.

D) - Changes in inexcitable nerves

TABLE 3

INEXCITABLE NERVES (in 213 patients dialysed for more than 3 years)

	No of patients	Peroneal	Tib. Post.
I - only at distal point (conduction block)	8	5	4
transient (< 3 m)		5	2
completed		0	1
unknown		0	1
II -both a distal and proximal point (total inexcitability)	32	25	27
transient (< 3 m)		9	12
slow recovery		5 (6 m-2 y)	5 (2 - 6 y)
no recovery		11 (1 - 9 y)	9 (1 - 8 y)
death		0	1

Table 3 summarises the results from patients with inexcitable nerves. Rarely (3,75 %) there is merely a proximal block to conduction wich is transient (i.e. observed at one examination but absent 1-3 months later). More often (8 %) there is total inexcitability of nerve both at the proximal and distal points. Sometimes such nerves recover promptly inside 3 months. Generally, however, the inexcitability is persistent with a delay of from 1-8 years, but sometimes the nerve may recover after long period of time. In one patient an inexcitable tibialis posterior nerve took 6 years to recover and NCV returned to normal value.

These data, along with those above mentioned, show that uraemic neuropathy may be completely reversed in some patients only with haemodialysis. Thus neuropathy is not a definitive complication of uraemia, but a manifestation whose recovery depends simply on adequate removal of the substance presumed to be toxic to nerves.

SUMMARY AND CONCLUSIONS

Motor nerve conduction velocities (NCV) in the median, ulnar, peroneal and tibialis posterior nerves have been systematically studied at regular intervals in 213 patients with end-stage renal failure treated by maintenance dialysis for more than 3 years.

The incidence of clinical signs of neuropathy and the distribution of affected nerves were variable but the slowing of motor NCV was the most frequent finding.

Transient episods of deterioration in motor NCV were seen which rapidly improved. They always related to extraneous incidents during dialysis treatment. Long term fluctuations on the other hand reflected the quality of dialysis. Slowing of motor NCV calls attention to inadequate treatment and the need to intensify dialysis programme.

Long term trends, in most cases, revealed stable motor NCV's, but in some patients there was a slow improvement occasionally leading to a normalization. Even in severe cases, the excitability of nerves may sometimes reappear.

Repeated measurements of the mean of 4 motors NCV's (or their sum) provides a usefull guide to the conduct of treatment, especially maintenance dialysis at home.

REFERENCES

1. Marin, O.S. and Tyler H.R. (1961) Neurology, 11, 999-1005.
2. Asbury, A.K., Victor, M. and Adamns R.D. (1963), Arch. Neurol., (Chicago), 8, 413-428.
3. Versaci, A.A., OLSEN, K.J., Mc Main, P.B., Nakamoto, S. and Kolf W.J. (1964), Trans. Amer. Soc. Artific. intern. Organs, 10,328-330.

4. Preswich, G. and Jeremy, D. (1964) Lancet, 11, 731-732.

5. Tenckhoff, H., Boen, F.S.T., Jebsen, R.H. and Spiegler, J.H. (1965), J. Amer. Med. Ass., 192, 1121-1124.

6. Williams, I.R., Davidson, A.M., Mawdsley, C. and Robson, J.S. (1973) in New developments in Electromyography and Clinical Neurophysiology, Desmedt, J.E. edit, Karger, Basel, pp. 390-399.

7. Rae, A.I., Rosen, S.N., Silva, H., Pomeroy, X., Bienenetock S. and Shaldon, s. (1963), Proc. Roy. Soc. Med., 56, 24.

8. Funck-Brentano, J.L., Chaumont, P., Mery, J.P., Vantalon, J. and Zingraff-kok, J. (1964), Proc. Europ. Dialysis Transplant Ass., 1, 23-29.

9. Héron, J.R., Konotey-Ahuluf, I.D., Shaloom, S. and Thomas, P.K. (1965), Proc. Europ. Dialysis and Transplant Ass., 2, 138-143.

10. Cadilhac, J., Daprés, G., Fabre, J.L. and Mion, Ch. (1973) in New developments in Electromyography and Clinical Neurophysiology, Desmedt, J.E. edit, Karger, Basel, pp. 372-380.

11. Coomes, E.N., Berlyne, G.M. and Shaw, A.R. (1965), Proc. Europ. Dialysis and Transplant Ass., 2, 133-137.

12. Jebsen, R.H., Tenckoff, H. and Honet, J.C. (1967), New. Engl. J. Med., 277, 327-333.

13. Van Der Most van Spijk, D., Hoogland, R.A. and Dijkstra, S. (1973), in New developments in Electromyography and Clinical Neurophysiology, Desmedt, J.E. edit, Karger, Basel, pp. 381-389.

14. Nielsen, V.K. (1967), Proc. Europ. Dialysis and Transplant Ass., 4, 279-284.

15. Guilheneuc, P. and Ginet, J. (1973) in New developments in Electromyography and Clinical Neurophysiology, Desmedt, J.E. edit, Karger, Basel, pp. 400-403.

16. Sodi, A., Campanella, G., Rizzo, M. and Durval, A. (1967, M.Nerva Nefrol., 14, 174.

17. Stanley, E., Brown, J.C. and Pryor, J.S. (1977), J. of Neurol. Neurosurg. and Psychiat., 40, 39-43.

18. Robson, J.S. (1968) in Symposium some aspects of neurology,Robertson, R.F. eds, pp. 74-84.

19. Tyler, R.H. (1970), Arch. Intern. Med., 126, 781-786.

20. Kominami, N., Tyler, R., Hampers, C.L. and Merrill, J.P. (1971), Arch. Intern. Med., 128, 235-239.

21. Nielsen, V.K. (1974), Acta Med. Scand., 195, 155-162.

22. Cambi, V., Arizi, L., Buzio, C., Rossi, F., Savazzi, G. and Migone, L. (1973), Proc. Europ. Dialysis Transplant. Ass., 10, 342-351.

23. Cadilhac, J., Mion, Ch., Daprés, G., Duday, H. and Jourfiet C. (1974), Rev. E.E.G. Neurophysiol., 4, 381-392.

24. Chadule (Groupe),(1974) Initiation aux méthodes statistiques en géographie, Masson et Cie, eds, Paris, 192 pp.

25. Reichman, W.J. (1964), Use and abuse of statistics, Pelican books, eds.

PERIPHERAL NEUROPATHIES IN DIABETES

Peripheral Neuropathies
N. Canal and G. Pozza, eds.
© 1978 Elsevier/North-Holland Biomedical Press

THE CLINICAL ASPECTS OF DIABETIC PERIPHERAL NEUROPATHY

MAX ELLENBERG, M.D.

Clinicl Professor of Medicine, Mt. Sinai Medical Center, New York, N.Y. U.S.A.

The recognition of diabetic neuropathy dates back almost two centuries.
However, it still remains the least understood and the most inadequately
studied of the degenerative complications of diabetes. This deficiency is
heightened by the fact that it is probably the most common complication of
diabetes with considerable clinical impact. Clinical aspects chiefly have
been exploited, but intensive efforts now are being devoted to the more
basic features.

The vasa vasorum have been shown to be involved in some cases of diabetic
neuropathy (1). The mononeuropathies have been attributed to ischemic
infarction (2). The motor end plate, which has been described previously as
being involved in diabetic neuropathy, now has been shown to be altered in
the early stages of juvenile diabetes (3). An outstanding new finding has
been the demonstration of segmental demyelination of peripheral nerve
fibers (4). Since the myelin sheath is formed by spiral folding of the
Schwann cell surface membrane, the implication is that diabetic neuropathy
may result from interference with the metabolic activity of the Schwann
cell. Thus, there is strong evidence for a metabolic basis for diabetic
neuropathy. An intriguing and as yet unexplained observation is the marked
discrepancy between the severity of the pathologic findings and the relative
paucity of the clinical findings in many instances (5). Differences in
the location of the pathology exist, including the anterior and posterior
horns, posterior root ganglion, peripheral nerves, and occlusion of the
vasa nervorum. All these changes have occurred independently and in
combination.

Recent investigations indicate definite metabolic aberrations as an
underlying factor in nerve affection. These include the dependence of
insulin response on the presence of an intact axon and myelin sheath (6);
the slowing of nerve conduction in the diabetic animal which is accompanied
by a decrease in in vitro incorporation of radioactive precursors into some
of the myelin lipids (7); and the involvement of the sorbitol pathway in
the intermediate metabolism of diabetic neural tissue (8). The last (i.e.,
the polyol pathway) has been studied in the alloxanized animal. Here,

the isolated nerve responds to significant elevations of blood sugar by increased formation of sorbitol and its retention within the nerve fibers, resulting in abnormal nerve function as measured by reduced motor nerve conduction velocity. Most exciting, this impairment is reversible in the experimental animal with lowering of the blood sugar to normal levels (9); this has not as yet been demonstrated in man.

Measurements of motor nerve conduction velocity as well as electromyography and sensory perception in the human have shown abnormalities present at the early onset of diabetes. This has been observed in juvenile diabetics (10), and tends to be more frequent, more consistent, and more marked with diabetes of longer duration. It has been demonstrated that sensory nerve conduction may be impaired at the onset of diabetes and may be the most sensitive index of peripheral neuropathy (11).

In the clinical field, the diversity of observation is even more in evidence, encompassing a polymorphous group of syndromes which range from an acute onset with a short duration and reversibility to an insidious onset which is inexorably progressive and irreversible. The symptoms also exhibit the widest range of manifestations.

One of the major disconcerting features of diabetic neuropathy is the diversity and seemingly contradictory nature of the findings as indicated. How may one reconcile these contradictory observations and hypotheses that obtain in the areas of etiology, pathology, and clinical manifestations? The discrepancies readily become concordant by appreciating that they are not necessarily mutually exclusive but, rather, represent different aspects of the problem, and that each may be correct. The implied conclusion, there-fore, is that diabetic neuropathy is not limited to a single entity but encompasses many different representations of varying etiology, pathology, and symptomatology. We therefore must speak of the diabetic neuropathies rather than diabetic neuropathy; this interpretation would harmonize the many incongruities and inconsistencies (12).

CLASSIFICATION

Many classifications of diabetic neuropathy have been proposed on the basis of the anatomic distribution of the lesions, the type of nerve involve-ment, the degree of associated vascular impairment, degenerative phenomena, etc.; no classification encompasses all aspects. The chief reason is that there are diabetic neuropathies of varying pathology and pathogenesis.

To achieve a sound clinical approach to the understanding of the neuropathic involvement, to aid diagnosis and treatment of the various syndromes, and for purposes of teaching, a working classification has been adopted (13). In this system, the manifestations of diabetic neuropathy are divided into two broad categories , somatic and visceral, and their subdivisions.

    I. Somatic (Peripheral) Neuropathy

        A. Lower extremities
            1. Peripheral neuropathy
            2. Neuropathic arthropathy
            3. Neuropathic ulcer
            4. Diabetic foot
        B. Upper extremities
        C. Asymmetric neuropathies
            1. Mononeuropathies
                a. Truncal
                b. Peripheral
                c. Extra-ocular muscle palsies
            2. Diabetic amyotrophy
        D. Diabetic neuropathic cachexia

   II. Visceral Neuropathy·

        A. Cranial nerves
            1. VII, VIII, XII
            2. Eyes
                a. Pupillary changes
        B. Gastrointestinal tract
            1. Esophageal neuropathy
            2. Gastroparesis diabeticorum
            3. Small bowel
                a. Diabetic enteropathy
                b. Malabsorption syndrome
                c. Pancreatic diarrheas
        C. Genitourinary tract
            1. Neurogenic vesical dysfunction
                a. Incipient neurogenic bladder
            2. Retrograde ejaculation
            3. Diabetic impotence
        D. Autonomic nervous system
            1. Orthostatic hypotension
            2. Anhidrosis
            3. Vasomotor instability

In keeping with the scope and purview of this symposium, the discussion will be limited to the diabetic peripheral neuropathies.

LOWER EXTREMITIES

Peripheral Neuropathy. The most common manifestation of peripheral neuropathy is bilateral, symmetric, predominantly sensory involvement of the lower extremities. There are two outstanding symptoms: pain and paresthesias. The pain may vary from dull or aching to cramplike, burning, lancinating, or crushing, and is usually in a root type of distribution. A distinguishing characteristic is the nocturnal intensification of the pain which is relieved by pacing the floor; this provides an added differentiating factor from peripheral vascular insufficiency. At times the skin is so sensitive that the patient cannot tolerate the touch of pajamas or bedclothes. The paresthesias are described as coldness, numbness, tingling, or burning. Occasionally patients complain that their feet feel dead and they seem to be walking on cotton or air. Another symptom worthy of note is anorexia, which may result in considerable loss of weight despite good diabetic control. Special mention should be made of the commonly present depression and irritability that may be a dominant factor in the clinical picture, a matter of grave concern to both the patient and family. Although this has been considered a reaction commensurate with the severe pain and associated inability to sleep, it is my impression that the depression is far more profound than can be explained on this basis and constitutes a symptom _sui generis_. Occasionally a lessening of the depression presages the clearing of the neuritis. As the neuropathy clears, the depression and anorexia simultaneously disappear (14).

On examination there may be tenderness of the calf muscles, but this is not constant. There is diminution of some of the modalities of sensation, particularly vibratory perception. The sensory findings, however, vary considerably and are unpredictable from patient to patient. The commonly observed disturbance of vibratory perception in the older nondiabetic population makes this finding by itself an unreliable diagnostic criterion.

The most reliable and consistent objective findings are the absence of knee jerks and/or ankle jerks, especially the latter. Furthermore, absence of deep reflexes is pathologic under any circumstances, including old age (15). With this as a background and with increasing experience, it has become evident that the most common cause of unexplained absent deep reflexes, especially ankle jerks, is diabetic neuropathy. Conversely, the unexplained absence of deep reflexes is enough to suggest strongly the diagnosis of diabetes and to make its exclusion mandatory. Thus, the sole finding of absence of ankle jerks may be a diagnostic clue to the presence of diabetes (16).

Neuropathic Arthropathy (Charcot's Joints). Since first reported as a complication of diabetes in 1936 (17) the number of cases of Charcot's joints has been on the increase. One of the outstanding clinical features of this syndrome is its remarkable painlessness. The foot slowly swells without fluid accumulation or signs of infection; it becomes shorter and wider, with a tendency to eversion and external rotation, and the longitudinal arch is completely flattened. The gait becomes abnormal. Eventually the foot may look like a clubfoot. The marked disturbance of normal configuration often leads to painless perforating ulcers at sites of abnormal pressure.

Normal peripheral pulses in the feet are characteristic and significant. The oscillometer readings and the filling time of the subpapillary venous plexus are normal. Thermocouple readings have been normal in patients in whom these were obtained. The toes and plantar surface of the foot are warm and pink.

The classic roentgenographic features are essentially those of bone lysis, with marked fragmentation and eburnation. There is a definite tendency to disarticulation and dissolution of the joints with overgrowth of bone and calcification in and around the involved joints. The small islets of fuzzy bone growing in the synovial membrane are reliable features of a neurogenic arthropathy.

Charcot-like joints occur in the presence of involvement of sensory components, specifically impairment of afferent pain and proprioceptive impulses; intact motor power; exposure of the joint to repeated, minor trauma, such as may occur in walking; and chronicity of the process. Involvement of the sensory component of the nerve and sparing of the motor portion occurs primarily in tabes and diabetes. The clinical picture of the Charcot joint occurs chiefly in tabes dorsalis and diabetes but also in the few, relatively rare conditions in which there may be neural impairment of the sensory fibers with intact motor component, e.g., hereditary sensory-loss syndrome, syringomyelia, leprosy, spinal dysraphia, and idiopathic myelodysplasia. This is a clear indication that neural involvement is an integral part of its pathogenesis.

The incidence of the Charcot joint is about the same in both sexes. It is more common in the fifth and sixth decades and in patients with long-standing diabetes, although it may occur in younger diabetics (e.g., it has been observed in a 22-year old) and in diabetes of recent onset. Infection has been suggested as playing a determining or contributory role, but this is incorrect. The arthropathy is the result of joint disorganization which causes abnormal pressure points, which in turn produce perforating ulcers. These may become infected and result in osteomyelitis, with loss of phalanges. Hence, infection, when present, is secondary to the underlying pathologic condition.

Differential diagnosis. The essential difference between the neuropathic arthropathy of tabes dorsalis and that of diabetes is the joint involved. In tabes, the knee is the most commonly involved joint; the vertebral column, the hip, and even the joints of the upper extremities may be affected. In diabetes, involvement of any but the tarsal and ankle joints is rare, so that arthropathy in these areas is most likely to be of diabetic orgin. Tabes was formerly the usual cause of these painless deformities; now the chief offender is diabetes.

Treatment. Although there is no cure for this condition, in our experience conservative management may halt progress in some cases, and in a few patients actual regression has occurred; some of these patients are able to get about with remarkable agility. Not only has arthrodesis not produced impressive results, but secondary infection and osteomyelitis have frequently followed the procedure. So far, the most satisfactory management has been the limitation of weight bearing by the use of orthopedic appliances (short leg braces, specially built or molded shoes, sponge rubber arch supports, prostheses, and crutches), thereby helping to prevent further deformity. The best results have been reported following the prolonged use of a walking cast (18). This has now become the treatment of choice and in our experience is most satisfactory.

Neuropathic Ulcer. The term neuropathic ulcer is used for a special type of lesion that may occur in a neuropathic foot, whatever the underlying disease--diabetes, tabes, leprosy, hereditary sensory syndrome, syringomyelia, etc. Synonyms include mal perforans, plantar ulcer, trophic ulcer, perforating ulcer, or pressure ulcer.

Plantar ulcer is the result of the stress of walking on a foot that has a reduced nerve supply. Neuropathy is an essential factor leading to the lesion and is characterized by the marked or complete loss of pain and temperature sensation; absent ankle jerks are the rule (19). The neuropathic disturbance results in weakness and atrophy of the intrinsic muscles which produce characteristic deformities. The toes are held dorsiflexed at the metatarsal phalangeal joints, with flexion at the interphalangeal joints; they are drawn into this cocked-up position (claw toes) by simultaneous contraction of the long flexors and extensors, since the normal balancing force of the intrinsic muscles is removed. This uncovers the metatarsal heads, as well as leading to thinning of the normal fat pad. As a result, the anterior arches soon become covered with a thick hard callus. In addition, there may be talipes valgus (splay foot) and hallux valgus. Because of the abnormal alignment, the thrust of the body weight is borne by areas not originally designed by nature to absorb these blows; the

The severity of the pain in some instances has required the use of narcotic drugs with the everpresent threat of addiction. This aspect has been alleviated to a degree with the introduction of diphenylhydantoin (Dilantin) in the treatment of the neuritis pain (25). The drug has proved to be moderately to highly successful in about 80% of the cases in which it has been tried. Although certainly not a panacea or the final answer in treating diabetic neuropathy, it clearly deserves a trial in controlling the painful aspects of this syndrome.

The use of the drug was predicated on the fact that it has been shown to have a direct action on peripheral nerves in addition to its central effect. It is used in the usual analeptic dose of o.1 gm. t.i.d. Although it takes 2-3 days for a demonstrable effect, if there is no response in a week, it is pointless to continue its use, since prolonged administration will be of no avail in such cases. If Dilantin proves ineffective, Carbamezapine (Tegretol) may be used in doses of 200 mg. q.i.d. (26); toxic manifestations are not uncommon.

Several other general measures are indicated. Good control of the diabetes is mandatory since it produces a sense of well-being. Warm baths and gentle massage, best carried out with lanolin, are indicated.

ASYMMETRIC NEUROPATHIES

These are characterized primarily by the predominance of motor involvement, relatively minor or even absent sensory involvement, sudden onset, frequency of severe pain, and a good prognosis.

Mononeuropathy. Mononeuropathy or mononeuropathy multiplex has all the above characteristics and is presumably a result of nerve infarction due to vascular involvement (27). Although the evidence is limited, the clinical picture is compatible with such a pathogenesis. Any nerve may be involved, including those of the eye muscles. Its importance is underscored by its frequent occurrence, mimicry of other syndromes (gall bladder, acute coronary artery disease, acute abdominal involvement, etc.) and frequent misdiagnosis.

Involvement of the cranial nerves (28) and nerves of the extremities (29) by this entity is well documented. More recently, diabetic mononeuropathy affecting the nerves of the trunk has been observed to be a relatively frequent and clinically important occurrence (30).

Of special interest is the recognitionof significant differences between truncal diabetic mononeuropathy and the known recognized forms. In our series there are several facts that stand out many of which indicate differentiating

characteristics between truncal mononeuropathy and the cranial and peripheral
nerve varieties:

....there is equal sex distribution; in the other peripheral neuropathies
there is a male predominance;

....the older age group is primarily affected; however, many of the patients
in our series were juvenile diabetics with long-standing disease;

....most had long duration, as distinguished from mononeuropathy of the
extremities or eye muscles, where not infrequently these may be the initial
clinical manifestation of the diabetes;

....there was virtually no motor involvement, in sharp contrast to the other
forms of diabetic mononeuropathy where motor involvement is not only more
prominent but at times the only abnormality;

....in truncal mononeuropathy the findings are almost entirely limited to
sensory abnormalities in a root distribution. This is best elicited by
stroking with a pin in a vertical direction both up and down, and in this
fashion a nerve distribution of hyperesthesia may be clearly outlined. Light
touch is often helpful, as in pinching the skin or pressure on it. When
there is doubt, electromyographic studies will help to corroborate the
diagnosis;

....the nerve involvement is almost always unilateral and asymmetric;

....there is a good prognosis, with most cases recovering in about three months;

....these clinical syndromes are almost invariably associated with the classic
manifestations of diabetic peripheral neuropathy;

....there is a nocturnal exacerbation of pain that can be helpful in
differential diagnosis.

Truncal mononeuropathy may simulate gall bladder disease, appendicitis,
coronary artery disease, intestinal pathology, pleurisy, and rib-cage
involvement, depending on which nerve is affected. Peripheral mononeuropathy
may affect the upper extremity and in the lower extremity may produce foot drop.

Extra-ocular muscle palsies. A very important aspect of peripheral
mononeuropathy is paralysis of the external ocular muscles. The paralysis is
usually preceded by severe ipsilateral pain which lasts for about 3-7 days
(31), follows the distribution of a branch of the trigeminal nerve, most
commonly the ophthalmic division, and is then followed by the rapid onset of
diplopia. The third, fourth, or sixth cranial nerve may be involved, the
third and sixth being the most commonly affected. Involvement of the third
cranial (occulmotor) nerve characteristically and diagnostically leaves
pupillary function undisturbed. There is a tendency to recurrence at

varying intervals, sometimes of years; such recurrence is not necessarily limited to the same muscle or even to the same side.

The syndrome of unilateral frontal headache and extraocular motor paralysis is suggestive of an aneurysm of the internal carotid artery, but increasing experience with the diabetic has altered this concept. In the absence of other focal neurologic features, the syndrome is most often due to diabetic neuropathy. With increasing recognition of this fact, arteriograms, which tend to produce an unusually high morbidity rate in diabetic patients, should be used less often as a diagnostic aid in this syndrome.

As a rule, the paralysis disappears spontaneously within 6-12 weeks, a fact of some significance in the differential diagnosis of the extraocular palsies, as well as being most encouraging. Of all the diabetic neuropathies, the extraocular palsies clear up the most consistently and most rapidly.

Diabetic amyotrophy. This syndrome was first clearly categorized and described as a progressive weakness and wasting of muscles accompanied by severe pain usually limited to the muscles of the pelvic girdle and thigh, the quadriceps being most commonly affected, little or no sensory involvement, and characteristically asymmetric distribution (32). Other components of the picture include: occasional extensor plantar response; reduced patella tendon reflex; increased total amount of protein in the cerebrospinal fluid; occurrence usually in older men; association with very mild diabetes which frequently does not require the use of insulin; and complete regression, usually in the course of several months. Amyotrophy may be the initial clinical manifestation of diabetes. Its essential difference from other peripheral diabetic neuropathic manifestations lies in its asymmetry, minimum to absent sensory impairment, and involvement of proximal masculature.

Diabetic Neuropathic Cachexia. The clinical picture, which has been observed only in male patients usually in the sixth decade of life, includes: profound weight loss up to 100 pounds and representing up to 60% of the total body weight (the picture of advanced cachexia), severe pain, the presence of bilateral symmetrical peripheral neuropathy, severe depression and anorexia, impotence, diabetes of a very mild nature usually controlled with diet and/or oral agents, simultaneous onset of the neuropathy with the clinical diagnosis of diabetes, and an excellent prognosis with uniformly satisfactory recovery in about one year (33).

One of the more remarkable features of this syndrome is that, in spite of the profound neurologic involvement, there are no accompanying evidences of nicroangiopathy, specifically no retinopathy or nephropathy. Blood pressures were uniformly normal. In addition, blood chemistries, including blood urea nitrogen, cholesterol, triglycerides, uric acid, electrolytes, blood count, bone marrow study, electrocardiogram, stool studies, and intensive x-ray examinations were normal.

Although there is no specific therapy available, all these patients spontaneously improved to the point of complete recovery with restoration of previous weight levels and virtual elimination of neuritis symptoms; occasionally there may be persistence of some paresthesias.

REFERENCES

1. Fagerberg, S.E.: Diabetic neuropathy: A clinical and histological study on the significance of vascular affections. Acta Med Scand. 164:1, 1959

2. Raff, M.D., Sangalang, V., Asbury, A.K.: Ischemic mononeuropathy multiplex associated with diabetes mellitus. Arch Neurol. 18:407, 1968

3. Reske-Nielsen, E., Lundback, K., Rafaelsen, O.J.: Pathological changes in the central and peripheral nervous system of young long-term diabetics. Diabetologia, 1:233, 1965

4. Thomas, P.K., Laescelles, R.G.: Pathology of diabetic neuropathy. Q.J. Med. 35:489, 1966

5. Dolman, C.L.: The morbid anatomy of diabetic neuropathy. Neurology 13:135, 1962

6. Field, R.A.: Altered nerve metabolism in diabetes. Diabetes 15:696, 1966

7. Eliasson, S.G.: Nerve conduction changes in experimental diabetes. J. Clin Invest. 42:2353, 1964

8. Gabbay, K.H., Merola, L.D., Field, R.A.: Sorbitol pathway. Science, 151:209, 1966

9. Gabbay, K.H., O'Sullivan, J.B.: The sorbitol pathway. Diabetes 17:239, 1968

10. Terkildsen, A.B., Christensen, M.J.: Reversible nervous abnormalities in juvenile diabetes with recently diagnosed diabetes. Diabetologia 7:113, 1971

11. Chochinov, R.H., Ullyot, G.L.E., Moorhouse, J.A.: Sensory perception thresholds in diabetic subjects and their close relatives. Diabetes 20 (suppl 1):26, 1971

12. Ellenberg, M.: Present status of diabetic neuropathy. Nord Med 78:921,1967

13. Ellenberg, M.: Diabetic neuropathy, in Ellenberg, M., Rifkin H. (eds): DIABETES MELLITUS: THEORY AND PRACTICE. New York, McGraw-Hill, 1970, ch 39

14. Ellenberg, M.: Diabetic neuropathy, in Dock, W., Snapper, I.(eds): ADVANCES IN INTERNAL MEDICINE, vol 12. Chicago, Year Book Press, 1964, p.11

15. Ellenberg, M.: Deep reflexes in old age. J.A.M.A. 174:468, 1960

16. Ellenberg, M.: Absent deep reflexes: Diagnostic clue in unsuspected diabetes. Am J. Med Sci. 242: 183, 1961

17. Jordan, W.R.: Neuritic manifestations in diabetes mellitus. Arch Intern Med. 57:307, 1936

18. Antes, E.H.: Charcot joint in diabetes mellitus. J.A.M.A. 156:6021, 1954.

19. Ellenberg, M.: Diabetic neuropathic ulcer. J. Mt. Sinai Hosp. 35:585,1968.

20. Kelly, P.J., Coventry, M.B.: Neurotrophic ulcers of the feet. J.A.M.A. 168:388, 1958

21. Coventry, M.B.: Resection of the metatarsal heads to relieve pain and deformity. Proc. Staff Meet. Mayo Clin. 40:240, 1965

22. McCook, J.P., Beauballet, P., Leanes, A., Charles, E.D.: Surgical treatment of the perforating ulcer of the foot. J. Cardiovasc. Surg. 7:101, 1966

23. Ellenberg, M.: Diabetic neuropathy of the upper extremities. J. Mt. Sinai Hosp. 35:134, 1968

24. Ellenberg, M.: Tactile impairment in diabetic neuropathy. (in prep.)

25. Ellenberg, M.: Treatment of diabetic neuropathy with Diphenylhydantoin. N.Y. State J. Med. 68:2653, 1968

26. Rull, J.A., Quibrera, R., Gonzalez-Millan, M., Castaneda, O.L.: Symptomatic treatment of peripheral diabetic neuropathy with Carbamezapine (Tegretol). Diabetologia 5:215, 1969

27. Raff, M.C., Asbury, A.K.: Mononeuropathies in diabetes mellitus. N. Eng. J. Med. 279:17, 1968

28. Zorilla, E., Kozak, G.P.: Ophthalmoplegia in diabetes mellitus. Ann. Int. Med. 67:968, 1967

29. Mulder, D.W.: The neuropathies associated with diabetes mellitus. Neurology 11:275, 1961

30. Ellenberg, M.: Diabetic truncal mononeuropathy - a new clinical syndrome. Diabetes care 1:10, 1978

31. Jackson, W.P.U.: Ocular nerve palsy with severe headache in diabetes. Br. Med. J. 2:408, 1955

32. Garland, H., Taverner, D.: Diabetic amyotrophy. Br. Med. J. 1:1405, 1953

33. Ellenberg, M.: Diabetic neuropathic cachexia. Diabetes 23:5, 1974

Peripheral Neuropathies
N. Canal and G. Pozza, eds.
© 1978 Elsevier/North-Holland Biomedical Press

HUMAN AND EXPERIMENTAL DIABETIC NEUROPATHY

P.K. THOMAS

Department of Neurological Science, Royal Free Hospital, Pond Street, London NW3
2QG, England.

ABSTRACT

The wide range of the clinical manifestations displayed by diabetic neuropathy
suggests that its causation is multifactorial. Clinically a subdivision may be
made into symmetrical polyneuropathies, and mononeuropathies or multiple mononeuropathies. A metabolic basis seems the likely explanation for the former but
its nature remains obscure. Osmotic damage secondary to sorbitol accumulation
has been suggested but has not been substantiated and it is not known what role
abnormalities of lipid metabolism may play. Vascular features are probably
unlikely to be important in the origin of symmetrical polyneuropathies but may be
involved in the causation of localized lesions, as may the so far unexplained
heightened vulnerability to pressure.

The cause of the reduced nerve conduction velocity in experimentally induced
diabetes remains in dispute. Structural changes may develop after prolonged
diabetes but have been disputed in the early stages. Electrophysiological
observations have suggested that this may depend upon alterations in the electrical properties of myelin but require substantiation. There is a reduced myoinositol content in diabetic peripheral nerve, but claims that dietary supplemen-
tation with myoinositol correct the reduced nerve conduction velocity have not
be validated. The neuropathy that may develop in genetic diabetes in animals
offers an additional experimental model.

INTRODUCTION

This contribution seeks to review the causation of diabetic neuropathy and
to assess how far experimental models have illuminated present knowledge concerning diabetic neuropathy in man.

Diabetic neuropathy in man

The wide variation in the types of peripheral nerve disturbance related to
diabetes mellitus suggests that their causation is multifactorial. Although
there have been suggestions that no useful classification is possible, a broad
subdivision into two general categories (see Table 1) is clinically helpful.
Mixed cases are admittedly frequent.

TABLE 1

CLASSIFICATION OF DIABETIC NEUROPATHY

Symmetrical polyneuropathy

    Sensory polyneuropathy

    Autonomic neuropathy

    Acute motor polyneuropathy

Mononeuropathy and multiple mononeuropathy

    Cranial nerve palsies

    Isolated nerve lesions of limbs and trunk

    Diabetic amyotrophy

The first category consists of symmetrical polyneuropathies with predominantly sensory or autonomic manifestations. The justification for including diabetic autonomic neuropathy in this category lies in the symmetry of involvement, manifested most clearly in the patterns of sensory loss.[1] Subdivision is probably possible within the category of sensory polyneuropathy. Brown et al.[2] in a survey of 40 cases found that they ranged continuously between two polar types. At one end of the spectrum were cases with painless distal sensory loss primarily involving vibration and position sense together with loss of tendon reflexes. This is the more familiar variety. At the other end were cases with severe burning pain, cutaneous hyperaesthesia, autonomic dysfunction, and relative preservation of the tendon reflexes and of sensory modalities mediated by large fibres. Cases of this type were found to display a predominant loss of unmyelinated and small myelinated fibres in sural nerve biopsies. Teased fibre preparations revealed little evidence of segmental demyelination and it was concluded that this was primarily an axonal disorder. In the former type, pathological studies have demonstrated a combination of axonal loss and segmental demyelination.[3,4]

A further type of sensory disturbance has so far not been studied in any detail. Occasional newly-diagnosed diabetics complain of troublesome tingling and burning paraesthesiae that promptly clear with the institution of diabetic control. The rapidity of this suggests that recovery is unlikely to have been related to axonal regeneration, or remyelination after segmental demyelination. Nerve biopsy studies have not yet been documented in this situation.

The second general category of diabetic neuropathy (Table 1) is that of mononeuropathies and multiple mononeuropathies, seen for example in isolated cranial nerve palsies or isolated peripheral nerve lesions in the trunk or limbs. The asymmetrical and often patchy nature of 'diabetic amyotrophy' indicates that it should be included in this category.

Numerous reports have indicated that many diabetics without symptoms of neuropathy have reduced conduction velocity. Presumably this partly reflects structural changes of the type that occur in overt neuropathy but of insufficient severity to give rise to symptoms or detectable signs. Another possible contributory factor has also to be considered. It is known that nerve conduction velocity tends to be reduced in newly diagnosed diabetics.[5,6] This may recover rapidly with treatment of the diabetic state, the time course suggesting that this is related to some process other than axonal regeneration, or remyelination after segmental demyelination, and which could be of a metabolic nature. It is of interest that Buchthal[7] could not explain the slowing of nerve conduction completely in diabetic neuropathy in terms of the structural alterations found in nerve biopsies.

The central question in diabetic neuropathy is that of causation. As suggested above, this is likely to involve multiple factors. It seems probable that the generalized polyneuropathies are of metabolic origin. The fact that they affect certain classes of neuron in the peripheral nervous system perhaps suggests parallels with system degenerations in the central nervous system related to metabolic differences between particular sets of neurons. The nature of the metabolic insult that gives rise to diabetic neuropathy remains elusive.

An attractive hypothesis was that related to sorbitol accummulation which is known to occur in diabetic nerve.[8,9] It has been generally accepted that the accummulation of sorbitol in the lens of the eye gives rise to cataracts through osmotic effects. It was therefore suggested that a similar process in peripheral nerve caused neuropathy. Alloxan-diabetic nerve was shown by Stewart et al.[8] to have an increased water content and this has recently been confirmed for strepto-zotocin-induced diabetes by Jakobsen.[41] Yet extensive ultrastructural studies on human and experimental diabetic nerve have failed to reveal any appearances that might indicate osmotic damage.[11] The situation with regard to cataract formation may also be more complicated than has been thought. Hutton et al.[12] have shown that cataract formation in streptozotocin-induced diabetes in rats can be reduced by as much as 85 per cent when administered dietary unsaturated fatty acid supplements, despite the fact that the concentration of sorbitol in the lens remains high. It seems therefore that dietary lipids can modify the long-term metabolic effects of diabetes. Fatty acid synthesis is known to be impaired in diabetic nerve,[13] but how far this might be related to the origin of diabetic neuropathy is uncertain.

It is now generally agreed that microangiopathy is not the explanation for
the whole spectrum of diabetic neuropathy, but it is a prominent feature in
cases of severe limb ischaemia with accompanying neuropathy. The accumulation
of PAS positive material around small vessels is seen on electron microscopy to
consist of multiple layers of reduplicated basal lamina. Such changes may be
important in the pathogenesis of isolated nerve lesions of sudden onset, such as
those of the third cranial nerve,[14] but how far 'diabetic amyotrophy' is due to
metabolic and how far to vascular factors is still uncertain. Timperley et al.[15]
have recently suggested that occlusion of the vasa nervorum by fibrin plugs may
be involved in the genesis of peripheral nerve damage.

The increased vulnerability of diabetic nerve to compression injury remains
unexplained. The studies of Gilliatt[16] and Ochoa[17] have illuminated the pathogenesis of tourniquet paralysis and entrapment neuropathy. Comparable studies on
diabetic nerve will be of interest, as will be the effect of any changes in endoneurial pressure consequent upon the increased water content of diabetic nerve.

Experimental diabetic neuropathy

Observations by Eliasson[18] and later workers on alloxan-induced diabetes, and
ourselves[19] and others on streptozotocin-induced diabetes, have repeatedly established that conduction velocity is reduced in diabetic animals. As yet, unanimity
has not been reached as to the explanation of this reduction. Apart from some
early observations to the contrary, it is now agreed that it is not associated
with paranodal or segmental demyelination. Sharma and Thomas[19] found that it was
unassociated with any reduction in nerve fibre diameter, whereas Jakobsen and
Lundbaek[20] reported that it was related to a reduction in fibre diameter, axon
diameter being affected to a greater extent than myelin thickness.[10] Later observations by Sharma et al.[21] confirmed that nerve fibre diameter was less in
diabetic animals than in age-matched controls. However, one of the problems in
working with rats is that they continue to grow until approximately 9 months of
age, this affecting both nerve conduction velocity[19] and fibre diameter. The
use of age-matched controls may therefore give fallacious results if the experimental procedure, such as the induction of diabetes, retards the growth of the
animal. For this reason, Sharma et al.[21] employed serial observations on the
same animals, before and after the induction of diabetes. Biopsies were taken
from the tibial nerve on one side before induction of diabetes and then on the
contralateral side after an interval of five weeks. For the diabetic animals,
the values both for maximal and average fibre diameter had increased slightly
although the difference was not statistically significant. For non-diabetic
control animals, maximal fibre diameter had increased significantly, the increase

in average diameter being non-significant over this interval. It was therefore concluded that the induction of diabetes does not reduce fibre diameter, but may produce a difference between diabetic and control animals because of retardation of nerve fibre growth in the former. From this it follows that the reduction in conduction velocity, which can be demonstrated by serial observations in the same animal, does not depend upon a reduction in nerve fibre diameter.

The explanation of the reduced nerve conduction velocity in experimental diabetes therefore remains to be established. The single fibre studies by Eliasson[18] suggested an abnormality in the myelin, because of 'leakiness' of the myelin sheaths, although an abnormality in the electrical properties of the nodes was not excluded. A conceivable mechanism for the increased electrical conductance of the myelin sheaths might be an opening-up of the Schmidt-Lanterman incisures. Hall and Williams[22] showed that these cytoplasmic clefts through the myelin sheath are labile and that they may open and close. If sorbitol accumulated in the Schwann cell cytoplasm - and there is some evidence that the sorbitol pathway in nerves is associated with Schwann cells[23] - this might lead to an overhydration of these cells and an opening of the Schmidt-Lanterman incisures. This possibility seems unlikely since Jakobsen[41] has shown that the amount of Schwann cell cytoplasm is not increased in diabetic animals. A further possibility might be an alteration in the protein particles that span the myelin lamellae and which could provide ion channels through the lamellae. Observations on myelin in diabetic nerve by freeze-fracture techniques will therefore be of interest. The nodes of Ranvier appear to be ultrastructurally normal on qualitative assessment.[19] Further observations on the electrical properties of the nodes using potential clamp techniques are required.

Another interesting speculation relates to the possible influence of myoinositol on nerve conduction. This substance is a precursor of the polyphosphoinositides which are present in plasma membranes, including those of neurons. They show a rapid turnover rate in nerve trunks and this led to the suggestion that they may be involved in nerve transmission.[24] Bi- and triphosphoinositides are present and both exhibit Ca^{2+} ion binding properties. It has been postulated that by interconversions between the different inositol lipids, the quantity of Ca^{2+} ions bound at specific sites on the plasma membranes might be altered and this might be involved in the generation and propagation of action potentials by controlling the opening and closure of axolemmal ion channels.

Myoinositol concentration is known to be reduced in diabetic nerve. Greene et al.[25] made the observation that the addition of 1 per cent myoinositol to the diet of rats with streptozotocin-induced diabetes prevented the reduction in nerve conduction velocity. Unfortunately, Jefferys et al.[26] were unable to confirm this finding.

An interesting feature of human and experimental diabetic neuropathy that is shared with a number of other neuropathies, such as that related to uraemia,[27] is an increased tolerance to ischaemia.[28] Conduction failure in diabetic nerve is substantially delayed during ischaemia.[29,30] The explanation for the conduction block is generally considered to be due to the accumulation of potassium ions around the nodal axolemma, leading to a reduced axolemmal resting potential. If periaxonal diffusion barriers were reduced in diabetes, the K^+ ions might diffuse away more readily and conduction failure would be delayed. Seneviratne et al.[31] claimed that the nodal gap substance was reduced in diabetic nerve. This substance is a polyanionic material surrounding the node and lying between the Schwann cell nodal processes. It exhibits strong cation-binding capacities. However, Sharma and Thomas[19] found that there were no differences in the appearances between diabetic and control nerve. The suggestion by Jakobsen[41] that over-hydration of the endoneurial space in diabetic nerve might be responsible is an interesting possibility. The peripheral nerves of galactose-fed rats also have an increased endoneurial water content,[32,33] and it will be of interest to establish whether they also display an increased tolerance to ischaemia.

Most of the observations on experimental diabetes have been made over a relatively short period of time. Our own[19] on the tibial nerve of the rat were made over a period of one year. Powell et al.[34] have recently reported that prominent morphological changes develop in the sciatic nerve of alloxan-diabetic rats after two years, and this may provide a useful experimental model for the study of morphological changes induced by diabetes. A note of caution has to be introduced, however, as Sharma[35] has recently found that striking morphological changes appear in the plantar nerves of normal rats with aging. At 15 months of age, no less than 40 per cent of the fibres exhibit evidence of demyelination, with a smaller number of fibres showing axonal degeneration. Any comparison with diabetic animals must therefore involve careful quantitative study.

A useful model is the mutant diabetic mouse db/db. Sima and Robertson[36] have recently reported that nerve conduction velocity is reduced and that this is associated with a reduction in nerve fibre size. It has not yet been established whether this reflects an atrophy of previously normal fibres or a retardation in normal growth. These mice show normal growth in limb length and become obese.

It would therefore be of considerable interest if there were a selective effect on axonal growth. Studies on the slow axonal transport system will therefore be important. Schmidt et al.[37] have found that there is probably a reduction in slow axoplasmic transport in the sciatic nerve of streptozotocin-induced diabetic rats.

Schlaepfer et al.[38] have reported morphological abnormalities in the spontaneously diabetic Chinese hamster, and this model requires more detailed studies. Preliminary observations by ourselves[39] have failed to detect the segmental demyelination described by these authors. We are therefore still lacking a satisfactory animal model for human diabetic neuropathy with comparable structural changes in the nerve fibres. The vascular changes with basal laminal thickening have also not been reproduced.[40] The animal models therefore may be more equivalent to the changes in newly diagnosed human cases.

ACKNOWLEDGEMENTS

Financial support from the Medical Research Council and National Fund for Research into Crippling Disease is gratefully acknowledged.

REFERENCES

1. Berge, K.G., Sprague, R.G. and Bennett, W.A. (1956) Diabetes, 5, 289.

2. Brown, M.J., Martin, J.R. and Asbury, A.K. (1976) Arch. Neurol. 33, 164.

3. Thomas, P.K. and Lascelles, R.G. (1966) Q. J. Med., 35, 489.

4. Chopra, J.S., Hurwitz, L.J. and Montgomery, D.A.D. (1969) Brain, 92, 391.

5. Gregersen, G. (1967) Neurology, 17, 972.

6. Ward, J.D., Barnes, C.G., Fisher, D.J., Jessop, J.D. and Baker, R.W.R. (1971) Lancet, i, 428.

7. Buchthal, F. (1978) This Symposium.

8. Stewart, M.A., Sherman, W.R. and Anthony, S. (1966) Biochem. Biophys. Res. Comm., 22, 488.

9. Gabbay, K.H., Merola, L.O. and Field, R.A. (1966) Science, 151, 209.

10. Jakobsen, J. (1976) Diabetologia, 12, 539 and 547.

11. Thomas, P.K. and Eliasson, S.G. (1975) in Peripheral Neuropathy, Dyck, P.J., Thomas, P.K. and Lambert, E.H. eds., Saunders, Philadelphia, 956.

12. Hutton, J.D, Schofield, P.J., Williams, J.F., Regtop, H.L. and Hollows, F.C. (1976) Br. J. Nutr., 36, 161.

13. Field, R.A. and Adams, L.C. (1964) Medicine (Baltimore), 43, 275.

14. Asbury, A.K., Aldredge, H., Hershberg, R. and Fisher, C.M. (1970) Brain, 93, 555.

15. Timperley, W.R. et al. (1975) Cited by Thomas, P.K. and Ward, J.D. in Complications of Diabetes, Keen, H., and Jarrett, J. Eds., 281. Edward Arnold, London, 1975.

16. Gilliatt, R.W. (1978) This Symposium.

17. Ochoa, J. (1978) This Symposium.

18. Eliasson, S.G. (1964) J. Clin. Invest., 43, 2353.

19. Sharma, A.K. and Thomas, P.K. (1974) J. Neurol. Sci., 23, 1.

20. Jakobsen, J. and Lundbaek, K. (1976) Br. Med. J., 2, 278.

21. Sharma, A.K., Thomas, P.K. and De Molina, A.F. (1977) Diabetes, 26, 689.

22. Hall, S.M. and Williams, P.L. (1970) J. Cell Sci., 6, 767.

23. Stewart, M.A., Passoneau, J.V. and Lowry, O.H. (1965) J. Neurochem., 12, 719.

24. Kai, M. and Hawthorne, J.N. (1969) Ann. N.Y. Acad. Sci., 165, 761.

25. Greene, D.A., De Jesus, P.V. and Winegrad, A.I. (1975) J. Clin. Invest., 55, 1326.

26. Jefferys, J.G., Palmano, K.P., Sharma, A.K. and Thomas, P.K. (1978) J. Neurol. Neurosurg. Psychiat., 41, 333.

27. Nielsen, V.K. (1978) This Symposium.

28. Steiness, I.B. (1959) Acta Med. Scand., 163, 195.

29. Seneviratne, K.N. and Peiris, O.A. (1968) J. Neurol. Neurosurg. Psychiat., 31, 348.

30. Seneviratne, K.N. and Peiris, O.A. (1969) J. Neurol. Neurosurg. Psychiat., 32, 462.

31. Seneviratne, K.N., Peiris, O.A. and Weerasuriya, A. (1972) J. Neurol. Neurosurg. Psychiat., 35, 149.

32. Gabbay, K.H. and Snider, J.J. (1972) Diabetes, 21, 295.

33. Sharma, A.K., Thomas, P.K. and Baker, R.W.R. (1976) J. Neurol. Neurosurg. Psychiat., 39, 794.

34. Powell, H., Knox, D., Lee, S., Charters, A.C., Orlott, M., Garrett, R. and Lampert, P. (1977) Neurology (Minneap.), 27, 60.

35. Sharma, A.K. (1978) Unpublished observations.

36. Sima, A.A.F. and Robertson, D.M. (1978) Acta Neuropath., 41, 85.

37. Schmidt, R.E., Matschinsky, F.M., Godfrey, D.A., Williams, A.D. and McDougal D.B. Jr. (1975) Diabetes, 24, 1081.

38. Schlaepfer, W.W., Gerritson, G.C. and Dulin, W.E. (1974) Diabetologia, 10, 541.

39. Grover-Johnson, N., Sharma, A.K. and Thomas, P.K. (1978) Unpublished observations.

40. Sharma, A.K. (1974) Ph.D. thesis, University of London.

41. Jakobsen, J. (1978) Diabetologia, 14, 113.

Peripheral Neuropathies
N. Canal and G. Pozza, eds.
© 1978 Elsevier/North-Holland Biomedical Press

THE RELATIONSHIP BETWEEN PERIPHERAL AND AUTONOMIC NEUROPATHY IN
INSULIN DEPENDENT DIABETES: A CLINICAL AND INSTRUMENTAL EVALUATION

N. CANAL[o], G. COMI[o], V. SAIBENE[oo], B. MUSCH[o], and G. POZZA[oo]
[o] Clinic of Nervous Diseases
[oo] Institute of Medical Pathology
University of Milan Medical School, Milan, Italy

Although autonomic neuropathy has been long recognized as a
complication of diabetes mellitus, it is far to be thoroughly investigated especially as far as its relation with peripheral neuropathy is concerned.

Literature on this problem is lacking of studies attempting to
evaluate the incidence of autonomic neuropathy in a diabetic population, both in terms of objective testing and of clinical features. Studies available so far had been planned in order to investigate the appearance of autonomic neuropathy in diabetics with
presenting signs and symptoms of peripheral neuropathy, or viceversa[1,2,3] ; in most of these studies the patients were unselected
as far as the type of diabetes is concerned. Moreover poor attention was drawn on other concomitant disorders (such as liver and
renal failure, ketoacidosis), able to alter both peripheral and
autonomic function.

We intended to approach the problem from a different point of
view, investigating in 105 consecutive insulin-dependent diabetics
attending at our metabolic unit evidence of autonomic and/or peripheral nerve involvement, irrespectively to the existence of
symptoms and signs. The admission criteria were: patients suffering from insulin-dependent diabetes, age below 55 years, no liver
or renal involvement, no hypertension or ischaemic heart disease.
No patients were admitted to our metabolic unit for ketoacidotic
coma.

PATIENTS AND METHODS
105 patients have been admitted to the study (65 males and 40
females); age ranged from 15 to 55 years (mean age 30.1). In 80

patients age ranged from 15 to 35 and in 25 from 35 to 55 years.
The mean duration of diabetes was 7.7 years, with a range from 1
week to 30 years.

25 patients had diabetes of less than 1 year duration, 23 between 1 and 5 years, whereas 57 were diabetics since 5 years or
more.

In order to evaluate autonomic cardiovascular function, Valsalva manoeuvre, handgrip-test and postural hypotension test were performed. All the tests were performed fasting in the morning and no
insulin administration was allowed in the 15 hours previous the
tests. Physical examination, EKG and chest X-ray were carried out
in order to exclude cardio-pulmonary diseases. Drugs acting on the
autonomic nervous function were not allowed. The response to the
Valsalva manoeuvre was expressed as Valsalva Ratio: values of 1.10
or less were considered as abnormal.

The postural hypotension test was defined as abnormal when a
fall in systolic blood pressure of 20 mmHg or more, 5 minutes after standing up from the supine position in standard condition,
was recorded.

The sustained handgrip-test was performed according to Ewing
et al. [4]. The absence of an increase in diastolic blood pressure
was considered as abnormal.

Normal ranges of instrumental tests were obtained from a group
of 50 healthy volunteers matched for sex and age.

The clinical features of autonomic dysfunction (symptoms of
postural hypotension, intermittent nocturnal diarrhoea,gustatory
sweating, altered sweating in the legs)-and of peripheral neuropathy (paresthesias, sensory disturbance and motor weakness) were
recorded and evaluated. At the time of the electrophysiological
study a neurological examination was performed.

Sensory conduction along the sural nerve (lateral malleolus to
140 mm proximal to it) and the median nerve (digit 11 to wrist),
mixed conduction along the median nerve (wrist-elbow) and motor
conduction (knee-ankle) of deep peroneal nerve were determined.
For stimulation and registration surface electrodes were employed.

Electromyography was performed in extensor digitorum brevis and
tibialis anterior muscles. Tests were carried out in a room at

constant temperature (24° - 26°C).

Fifty healthy volunteers, matched for sex and age, formed the control group. The significance of the results was assessed by standard statistical analysis.

RESULTS

Clinical evidence of peripheral neuropathy (Fig. 1) has been

Muscle wasting	13%	
Muscle weekness	21%	
Sensory involvment	36%	} 45%
Diminished or absent deep tendon reflexes	43%	

Fig. 1. Signs of peripheral neuropathy in 96 insulin-dependent diabetics.

observed in 45% of our patients. Impairement of deep tendon reflexes was the sign of peripheral neuropathy most frequently encountered. It has to be pointed out that we have never observed mononeuropathy or proximal amyotrophy: this was expected however as the latter are late complications of diabetes. A high percentage of patients had one or more abnormalities of the electrophysiological tests. (Fig. 2). If the tests employed are examined in details it has to be noticed that abnormalities in the lower limbs are more frequent, nevertheless the evidence of nerve function impairement was frequent in the upper limbs as well.

Needle EMG	33.8%	
Median Nerve DSL	28.0%	
Median Nerve MxCV	33.3%	} 63.5%
Peroneal Nerve MCV	39.6%	
Sural Nerve SCV	42.7%	

Fig. 2. Electrophysiological abnormalities in 96 insulin-dependent diabetics

Needle EMG showed signs of denervation in a high percentage of patients. Symptoms of peripheral neuropathy (Fig. 3) were present in 35% of cases, while signs in 45%.

Comparison between these data and the results obtained from e-lectrophysiological tests leads to the conclusion that 18% of our patients were suffering from sub-clinical neuropathy. The inci-dence of peripheral neuropathy increases together with the dura-tion of diabetes (Fig. 4).

It is noteworthy that signs of peripheral neuropathy were pre-sent in 41.8% of patients with diabetes of 1 year or less dura-tion. A remarkable percentage (50%) of these early neuropathies were assessable only by means of instrumental tests (sub-clinical neuropathies).

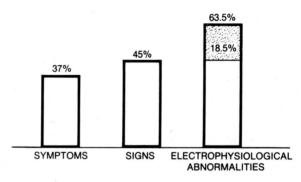

Fig. 3. Diagnostic steps of peripheral neuropathy in insulin-de-pendent diabetics.

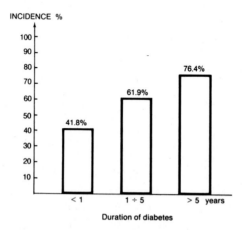

Fig. 4. Incidence of instrumental signs of peripheral neuropathy as a function of duration of diabetes.

In longer standing diabetes a progressive increase in percentage of clinical neuropathies was observed (Fig. 5)

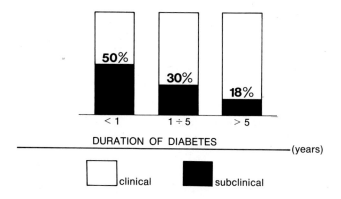

Fig. 5. Percentage of patients with sub-clinical peripheral neuropathy according to duration of diabetes.

Tests for cardiovascular autonomic function were altered in
46.5% (Fig. 6).Valsalva manoeuvre appeared to be the most frequently altered test (36.3%) whereas postural hypotension (19.3%)
and abnormal handgrip-test (3.6%) were less frequently observed.

VALSALVA MANOEUVRE   36.3%
POSTURAL HYPOTENSION   19.3%   **46.5%**
HANDGRIP-TEST   3.6%

Fig. 6. Incidence of abnormal tests of cardiovascular autonomic
function in insulin-dependent diabetics.

A direct, statistically significant correlation (Fig. 7) was
also noticed between the severity of the electrophysiological aspects of the peripheral neuropathy (assessed according to a conventional score [5]) and the duration of diabetes. Symptoms of autonomic involvement are rare in the first year of the disease, and
their incidence tends to increase in parallel with the duration
of diabetes (Fig. 8), whereas instrumental tests for autonomic
cardiovascular function were abnormal in a high percentage of patients (52.4%) already in diabetes of less than 1 year duration.

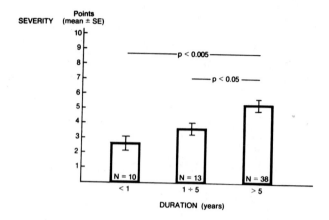

Fig. 7. Grading of electrophysiological abnormalities according to duration of diabetes.

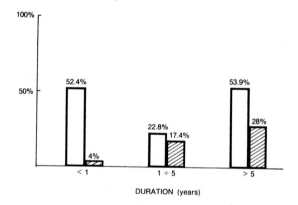

Fig. 8. Abnormal tests for autonomic cardiovascular function (white columns) and symptoms of autonomic dysfunction (barred columns) as a function of duration of diabetes.

These data suggest the existence in this time interval of a sub-clinical autonomic neuropathy. 85 patients were tested for both autonomic and peripheral involvement: the correlation between these two entities (Fig. 9) is statistically significant ($p < 0.05$).

The patients having positive tests for autonomic neuropathy have a somewhat more severe peripheral involvement than the patients without evidence of autonomic involvement (Fig. 10). The two groups considered are not biased by a different duration of diabetes as the difference observed is not statistically significant.

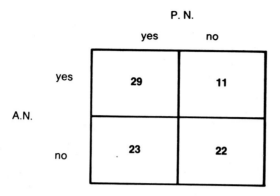

$$\chi^2 = 4.036 \qquad 0.02 < P < 0.05$$

Fig. 9. Patients with instrumental findings of autonomic and peripheral neuropathy.

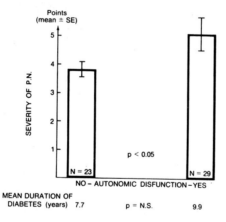

Fig. 10. Relationship between severity of peripheral neuropathy and autonomic dysfunction.

DISCUSSION

Peripheral and autonomic diabetic neuropathy have been extensively investigated [6,7,8] both from the clinical and instrumental point of view; nevertheless in the literature few reports are available concerning the relationship between these two entities [1,2,3].

Studies carried out so far in order to investigate the appearance
of peripheral neuropathy in patients with evidence of autonomic
neuropathy and viceversa have proved an association between these
two entities [2,3].

Nevertheless this approach leaves many problems unresolved such
as the trend of this association in relation to the duration of
diabetes: some of the Authors consider the autonomic neuropathy
as a late and uncommon complication of diabetes [9], claiming that
its appearance is correlated with a high mortality risk [10]. A
more accurate epidemiological approach to the study of autonomic
and peripheral involvement in diabetes is needed in order to exclude factors, not related to the metabolic disorder, which can
alter the results.

Consequently we studied patients with a mean age of 30.1 years,
half of them suffering from diabetes for less than 5 years. This
criteria enabled us to evaluate the incidence of peripheral and
autonomic involvement even in the early stages of diabetes. We
observed a remarkably high incidence of both peripheral and autonomic dysfunction already in patients with a less than 1 year history of diabetes.

This involvement was represented by alterations in the instrumental tests in patients without presenting symptoms and signs of
neuropathy. In the later stages of diabetes the incidence of
nerve dysfunction (both peripheral and autonomic) together with
the evidence of clinical features of neuropathy, was higher. This
observation leads to the hypothesis that at the beginning the
nerve disorder could be only functional as suggested by Ward et
al. [11].

Abnormal tests for cardiovascular autonomic function have been
observed in some patients without evidence of peripheral nerve involvement (regardless the duration of diabetes); on the other
hand in patients with concomitant evidence of autonomic and peripheral involvement, the latter was more severe.

These results and a statistically weak association between the
two entities are suggestive of pathogenetic pathways only partially common.

A more accurate definition of these correlations can be reached
only with a follow-up study of our patients.

In juvenile-onset insulin-dependent diabetes the observation of such a high incidence of autonomic cardiovascular dysfunction cannot be suggestive of a high mortality risk, as reported in long standing diabetes with clinical features of autonomic neuropathy [10].

Nevertheless the observation of an autonomic dysfunction deserves particular caution in situation such as the administration of drugs acting on autonomic nervous system and general anaesthesia.

REFERENCES

1. Martin M.M. (1953) Lancet 1, 560-565
2. Bishnu S.K., Berenyi M.R. (1971) J. Amer. Geriatr. Soc. 19, 159-166
3. Ewing D.J., Burt A.A., Williams I.R., Campbell I.W. Clarke B.F. (1976) J. Neurol. Neurosurg. Psychiat. 39, 453-460
4. Ewing D.J., Irving J.B., Kerr F., Wildsmith J.A.W., Clarke B.F. (1974) Sci. molec. Med. 46, 295-306
5. Lamontagne A., Buchthal F. (1970) J. Neurol. Neurosurg. Psychiat. 33, 442-452
6. Pirart J. (1965) Diabetes 14, 1
7. Thomas P.K., Ward J.D. (1975) Diabetic neuropathy in peripheral neuropathy - Vol. II, pp 151-177, Eds. Dyck, Thomas, Lambert W.B. Saunders CO.Philadelphia,London, Toronto
8. Ellenberg M. (1976) Metabolism 25, 1627-1655
9. Campbell I.W., Ewing O.I.,Harrower A.B.D., Neilson J.M.N., Fraser D.M., Baldwa V.S., Murray A., Clarke B.F. (1976) Lancet 2, 167-169
10. Ewing D.J., Campbell I.W., Clarke B.F. (1976) Lancet 1, 601-603
11. Ward J.D., Barnes C.G., Fisher D.J., Jessop J.D., Baker R.W.R. (1971) Lancet 1, 428-430

Peripheral Neuropathies
N. Canal and G. Pozza, eds.
© 1978 Elsevier/North-Holland Biomedical Press

DIABETIC PROXIMAL AMYOTROPHY

S. CHOKROVERTY, MBBS, MRCP

From the Neurology Service and the Neurology Research Laboratory, Veterans
Administration Hospital Hines, Illinois, USA

ABSTRACT

Clinical, electrophysiological and morphological observations in 16 cases
of diabetes mellitus presenting with a motor syndrome affecting the pelvifemoral muscles suggested that diabetic proximal amyotrophy is a distinct clinical entity and most likely results from proximal crural motor neuropathy.
Neuropathic electromyograms in the proximal leg muscles, prolonged femoral
nerve motor latencies and reduced F-wave conduction velocities in the deep
peroneal nerves supported the above suggestion. Light and electronmicroscopic findings in the vastus medialis muscle, motor point biopsy samples
and the intramuscular branches of the femoral nerves further corroborated
the above conclusion. Insidious onset and subacute progression, improvement
concomitant with good control of hyperglycemia, onset simultaneous with or
early in the course of diabetes mellitus in most cases and presence of autonomic deficits in some suggested a metabolic rather than an ischemic cause
for diabetic proximal amyotrophy.

INTRODUCTION

In 1953, Garland and Taverner[1] under the heading of "diabetic myelopathy"
described a motor syndrome of proximal muscle wasting and weakness affecting
the legs in 5 patients with diabetes mellitus. Later in 1955, Garland[2]
coined the noncommittal term "diabetic amyotrophy" for this syndrome because
of uncertainty about the role of spinal cord in the pathogenesis of this
entity. This syndrome, in fact, was originally described by Bruns[3] in 1890
under the title of "neuritic paralysis in diabetes mellitus". Bruns described
4 patients, aged 59-70 years with diabetes mellitus, who had subacute onset
and gradual progression of pronounced paralysis of the proximal muscles of the
legs associated with pain. The manifestations were unilateral in 2 and bilateral but asymmetrical in the other 2 patients. All his patients improved
after dietetic treatment. Between then and Garland's publication, there were
occasional references to a motor syndrome in diabetes mellitus[4-6]. In 1961,
Garland[7] summarized the data on 27 patients and stated that the manifestations

were mostly limited to the thigh muscles and although bilateral, were usually asymmetrical.

Since Garland's publications,[1,2] many reports appeared in the literature.[8-17] Controversies and confusion have surrounded the entity over the years. Certain authors[10,14] used the term to include cases of diabetes mellitus with marked muscle atrophy in the distal limbs while others[18-20] suggested that the term diabetic amyotrophy be discarded altogether and the entity included under the heading of ischemic mononeuropathy multiplex associated with diabetes mellitus. Based on clinical, electrophysiological and morphological observations in 16 personally observed cases and examining critically the data of patients described by Garland,[7] Locke,[11] and others,[9,15,16] I provide evidence that the syndrome of diabetic proximal amyotrophy has a characteristic clinical picture which can be differentiated from the common diabetic distal polyneuropathy or mononeuropathy multiplex, and is secondary to certain metabolic defects of diabetes mellitus rather than due to diabetic microangiopathy.

MATERIALS AND METHODS

Table 1 summarizes the clinical data in 16 cases of diabetic proximal amyotrophy, 12 of which have recently been published in details.[17] All presented with moderate to marked pelvifemoral muscle wasting and weakness with no distal affection except in 4 patients (cases 4,5,11, and 14), who had mild weakness of foot dorsiflexors. Six patients had symmetrical, 4 asymmetrical, and 6 unilateral pelvifemoral muscle weakness and wasting insidiously over a period of 1 month to 1 year. All but 2 had pain in the thigh or low back area. Sensation was normal except for mild impairment distally in 2 patients (cases 2 and 3) and along the left femoral nerve in patient 5. Only 1 patient (case 5) had diabetic retinopathy. Fasting blood glucose levels ranged from 134 to 290 mg/dl. There was no laboratory evidence of nephropathy. All had functional improvement after good control of hyperglycemia during a follow-up period of 1 1/2 - 4 1/2 years.

Electrophysiological Study. Motor conduction velocities of the ulnar, median, common peroneal, and posterior tibial nerves were determined bilaterally by use of surface electrodes and standard methods. In all patients, femoral nerve latencies were measured from the inguinal region to the active surface electrode in the vastus medialis muscle. I obtained F-wave conduction velocity in the proximal segment of the deep peroneal nerve in 6 patients (cases 7,8,10,11,15 and 16) according to the method of Panayiotopoulos.[21]

Electromyographic examinations of the quadriceps, gluteal, hamstrings,

TABLE I

CLINICAL DATA AND FASTING BLOOD GLUCOSE IN 16 CASES OF DIABETIC PROXIMAL AMYOTROPHY

Patient No. & Age(yrs)	Duration of Diabetes	Duration of Amyotrophy & Weakness	Low Back or Thigh Pain	Pelvifemoral Muscle Wasting & Weakness Moderate	Marked	Muscle Symmetry	Knee Jerk	Ankle Jerk	Fasting Blood Glucose mg/dl
1: 59	6 mos.	3 mo.	+		+	S	A	D	154
2: 62	new	6 mo.	+		+	S	N	N	162
3: 53	20 yrs.	1 mo.	+		+	AS(L>R)	L:A R:D	A	290
4: 68	8 mo.	5 mo.	+	+		S	A	A	170
5: 61	new	1 mo.	+	+		U(L)	L:A R:D	L:A R:D	155
6: 57	2 1/2 yrs.	6 mo.	+		+	AS(L>R)	D	D	150
7: 29	3 yrs.	4 mo.	−		+	S	D	A	286
8: 56	4 1/2 yrs.	7 mo.	+		+	AS(R>L)	R:A L:D	A	134
9: 67	1 1/2 yrs.	4 mo.	+	+		U(R)	R:A L:N	N	179
10: 58	new	1 mo.	+		+	U(R)	R:A L:N	N	269
11: 61	10 mo.	6 mo.	+		+	U(L)	N	N	135
12: 52	10 mo.	2 mo.	+	+		S	A	N	135
13: 59	new	2 mo.	+	+		U(L)	L:A R:D	N	240
14: 58	20 yrs.	8 mo.	+		+	AS(L>R)	A	A	157
15: 79	new	1 yr.	−		+	S	A	N	143
16: 60	2 yrs.	6 mo.	+		+	U(L)	L:A R:N	N	151

+ = Present S = Symmetrical L = Left

− = None AS = Asymmetrical R = Right

U = Unilateral N = Normal

D = Diminished

A = Absent

anterior tibial, gastrocnemius, biceps, deltoid and lumbar paraspinal muscles
were obtained by use of coaxial needle electrode.

Muscle and motor point biopsy. In 12 patients biopsies of the vastus
medialis muscles on one side in the region of the motor points were obtained.
Histological staining and histochemical reactions of a piece of quick-frozen
muscle and esterase activities at the myoneural junctions of a second strip of
muscle, fixed in 3% glutaraldehyde, were obtained according to the methods
used in this laboratory.[17]

Fine structural observations of the muscles and motor endplates were made
according to the technique described previously.[17,22] The basement membrane
thickness of the intramuscular capillaries observed in the longitudinal section of the muscles under the electronmicroscope was measured by the method of
Williamson et al[23] in 7 patients (cases 3,6-10,14). Intramuscular nerve filaments near the neuromuscular junctions were examined under electronmicroscope
in 4 patients (cases 7-10).

Autonomic function study. In 6 patients (cases 7,11,12 and 14-16) circulatory responses after tilting the table upward, immersion of hand in ice cold
water, and Valsalva maneuver and plasma renin in supine and erect positions
were determined according to the standard methods.

RESULTS

Electrophysiological observations. Electromyograms of the pelvifemoral
muscles showed changes consistent with chronic neurogenic lesions, as described previously[17]. Fibrillations at rest were present in the lumbar
paraspinal muscles in 4 patients, (cases 5,6,8 and 16), one of whom had had
a lumbar laminectomy previously. In the distal leg muscles, fibrillations at
rest and mildly reduced interference pattern and motor unit amplitudes were
seen in 5 patients (cases 2,6-8 and 10). Electromyograms of the upper limb
muscles were normal.

Nerve conduction data. Table 2 summarizes the results of nerve conduction
study. The median and ulnar nerve conduction velocities were mildly reduced
in 2 patients (cases 4 and 7). The motor conduction velocities of the common
peroneal and the posterior tibial nerves were slightly reduced in all patients.
The femoral nerve latencies to vastus medialis muscles were prolonged in 11
patients (cases 1-3,5,7-9,12,14-16) in the affected limbs. F-wave velocities
in the proximal segments of the peroneal nerve, measured between first lumbar
vertebra and the knee, were disproportionately more reduced than the motor
conduction velocities in the distal segments between knee and ankle in all 6

TABLE 2

MOTOR NERVE CONDUCTION VALUES IN 16 CASES OF DIABETIC PROXIMAL AMYOTROPHY

Patients No.	Ulnar Velocity (meters/sec)	Peroneal Velocity (meters/sec)	Femoral latency (millisec) From inguinal region to Vast. Medialis Muscle		F-Wave (peroneal) Velocity (meters/sec)
1:	52	32	8.2	(D 28 cm)	
2:	50	35	8.1	(D 26 cm)	
3:	48	36	L14.0	(D 28 cm)	
4:	39	25	5.5	(D 21 cm)	
5:	52	37	7.0	(D 22 cm)	
6:	48	35	L4.5	(D 21 cm)	
7:	40	32	7.8	(D 34 cm)	36
8:	49	R31	R7.0	(D 29 cm)	R35
9:	60	36	R6.5	(D 27 cm)	
			L5.0	(D 28 cm)	
10:	–	R36	R5.0	(D 27 cm)	R42
		L40	L4.5	(D 27 cm)	L44
11:	61	R40	R4.0	(D 29 cm)	R50
		L38	L4.8	(D 27.5 cm)	L45
12:	50	33	R6.5	(D 30 cm)	
			L6.0	(D 34 cm)	
13:	54	35	R5.0	(D 30 cm)	
			L4.5	(D 29 cm)	
14:	–	33	R7.3	(D 28 cm)	
			L9.0	(D 29.5 cm)	
15:	58	R41	R5.8	(D 27 cm)	R38
		L38	L10.0	(D 28 cm)	L37
16:	53	R39	R5.3	(D 31 cm)	R43
		L36	L6.0	(D 31 cm)	L41

D = Distance from cathode to the active electrode

R = Right   – = Not measured

L = Left

patients.

<u>Muscle and motor point biopsy findings</u>. Histological and histochemical
examination of the vastus medialis muscles in the affected limbs showed groups
of angular atrophic type I and type II fibers (Fig. 1a), atrophic single
fibers and targets in type I fibers (Fig. 1b). Intramuscular nerve fibers
had patchy demyelination and axonal degeneration in 3 patients (Fig. 1e and
1f).

Histochemical reactions of the myoneural junctions for cholinesterase
activities showed many complex subneural apparatuses (Fig. 1c), beaded and
thickened terminal axons, axonal spheroids, collateral ramifications, (Fig.
1d), ultraterminal sprouts and multiple endplates).

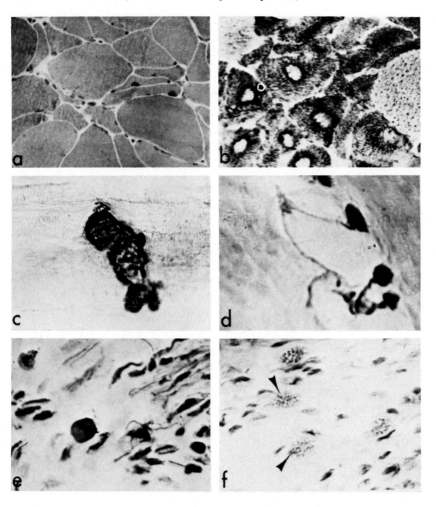

Electronmicroscopic examination of 56 motor endplate regions in 4 patients (cases 7-10) disclosed many degenerated and small nerve terminals. In many regions, the nerve terminals were missing and the regions were occupied by the Schwann cell processes (Fig. 2). The junctional folds underlying the degenerated or missing nerve terminals were atrophic and showed residual deposits of dense materal and basement membrane remnants (Fig. 2).

Fine structural observations of the muscles showed nonspecific myofibrillar degeneration, Z-band streaming, lipofuscin bodies, dilatation of elements of the sarcoplasmic reticulum, prominent Golgi complex, many vesicles with or without limiting membranes and in one patient tubular aggregates and mitochondrial paracrystalline inclusions.

Fine structure of the nerve filaments near the neuromuscular junctions in the vastus medialis muscles in 4 patients (cases 7-10) demonstrated axonal degeneration and changes in the Schwann cell organelles.

Autonomic function data. Tilt table study showed orthostatic hypotension in 3 patients (cases 11,14 and 16) with no rise of heart rate in 2 (cases 14 and 16) in the erect posture. Valsalva responses were impaired in all these 3 patients. Cold pressor test showed normal rise of blood pressure and heart rate in patient 11 but impaired response in patients 14 and 16. Plasma renin activity increased normally in the erect position in all patients. Therefore, these studies suggested that the autonomic deficits in patient 11 were due to a lesion in the afferent arc while those in patients 14 and 16 were related to a lesion in the efferent arc of the baroreceptor reflex mechanism.

Figure 1:

a. Groups of angular atrophic fibers in patient 9. Modified trichrome, X77

b. Targets in type I fibers (Patient 9). Reduced nicotinamide adenine dinucleotide tetrazolium reductase, X78

c. Degenerated subneural apparatus (soap bubble appearance) in Patient 2. Lehrer-Ornstein (alpha-naphthyl acetates as substrate). X400

d. Collateral sprouts in Patient 2. Karnovsky technique with butyrylthiocholine (ph 6), X245

e. Axonal swellings in intramuscular nerves of vastus medialis muscle in Patient 9. Bodian, X201

f. Loss of myelinated fibers and remnants of myelin (arrows) in intramuscular nerves of vastus medialis muscle in Patient 9. Modified trichrome, X195

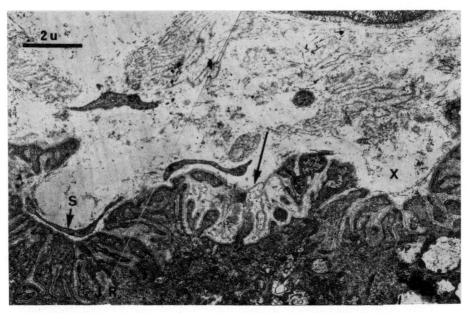

Figure 2

Three immediately adjacent regions of one endplate in the vastus medialis muscle of Patient 9 are shown. Note the missing nerve terminal (X) and Schwann cell process (S with arrow) occupying a missing nerve terminal area. Arrow points to atrophic residues of junctional folds and basement membrane remnants in a region denuded of nerve terminal.

DISCUSSION

Clinical features. An analysis of the clinical features of 16 personally observed cases and those in the literature shows that the syndrome of diabetic proximal amyotrophy comprises a motor manifestation of moderate to marked weakness and wasting of the pelvifemoral muscles, mostly accompanied by diffuse thigh and low back pain but without sensory impairment. Its insidious and slowly progressive onset differentiates it from the relatively sudden beginning of ischemic mononeuropathy multiplex. Its proximal motor manifestations are in contrast to the distal sensory-motor features of the common diabetic polyneuropathy. This syndrome usually is recognized in a middle aged or elderly patient shortly after or simultaneously with the onset of diabetes mellitus, occasionally also in younger individuals and in cases of long standing diabetes. While the distal leg muscles are normal or midly weak in some patients, the pelvifemoral muscles are disproportionately weaker.

Maximal wasting and weakness begin in the quadriceps femoris and then proceed to the gluteal, hamstring, adductor and iliopsoas muscles. The manifestations may be symmetrical, asymmetrical or unilateral, but unilateral features may later become bilateral. Patellar reflexes are usually diminished or absent, and the ankle reflexes may be normal or diminished. The bulbar muscles are spared and the scapulohumeral muscles are rarely involved and then usually after involvement of the pelvifemoral muscles. Most but not all patients fail to show evidence of nephropathy, diabetic retinopathy and peripheral vascular disease. Tests for autonomic functions may reveal evidence of autonomic neuropathy in some cases as noted in 3 of 6 patients studied in the present series. These findings of autonomic deficits in diabetic proximal amyotrophy are in contrast to the statement made by Bruyn and Garland[24] that they had never seen any of the autonomic syndromes in association with diabetic amyotrophy.

Electrophysiological findings. The electromyograms in all patients showed evidence of chronic neurogenic lesions in the pelvifemoral muscles suggesting involvement of the lower motor neurons. Absence of fasciculations and large motor units makes anterior horn cells unlikely but not improbable sites of lesions. In some patients (cases 5,6,8 and 16), lumbar paraspinal muscles may show fibrillations indicating the presence of lumbar rediculopathy.

The prolonged femoral nerve motor latencies and reduced F-wave conduction velocities in the proximal segments of the peroneal nerves indicated that the lesions occurred most frequently in the proximal motor nerves, although nerve conduction study showed evidence of subclinical mild distal neuropathy. (Table 2).

Morphological changes. The presence of groups of angular atrophic type I and type II fibers and target fibers clearly indicated that muscle changes in diabetic proximal amyotrophy were neurogenic. Light and electronmicroscopic findings of motor endplates were consistent with denervation and reinnervation. Morphological changes in the intramuscular nerve filaments in vastus medialis muscles further convinced me that changes resulted from an affection of the nerves in these muscles. I would agree with Bloodworth and Epstein[12] and Hamilton et al[13] that intramuscular capillary basement membrane thickening is not primarily responsible for diabetic proximal amyotrophy.

Anatomical site of the lesions. The most probable sites of lesions in diabetic proximal amyotrophy seem to be either the proximal nerve trunks in a patchy fashion or the intramuscular branches of the proximal crural nerves or their terminal portions. In support of this hypothesis, I would point to the pathological changes observed by light and electronmicroscopic examination

of the intramuscular nerves and the motor endplates and the electrophysiological findings of prolonged femoral nerve latencies and reduced F-wave conduction velocities in the peroneal nerves. In some patients, lumbosacral radicu-
lopathy may be the responsible lesions. In absence of careful pathological
examination of a number of cases of diabetic proximal amyotrophy the role of
the ventral horn cells of the spinal cord in the pathogenesis of this syndrome
cannot be ascertained.

Pathogenesis: Ischemia vs. metabolic cause. The role of ischemic lesion
and metabolic dysfunction in the pathogenesis of diabetic proximal amyotrophy and in diabetic neuropathies in general has not been settled. Raff and
Asbury[18] and Raff et al[19] advocated that diabetic amyotrophy is a type of
ischemic mononeuropathy multiplex. They based their opinion mainly on the
postmortum[19] evidence of multiple small infarctive lesions of the proximal
major nerve trunks of the leg in a man who developed rapid onset of left leg
weakness, both proximal and distal, with minimal affection of the right leg
and died 6 weeks later. In my opinion the onset, progression and the total
clinical picture of this patient did not fit well with the usual case of
diabetic proximal amyotrophy.

In my patients, the insidious onset, subacute progression, absence of evidence of nephropathy, retinopathy or diabetic peripheral vascular disease in
most cases mitigate against ischemic theory in the pathogenesis. Furthermore, thickness of muscle capillary basement membranes has been noted in
many nondiabetic elderly individuals and in diabetic patients with or without neuropathy or amyotrophy.[17]

Following points would support the metabolic theory in the pathogenesis
of diabetic proximal amyotrophy: Improvement concomitant with good control
of hyperglycemia in most of the patients; onset simultaneous with or early
in the course of diabetes mellitus rather than in long standing cases; symmetry of the affection in many; and the presence of autonomic dysfunction
early in course of the illness as noted in 3 of the 6 patients studied in
the present series. It is well known that the autonomic fibers are relatively
resistant to ischemia. However, occasional patients particularly those with
asymmetrical or unilateral manifestations and relatively sudden onset may
have an ischemic basis for diabetic proximal amyotrophy.

What is the nature of the metabolic defect? Hyperglycemia, active sorbitol
pathway, enzyme deficiency, abnormalities of membrane transport mechanism and
an excessive lipid accumulation in Schwann cells have all been suggested[2,25]
but hyperglycemia appears to be the most important factor[2] in the pathogenesis
of diabetic proximal amyotrophy and diabetic neuropathies in general.

In conclusion, I would suggest that in order to avoid confusion with the more common diabetic polyneuropathy presenting with marked distal amyotrophy, we use the term "diabetic proximal amyotrophy" to define a characteristic clinical syndrome in diabetes mellitus.

ACKNOWLEDGEMENTS

Supported in part by the Medical Research Service of the Veterans Administration. I thank M.G. Reyes, M.D., for the histochemical study of the muscles and H. Tonaki and N. Nishamura for assistance with electronmicroscopic study.

REFERENCES

1. Garland, H. and Taverner, D. (1953) Diabetic myelopathy. Br. Med. J., 1, 1405-1408.

2. Garland, H. (1955) Diabetic Amyotrophy. Br. Med. J., 2, 1287-1290.

3. Bruns, L. (1890) Ueber Neuritische Låhmungen beim diabetes mellitus. Berl. Klin. Wochenschr., 27, 509-515.

4. Kraus, W.M. (1922) Involvement of the peripheral neurons in diabetes mellitus. Arch. Neurol. Psychiat., 7, 202-209.

5. Root, H.F. and Rogers, M.H. (1930) Diabetic neuritis with paralysis. N. Engl. J. Med., 202, 1049-1053.

6. Alderman, J.E. (1938) Diabetic anterior neuropathy - clinical and pathological observations. J. Mt. Sinai Hosp., 5, 396-402.

7. Garland, H. (1961) Diabetic amyotrophy. Br. J. Clin. Pract., 15, 9-13.

8. Skanse, H. and Gydell, K. (1956) A rare type of femoral-sciatic neuropathy in diabetes mellitus. Acta Med. Scand., 155, 463-468.

9. Bischoff, V.A. (1959) Zur diabetischen amyotrophie (neuromyopathie). Schweiz. Med. Wochenschr., 89, 519-525.

10. Isascs, H. and Gilchrist, G. (1960) Diabetic amyotrophy. S. Afr. Med. J. 34, 501-505.

11. Locke, S., Lawrence, D.G., and Legg, M.A. (1963) Diabetic amyotrophy. Am. J. Med., 34, 775-785.

12. Bloodworth, J.M.B., Jr. and Epstein, M. (1967) Diabetic amyotrophy: light and electron microscopic investigation. Diabetes, 16, 181-190.

13. Hamilton, C.R. Jr., Dobson, H.L., and Marshall, J. (1968) Diabetic amyotrophy: Clinical and electron microscopic studies in 6 patients. Am. J. Med., 256, 81-90.

14. Gregersen, G. (1969) Diabetic amyotrophy - a well defined syndrome? Acta Med. Scand., 185, 303-310.

15. Casey, E.B. and Harrison, M.J.G. (1972) Diabetic amyotrophy: a follow-up study. Br. Med. J., 1, 656-659.

16. Williams, I.R. and Mayer, R.F. (1976) Subacute proximal diabetic neuropathy. Neurology (Minneap), 26, 108-116.

17. Chokroverty, S., Reyes, M.G., Rubino, F.A. and Tonaki, H., (1977) The syndrome of diabetic amyotrophy. Ann. Neurol., 2, 181-194.

18. Raff, M.C. and Asbury, A.K. (1968) Ischemic mononeuropathy and mononeuropathy multiplex in diabetes mellitus. N. Engl. J. Med., 279, 17-22.

19. Raff, M.C., Sangalang, V., and Asbury, A.K., (1968) Ischemic mononeuropathy multiplex associated with diabetes mellitus. Arch. Neurol., 18, 487-499.

20. Asbury, A.K. (1977) Proximal diabetic neuropathy. Ann. Neurol., 2, 179-180.

21. Panayiotopoulos, C.P., Scarpalezos, S. and Nastas, R., (1977) F-wave studies on the deep peroneal nerve. Part 1. Control subjects. J. Neurol. Sci., 31, 319-329.

22. Chokroverty, S., Reyes, M.G., Chokroverty, M. and Kaplan, R., (1978) Effect of prednisolone on motor end-plate fine structure: A morphometric study in hamsters. Ann. Neurol., 3, 358-365.

23. Williamson, J.R., Vogler, N.J., and Kilo, G., (1969) Estimation of vascular basement membrane thickness: Theoretical and practical considerations. Diabetes, 18, 567-578.

24. Bruyn, G.W. and Garland, H. (1970) Neuropathies of endocrine origin, in Handbook of Clinical Neurology, Vinken, P.J. and Bruyn, G.W., Eds., North Holland, Amsterdam, Vol. 8, pp. 29-52.

25. Thomas, P.K. and Eliasson, S.G. (1975) Diabetic neuropathy, in Peripheral Neuropathy, Dyck, P.J., Thomas, P.K. and Lambert, E.H., Eds., W.B. Saunders, Philadelphia, pp. 956-981.

Peripheral Neuropathies
N. Canal and G. Pozza, eds.
© 1978 Elsevier/North-Holland Biomedical Press

MORPHOMETRY OF PERIPHERAL NERVES IN STREPTOZOTOCIN DIABETIC RATS

JOHANNES JAKOBSEN

University Institute of Anatomy and Pathology and Second Clinic
of Internal Medicine, Kommunehospitalet, DK-8000 Aarhus C, Denmark

INTRODUCTION

Nerve function is decreased quite early in patients with
juvenile diabetes mellitus. Gregersen (1967) showed that motor
nerve conduction velocity is reduced at the time of diagnosis
and that the velocity gradually declines with the duration of
the disease[1].

Histological studies of peripheral nerves after several years
of diabetes have demonstrated loss of myelin sheaths and axons,
particularly segmental demyelination[2]. There is one ultrastructural study of peripheral nerves in early juvenile diabetes
(Bischoff, 1973)[3]. In that study signs of primary axonal degeneration was found in biopsies from six patients. However,
no structural correlate to the functional abnormality of nerve
conduction in early diabetes is known at present.

In experimental diabetes in the rat nerve conduction velocity is decreased after one or two weeks duration of the disease[4,5]. A few histological studies from the sixties have reported myelin sheath abnormalities in peripheral nerves of
rats several months after the induction of diabetes [6,7]. However,
an extensive morphometric study by Sharma and Thomas (1974)
failed to define any pathological alteration at all in strept-
zotocin as well as in alloxan diabetic rats with a diabetes
duration of up to one year[5].

To further investigate the structural background of the
early functional nerve changes in the streptozotocin diabetic
rat the present study was undertaken.

MATERIALS AND METHODS

Ten male wistar rats weighing between 330 and 380 gm were injected intravenously with streptozotocin and sacrificed after

a diabetes duration of four weeks at the age of 23-24 weeks. Ten age and weight-matched animals were used as controls.

The hind limbs were fixed by vascular perfusion and a specimen of the common peroneal nerve was taken for the various morphometric analyses.

For each animal an average of 250 myelinated nerve fibres were counted and measured within two circle sectors placed at random on a light microscopic projection of a nerve cross section Fibre size, axon size and fractional "endoneurial area" within the sectors were estimated by a point-counting technique.

Internodal length and fibre thickness were measured in 20 isolated fibres from each animal.

A random sample including nearly 200 cross sectioned myelinated nerve fibres from each animal was used for a morphometric analysis of the ultrastructure. Electron micrographs at a magnification of 13,500 were pasted together to one composite picture and the various fractional areas were obtained by point-counting. The absolute areas were calculated by multiplying the fascicular area by the various fractional areas.

RESULTS

Diabetic rats all lost weight and blood sugars ranged between 300 and 600 mg per 100 ml.

Histological studies. The number of myelinated nerve fibres was unchanged in the group of diabetic rats as compared to the group of controls, being 1881 +/- 111 (SD) in diabetics and 1870 +/- 108 in controls.

Mean fibre size for each rat is shown in Figure 1. The mean fibre size in diabetic rats and controls were 36.15 μm^2 +/- 2.12 and 42.08 +/- 3.44, respectively. This difference which amount to 14% is statistically significant (2p < 0.001).

The mean axon size in diabetic rats and controls were 16.00 μm^2 +/- 1.52 and 19.96 μm^2 +/- 2.34, respectively. In diabetic rats this decrease of the axon area of 20% was followed by a decrease of 9% of the cross sectional myelin sheath area. The differences of axon and myelin sheath areas were both statistically significant, the 2p-values being smaller than 0.001 and 0.01, respectively. Axon-myelin ratios were calculated for each animal. The individual values are shown in Figure 2.

mean fibre size   axon/myelin ratio

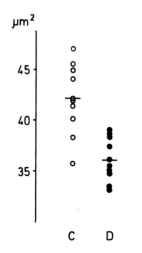

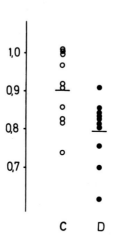

Fig. 1. Mean fibre size in   Fig. 2. Axon/myelin ratio in
each of ten diabetic rats (●)   each of ten diabetic rats (●)
and in ten age-matched con-   and in ten age-matched controls (o).   trols (o).

The axon-myelin ratio was decreased in diabetic rats as compared to controls (2p < 0.02).

   To obtain information about the involvement of small as well
as large fibres in the reduction of fibre size ten percentiles
of cumulative frequency-size distributions from each of the two
groups were compared. For all percentiles examined the diabetic
values were lower indicating that all fibres are thinner in diabetic rats.

   The area between myelinated fibres - the "endoneurial area" -
is shown for each animal in Figure 3. In the diabetic group the
area was increased by nearly 30% as compared to controls
(2p < 0.02).

   Neither segmental demyelination nor remyelination was observed
in the study of isolated fibres. Regression lines between length
and thickness of internodes were calculated for each animal.
The slope coefficients of the regression lines in diabetic rats
and controls were 0.104 +/- 0.011 and 0.095 +/- 0.011, the 2p
value being between 0.1 and 0.05. Internodal length and thick-

'endoneurial' space

structureless endoneurial space

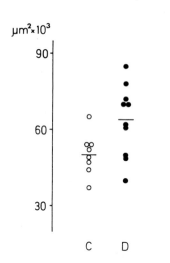

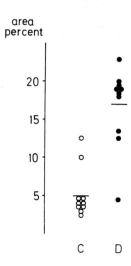

μm²×10³

area
percent

Fig. 3. "Endoneurial" space – area between myelinated nerve fibres – in each of ten diabetic rats (●) and in ten age-matched controls (o).

Fig. 4. Structureless endoneurial space measured from electron micrographs in each of ten diabetic rats (●) and in ten age-matched controls (o).

ness of the five thickest fibres of each animal were examined. Internodal thickness was decreased in diabetic rats ($2p < 0.05$), whereas, internodal length was unchanged. Internodal length in the diabetic group was 1.26 mm +/- 0.10 as against 1.25 mm +/- 0.10 in controls.

Electron microscopic studies. The morphometric analysis of the electron microscopic photomontages showed that the myelinated fibre area of the common peroneal nerve was 75,800 μm^2 +/- 7,700 in diabetic rats as against 87,500 μm^2 +/- 11,100 in controls. The difference was statistically significant ($2p < 0.01$). The amount of Schwann cell cytoplasm of myelinated nerve fibres was also decreased, being 7,400 μm^2 +/- 1,100 in diabetic rats and 10,300 μm^2 +/- 2.100 in controls ($2p < 0.01$).

As to the endoneurial space there was a 3-4 fold increase of the structureless endoneurial area. Values for each animal are shown in Figure 4. The mean value for the diabetic group was 22,500 μm^2 +/- 7,900 as compared to 6,600 μm^2 +/- 4,400 in controls ($2p < 0.001$).

DISCUSSION

After four weeks of streptozotocin diabetes in the rat the calibre of myelinated fibres is decreased as compared to age-matched controls[8,9]. A similar change of fibre calibre has recently been reported to occur in the obese hyperglycemic (db/db) mouse[10].

It has been suggested that the reduction of the calibre can be explained by decreased skeletal growth. However, tibial length did not differ between a group of controls and a group of diabetic rats who had the same age and the same degree and duration of diabetes as the rats used in the present study. Furthermore, internodal length of thin diabetic fibres does not differ from the length of internodes of age-matched control rats.

The difference in fibre size may arise in several ways. It might either be due to a larger increase of the calibre in controls than in diabetics during the experiment or to axonal dwindling or to a combination of both. However, the decisive finding of the present experiment is the one of a predominant decrease of the axon calibre. It is suggested that nerve conduction velocity is dependent upon fibre calibre[11]. If this suggestion is correct the slowing of the nerve impulse in experimental diabetes is at least partially explained by the decrease of the fibre calibre.

It has been suggested by Gabbay (1968) that the increased amount of sorbitol found in peripheral nerve of streptozotocin diabetic rats is localized within the schwann cell cytoplasm leading to overhydration and swelling and thereby to osmotic damage to the myelin sheath[12]. However, the finding of the present study of a 30% decrease of the amount of schwann cell cytoplasm of myelinated fibres is in conflict with the sorbitol theory.

The enlargement of the endoneurial space indicates the existence of an endoneurial oedema in peripheral nerve of streptozotocin diabetic rats. This suggestion is further supported by the finding of an increased water content in peripheral nerve of the same rats[13]. Such an oedema might be due to extravasation of serum proteins through vasa nervorum. In fact, an increased extravasation of Evans blue albumin into the sciatic nerve of alloxan diabetic rats has been found by Seneviratne

274

(1972)[14]. However, in a recent study by Jakobsen, Malmgren and Olsson (1978) it is reported that in sciatic nerves no difference in vascular permeability could be detected between controls and streptozotocin diabetic rats even though new and more sensitive tracer techniques were used[15].

REFERENCES

1. Gregersen, G. (1967) Neurology, 17, 972-980.
2. Thomas, P.K., and Lascelles, R.G. (1965) Lancet I, 1355-1357.
3. Bischoff, A. (1973) in Vascular and Neurological Changes in Early Diabetes. Advances in Metabolic Disorders, Suppl 2, Camerini-Dávalos, R.A., and Cole, H.S. eds., New York and London, Academic Press, pp. 441-449.
4. Eliasson, S.G. (1964) J. clin. Invest., 43, 2353-2358.
5. Sharma, A.K., and Thomas, P.K. (1974) J. neurol. Sci., 23, 1-15.
6. Preston, G.M. (1967) J. Physiol., 189, 49P-50P.
7. Hildebrand, J., Joffroy, A., Graff, G., and Coërs, C. (1968) Arch. Neurol., 18, 633-641.
8. Jakobsen, J. (1976) Diabetologia, 12, 539-546.
9. Jakobsen, J. (1976) Diabetologia, 12, 547-553.
10. Sima, A.A.F., and Robertson, D.M. (1978) Acta neuropath., 41, 85-89.
11. Rushton, W.A.H. (1951) J. Physiol., 115, 101-122.
12. Gabbay, K.H., and O'Sullivan, J.B. (1968) Diabetes, 17, 239-243.
13. Jakobsen, J. (1978) Diabetologia, 14, 113-119.
14. Seneviratne, K.N. (1972) J. Neurol. Neurosurg. Psychiatry, 35, 156-162.
15. Jakobsen, J., Malmgren, L., and Olsson, Y. (1978) Exp. neurol., 60, in press.

Peripheral Neuropathies
N. Canal and G. Pozza, eds.
© 1978 Elsevier/North-Holland Biomedical Press

ASSESSMENT OF DIABETIC AUTONOMIC NEUROPATHY BY MEASUREMENT
OF HEART RATE RESPONSES TO DEEP BREATHING AND TO STANDING.

J.D. MACKAY AND P.J. WATKINS

Department of Diabetes, King's College Hospital, London SE5 9RS, England.

INTRODUCTION

Autonomic neuropathy in diabetics can be detected by demonstrating the
presence of abnormal cardiovascular reflexes.   In recent years instantaneous
heart rate (H.R.) monitoring has provided a convenient and simple technique
for doing this by measuring the degree of autonomic denervation of the heart.

In 1973, using this technique in diabetics for the first time [1], we showed
that diabetics with autonomic neuropathy have loss of the normal H.R.
variation on deep breathing, or sinus arrhythmia (fig. 1).   Atropine has the
same effect and loss of H.R. variation is due to vagal neuropathy - a
parasympathetic defect.

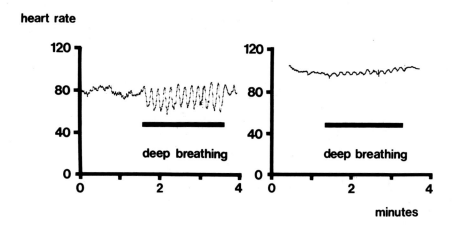

Fig. 1.   H.R. variation on deep breathing in a normal subject (left), and in a
diabetic with autonomic neuropathy (right).
The H.R. monitor detects each R wave from the E.C.G. and each RR interval
is converted into the equivalent heart rate in beats/min.

Diabetics with autonomic neuropathy may have abnormal H.R. responses
to standing [2,3]. When normal subjects stand up H.R. increases rapidly and
then overshoots (fig. 2), but in patients with autonomic neuropathy there is a
more gradual increase in H.R. and loss of the overshoot. In rare cases
cardiac denervation is complete and H.R. does not alter on standing.
Atropine modifies but does not abolish the normal H.R. response to standing
which has both parasympathetic and sympathetic components.

heart rate

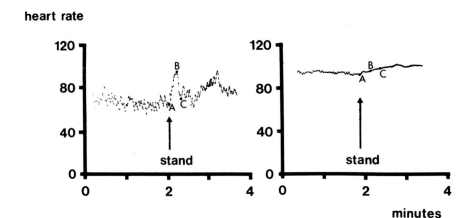

Fig. 2. Standing H.R. responses in a normal subject (left), and in a diabetic
with autonomic neuropathy (right) showing loss of the normal peak and overshoot.
H.R. increase = B-A.   H.R. ratio = B/C.

We have compared our results from these two tests, the H.R. responses
to deep breathing and to standing, testing a wide range of diabetics.

PATIENTS AND METHODS
We tested 301 diabetics and 54 normal subjects. They were between 20
and 49 years old. Subjects 50 years old and over were excluded because

of a marked decline in the normal H.R. responses to these manoeuvres in older subjects. Diabetics were allocated to one of 3 groups depending on the degree of neuropathy detected clinically.

Diabetics without neuropathy (143 patients) were defined by the presence of intact leg reflexes. Nerve conduction studies were not performed. Diabetics with peripheral neuropathy (94 patients) at least had absent ankle jerks, and they had no autonomic symptoms. Diabetics with autonomic neuropathy (64 patients) had symptoms and/or signs as noted in table 1. More than half of the patients had two or more of these autonomic features. Impotence was excluded as a symptom because of difficulties with its assessment.

TABLE 1   TOTAL NUMBERS OF SYMPTOMS AND SIGNS IN 64 DIABETICS WITH AUTONOMIC NEUROPATHY

Postural hypotension a	Diarrhoea b	Gustatory sweating c	Oesophageal and gastric atony d	Bladder atony d	Cardio-respiratory arrests e
25	43	37	9	8	4

a: defined by the presence of postural symptoms and a fall in systolic pressure on standing of 30mmHg or more.
b: pattern of diarrhoea thought to be typical of "diabetic diarrhoea".[4]
c: facial sweating with tasty meals.
d: detected radiologically.
e: unexpected arrests associated with anaesthesia.[5]

H.R. changes were recorded using a Hewlett-Packard instantaneous H.R. monitor. With the subject supine regular deep breathing was performed at a rate of 6 breaths per minute. H.R. variation on deep breathing (fig. 1.) was assessed by measuring the difference between maximum and minimum heart rates over 10 breaths; and a mean of 20 readings gave the deep breathing score. After resting supine for a few minutes subjects stood up by the bedside for at least one minute. Two measurements of the standing H.R. response were taken (fig. 2). 1) The standing H.R. increase is the difference between the H.R. at peak (B) and the resting H.R. (A). 2) The

TABLE 2   GROUPED DATA FOR THE 3 H.R. TESTS IN THE NORMAL
SUBJECTS AND THE 3 GROUPS OF DIABETICS.

	Mean $\pm$ ISD	Range	Lower limit of normal
			% abnormal in diabetics
Normal subjects			
D.B. response (54)	24.6 $\pm$ 7.8	9.5-43.4	less than 9.0
H.R. increase (53)	27.1 $\pm$ 7.8	12-48.0	less than 12.0
H.R. ratio (51)	1.37 $\pm$ 0.167	1.08-1.73	less than 1.04
Diabetics without peripheral neuropathy			
D.B. response (143)	22.1 $\pm$ 9.3	1.7-43.8	7%
H.R. increase (140)	26.0 $\pm$ 7.8	10.0-48.0	3%
H.R. ratio (139)	1.24 $\pm$ 0.16	1.01-1.69	4%
Diabetics with peripheral neuropathy			
D.B. response (94)	26.0 $\pm$ 7.8	1.0-36.3	30%
H.R. increase (88)	19.9 $\pm$ 7.6	3.0-41.0	13%
H.R. ratio (88)	1.16 $\pm$ 0.14	0.15-1.64	10%
Diabetics with autonomic neuropathy			
D.B. response (64)	4.8 $\pm$ 3.8	1.0-17.6	84%
H.R. increase (58)	10.5 $\pm$ 7.7	0-27.0	57%
H.R. ratio (58)	1.03 $\pm$ 0.07	0.85-1.29	57%

D.B. = deep breathing.   Numbers of subjects tested given in brackets. The
total number of standing responses is slightly reduced because only D.B.
responses were obtained in some subjects.

standing H.R. ratio is the H.R. at peak (B) divided by the H.R. at the end of the overshoot (C). In those diabetics with autonomic neuropathy who had loss of the peak the H.R. increase at 15 seconds after standing was taken instead, and the H.R. ratio was the H.R. at 30 seconds after standing divided by the H.R. at 15 seconds after standing.

RESULTS

These are summarized in table 2. In all three tests the range of normal was wide. Abnormal scores were defined as those more than 2 S D below the mean value in normal subjects.

DISCUSSION

Loss of normal H.R. variation on deep breathing is found in a high proportion (84%) of diabetics with autonomic symptoms and scores are low in almost all of them, so that the deep breathing test is useful for confirming the presence of autonomic neuropathy when it is suspected clinically. Also a significant proportion, 30%, of diabetics with peripheral neuropathy have abnormal scores, and even 7% of diabetics without neuropathy. We suggest that these diabetics have asymptomatic autonomic neuropathy. Three of these diabetics had symptoms suggestive of autonomic neuropathy (mild postural hypotension), and one diabetic later developed definite autonomic symptoms.

In all groups of diabetics the standing H.R. increase and the standing H.R. ratio were less frequently abnormal than the deep breathing test, and in diabetics with autonomic neuropathy both tests were abnormal in only 57% of cases. We believe that this is so, particularly for the H.R. increase on standing, because H.R. changes on standing include both sympathetic and parasympathetic components and, in diabetics with autonomic neuropathy, parasympathetic denervation occurs earlier than sympathetic denervation. In 21 diabetics with postural hypotension (and more severe sympathetic denervation) who had standing responses the H.R. increase was abnormal in 16, or 76% of them.

Interpretation of the standing H.R. ratio is more complex, but its value is largely dependant on the size of the H.R. overshoot (fig. 2:B-C) which is a vagally mediated response. Despite this it was less frequently abnormal than the deep breathing response and this would limit its use - and the use of similar ratios from a simple E.C.G. rhythm strip [3] - as a confirmatory test for clinical autonomic neuropathy.

SUMMARY

1. Loss of normal H.R. variation on deep breathing, due to vagal neuropathy is frequently detected in the presence of autonomic symptoms, and it is therefore a good diagnostic test for clinical autonomic neuropathy.
2. The H.R. responses to standing are less sensitive tests for detecting autonomic neuropathy in diabetics than the deep breathing test.
3. Autonomic (vagal) neuropathy is present in some diabetics without autonomic symptoms and a few of these are without clinical peripheral neuropathy.

ACKNOWLEDGEMENTS

We are grateful to Dr. D.A. Pyke for his encouragement, and to Mrs. J. Cambridge for technical assistance. This work was supported by the Research Committee, King's College Hospital, and Winthrop Laboratories.

REFERENCES

1. Wheeler, T. and Watkins, P.J. (1973) British Medical Journal, 4, 584-586.
2. Page, M.M. and Watkins, P.J. (1977) Clinics in Endocrinology and Metabolism, 6, 380-381.
3. Ewing, D.J. et al. (1978) British Medical Journal, 1, 145-147.
4. Watkins, P.J. (1973) British Medical Journal, 1, 583-587.
5. Page, M.M. and Watkins, P.J. (1978) Lancet, 1, 14-16.

Peripheral Neuropathies
N. Canal and G. Pozza, eds.
© 1978 Elsevier/North-Holland Biomedical Press

CLINICAL AND ELECTROMYOGRAPHICAL OBSERVATION ON 83 CASES OF DIABE-
TIC NEUROPATHY.

P. NEGRIN, P. FARDIN, D. FEDELE, A. TIENGO and L. BATTISTIN

P.N., P.F. and L.B.: Department of Neurology; D.F. and A.T.: Department of Gerontology and Metabolic Diseases, University of Padova
Medicl School, Padova, Italy.

INTRODUCTION

Among the majority of the Authors there is already an agreement
that in diabetes mellitus a diminution of nervous motor conduction
velocity (MCV) is present; on the other hand we are still discussing on the relationship between such diminution and the duration
of the illness and the entity of the metabolic change.

For this reason we considered it useful to study the MCV in a
group of diabetic patients relating it to the clinical findings,
the age of the patient, the duration of the illness and the entity of the metabolic damage.

MATERIALS AND METHODS

83 patients, 46 males and 37 females, whose ages ranged from
14 to 71 years, 50 affected by insulin-independent diabetes and
33 insulin-dependent diabetes, with the illness dating from a minimum of one month to a maximum of 32 years, were submitted to MCV
examination of peroneal nerve. The examination was carried out in-
dipendently of the presence of clinical signs of peripheral neuro
pathy.

Clinically we placed the patients in three groups defined with
the terms of absent, sub-clinical and clinical neuropathy. In the
first group of 19 subjects there were no signs of neuropathy either subjective (weakness, paresthesias, pain) or objective (depression, loss of the deep jearks, impairment or loss of vibration
sense). In the second group, comprising 25 patients, we were able
to show a slight diminution of the tendon reflexes and/or impairment of vibration sense. In the third group of 39 diabetics both
subjective and objective symptoms were present in a marked degree.

The metabolic control was evaluated by various tests: insulin-
dependence, presence or absence of acetonuria, glycosuria through

24 hours, fasting glycemia and glycemia 2 hours after a.meal; finally the average between these two glycemic measurement as a value indicating the average daily glycemia. In order to obtain data referring to a fairly long period, all these parameters have been referred on the average to results obtained on three consecutive and distinct days.

The MCV values were compared with those of a group of 43 control subjects free from metabolic illness, or family diabetic tendency and without neurological illness.

RESULTS AND DISCUSSION

As already illustrated in the literature, the MCV in the group of diabetic subjects is significantly impaired compared with normal subjects, with average values of 42.2 m/sec. in the diabetics against 51.2 m/sec. in the normal group (fig. 1)

Considering the behaviour of the MCV according to the presence or absence of clinical neuropathy, we can state that the MCV is significantly impaired even in the absence of subjective and objective signs of neuropathy and that it is further reduced by the appeerence of clinical neuropathy (fig. 2).

The impairment of MCV significantly increased with the age of the patient.

The evaluation of MCV in relation to the duration of diabetic illness indicated that there is not a clear correlation between these two parameters, but confirms that the MCV is significantly reduced already in the early stages of the illness. In fact, in patients suffering from the disease for less than one year the MCV was 43 m/sec; particularly, a 14 year-old patient had an MCV of 42 m/sec after a month's illness, while another patient of 37 showed a MCV of 39 m/sec after two months. The duration of the diabetes showed further effects after ten years, probably on account of the influence of age of the patients.

However, the duration of the illness is on the other hand very important in the clinical evidence of peripheral neuropathy. In fact, the longer the duration of the illness the more we found a significant reduction of patients with absence of symptomatology and a progressive increase in clearly diabetic neuropathy; in the cases of diabetes with a duration of ten years we found no absent cases, but 8 subclinical and 12 clinical cases of neuro-

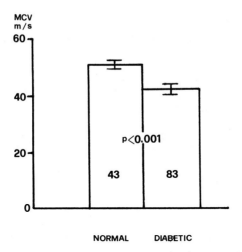

Fig. 1

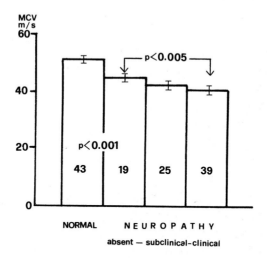

Fig. 2

pathy.

With regard to the metabolic control a primary distinction was made between insulin-dependent diabetes and insulin-independent, and between acetonuric and non acetonuric patients. Differences existed between the two groups even if not particularly significant, especially between the acetonuric and non, yet evidencing a certain influence of metabolic control on the MCV.

The presence or absence of glycosuria did not significantly influence the MCV.

The evaluation of the metabolic control with average glycemic values, fasting and hours after a meal, did not show significant correlation between these two parameters and MCV. When we divided the diabetic patients into three groups according to the glycemic values medi/die, we found that also patients with daily glycemia less than 150 mg/die (and therefore presumably with a satisfactory metabolic balance) presented a significant impairment of the MCV. It should also be noticed that in poor metabolic control such as that represented by glycemia above 250 mg/die, the MCV was further reduced.

As to the duration, the metabolic control is important in conditioning the appearence of the peripheral neuropathy; in fact, with glycemic values of more than 250 mg/die, the majority of diabetics showed a marked clinical neuropathy.

CONCLUSIONS

We may conclude that:
1) the MCV is impaired in diabetic illness
2) the impairment of conduction is precocious even in the absence of clinical neuropathy
3) the impairment of conduction is directly related to the age also in diabetic patients
4) the duration of diabetes is not correlated to the MCV, but may influence the appearence of the neuropathy symptoms
5) the MCV is impaired also in the presence of a fair metabolic control.

This, however, does not mean that metabolic control has no importance in influencing the appearence and development of diabetic neuropathy, but only that the MCV is impaired also in the presence of only slightly increased glycemic values and that, in order to obtain its normalisation, a through glycemic control is necessary.

Thus in agreement with the data of Green et al. (1975)[1] who succeded on hindering in streptozotocinized cats the impairment of the MCV, with only one insulin treatment able to maintain an average daily glycemia of 75 mg/die.

We may therefore conclude by afferming that the MCV is a valuable parameter in diabetes because it allows the diagnosis of peripheral neuropathy long before it becomes clinically manifested.

SUMMARY

The MCV of the peroneal nerve was studied in 83 diabetics to see if the impairment usually noticed is in relation to clinical symptomatology, to the age of the patient, to the duration of the illness or to the metabolic control.

A comparison with 43 normal patients confirm tha significant impairment of the MCV in diabetics, evident even in the absence of clinical signs of neuropathy; its gravity is directly correlated to the age of the patient.

The duration of the illness has little influence on the impairment of the MCV already present in the early stages, while it is very important in the clinical appearence of the peripheral neuropathy.

Insulin-dependence and the presence of acetonuria or glycosuria do not influence the MCV; hyperglycemia is important in the clinical appearence of peripheral neuropathy, while it is less important in the impairment of the MCV, present also in patients with a fair metabolic control.

REFERENCE

1) Green, D.A., De Jesus, P.V., Winegard, A.J.: Effects of insulin and dietary myoinositol on impaired peripheral motor nerve conduction velocity in acute streptozotocin diabetes. J. Clin. Invest. 55, 1326-1336 (1975).

Peripheral Neuropathies
N. Canal and G. Pozza, eds.
© 1978 Elsevier/North-Holland Biomedical Press

EVALUATION OF THE MOTOR AND SENSORY CONDUCTION VELOCITY (MCV, SCV) IN DIABETIC PATIENTS BEFORE AND AFTER A THREE DAYS TREATMENT WITH THE ARTIFICIAL BETA CELL (BIOSTATOR).

V.GALLAI[*], L.AGOSTINI[*], A.ROSSI[*], M.MASSI-BENEDETTI[**], G.CALABRESE[**], A.PUXED-DU[**] and P.BRUNETTI[**].

Istituto di Clinica Neurologica[*]

Istituto di Patologia Speciale Medica, Università , Perugia, Italy [**]

INTRODUCTION

The patogenesis of diabetic neuropathy is dependent, at least in part, on hyperglycemia per se as was shown in nely or recently diagnosed diabetic patients. In fact, someAA showed a regression of electromyographical signs after a few days of treatment, parallel with improvement or normalization of blood glucose levels [1,2].

The aim of our study was to verify if the motor and sensory conduction velocity (MCV, SCV) could be modified after short-term glyco-metabolic control obtained with artificial bet cell (or Biostator).

MATERIALS AND METHODS

Sixteen diabetic patients were studied, divided into two groups.

In the first group, consisting of eight diabetic patients with neuropathy, the MCV and/or SCV was decreased in at least two peripheral nerves (Table 1).

The mean age of the patients studied was 34 years - the youngest was 19 and the oldest was 53.

The mean duration of diabetes was about 22 months, not considering case n.6, in which it had lasted 20 years. The control group consisted of 8 diabetics with no decrease in MCV and/or SCV, who had the same characteristics for age and duration of disease. To evaluate physiological fluctuations in nerve conduction velocity, 8 normal subjects were examined at 3 day intervals. No significant differences were registered.

The MCV of the two peroneals and tibials and the SCV of the right median were determined twice, before and after treatment with biostator.

The nerves were stimulated with supermaximal impulses and the muscle response was recorded with a lower than 2 K ohm skin resistance.

All measurements were made by the same investigator in the same environment, with skin temperature maintained at or above 30ºC.

Our normal laboratory values were:

for MCV: Right and left peroneal = 47.7 ± 4.5

M.C.V. AND S.C.V. m/s

	AGE YEARS	DURATION OF DIABETES	before treatment with B Cell					after treatment with B Cell				
			R.P.	L.P.	R.T.	L.T.	R.M.	R.P.	L.P.	R.T.	L.T.	R.M.
1	33	2 MONTHS	48,3	48	37,1	34,1	.69	46,1	48,3	44,2	43	65,9
2	49	1 YEAR	32,8	45,1	42,3	41,6	52,1	44,3	47,2	48	42,5	61,4
3	37	2 YEARS	39,6	45,8	40,9	41,1	55,3	44	45,2	46,1	42,9	56,4
4	23	5 YEARS	44,5	52,4	35,2	38,4	62,5	51,7	55,3	42,7	47,4	61,4
5	50	3 YEARS	42,6	38,7	46,6	37,9	67,5	45,3	44,3	45,4	46	68,9
6	53	20 YEARS	34,2	39,4	43,4	38,1	48,9	38,6	38,2	46,4	39	54,6
7	46	4 YEARS	38,3	44,1	45,1	40,1	52,1	46,1	47,5	44,3	43,1	62,1
8	19	2 MONTHS	41,5	42,3	38,1	46,1	50	54	49,2	45	50	68,5

R.P. and L.P. = RIGHT and LEFT Peroneal

R.T. and L.T. = RIGHT and LEFT Posterior Tibial

R.M.　　　　　 = RIGHT MEDIAN

MOTOR AND SENSORY CONDUCTION VELOCITY IN PERIPHERAL NERVES IN 8 DIABETICS
WITH NEUROPATHY BEFORE (B) AND AFTER (A) THREE DAY TREATMENT WITH ARTIFICI
β-CELL (BIOSTATOR)

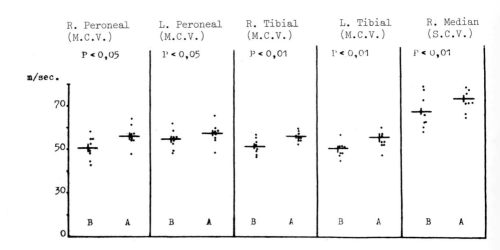

Right and left tibial = 45.1 + 3.8
for SCV of median = 62.7 + 4.3

RESULTS

The results obtained are indicated in Tables 1 and 2. Of the 21 pathological nerves examined there was an increase in the CV in 16 of the nerves(6 peroneal nerves, 7 post-orbital nerves, 3 right median nerves), while in five, four of which belonging to patient n.6 whose diabetes had lasted for 20 years, there was no improvement.

Therefore in patients in which the diabetes had a shorter duration (22 months) there was an improvement in the MCV and/or SCV.

This improvement was more apparent in patient n.4, who had been diagnosed a diabetic only two months before and in who there was a severe initial glyco-metabolic imbalance.

Instead no significant changes of nerve conduction velocity was observed in the patients of the second group.

CONCLUSIONS

Our study therefore demonstrates that in a group of patients with an alteration of CV, the MCV and SCV increase significantly after strict glyco-metabolic control.

These findings are compatible with the hypothesis that diabetic neuropathy derives from hyperglycemia [3,4].

The correction of the glyco-metabolic imbalance can, therefore, be the best way to prevent or improve diabetic neuropathy, at least in its initial phases, when the alterations of the nerves are still reversable because they are caused only by metabolic disorders.

REFERENCES

1. Ward, J.D., Barnes, C.G., Fisher, D.J., Jessop, J.D., Baker, R.W.R. (1971) Lanced 1, 428-431.

2. Fraser, D.M., Campbell, I.W., Ewing, D.J., Murray, A., Nielson, J.M.M., Clarke, B.F. (1977) Diabetes, 6, 546-550.

3. Gabbay, K.H., Tze, W.J. (1972) Proc.Natl.Acad.Sci.USA, 69, 1435.

4. Ward, J.D. (1974) Diabetes Proc. 8th Congr.Inter.Fedn., Bruxelles 1973 - Excerpta Medica, Amsterdam, pp. 419.

Peripheral Neuropathies
N. Canal and G. Pozza, eds.
© 1978 Elsevier/North-Holland Biomedical Press

DIABETIC NEUROPATHY IN CHILDREN

V.GALLAI,[*] F.MASSI-BENEDETTI,[**] C.FIRENZE,[*] A.ROSSI,[*] L.AGOSTINI[*] and G.LANZI[***]

Istituto di Clinica Neurologica - Università di Perugia Italy[*]

Istituto di Clinica Pediatrica - Università di Perugia - Italy [**]

Cattedra di Neuropsichiatria Infantile - Università di Pavia - Italy [***]

INTRODUCTION

Diabetic neuropathy in children has been studied much less than in adults, even though it presents very interesting aspects. In fact, in children it is much easier to establish the real onset of the diabetes and the ischemic vascular disturbances are far less important than those in adults.

MATERIALS AND METHODS

The object of this work was to study 30 diabetics between the ages of 3 and 16 who were admitted consecutively to our hospital within the last year. The patients were examined clinically and the M.C.V. of peroneal, tibial and S.C.V. median both sides was determined in each one. The velocity was determined with a Medelic Electromyography, the stimulus consisted of supermaximal impulses and the recording was done using surface electrodes with lower than 2 K ohm resistance. The room temperature was always constant. The mean values in our laboratory for the single nerves were R.P. 48.4 $\pm$ 4.2; L.P. 50.2 $\pm$ 6.3; R.T. 46.5 $\pm$ 5.2; L.T. 45.7 $\pm$ 4.8; R.M. 65.7 $\pm$ 5.4; L.M. 64.8 $\pm$ 4.5.

The degree of metabolic control in diabetes was established by periodic hemato-chemical and urinary controls according to White's data [1].

RESULTS

The diagnosis of neuropathy was made only on the basis of clinical signs (deep reflex, vibration, position sense, pin-prick and temperature sensation): mild, if there were at least 2 objective symptoms, moderate-severe if there were objective signs.

In all cases of neuropathy the conduction velocity was decreased in at least two nerves; where there were no clinical signs, but only electrophysiological ones, we did not diagnose it as neuropathy; in this latter case one could, however, speak of subclinical neuropathy.

The total of neuropathy in our 30 patients is reported in Table 1. The relationship to age was not statistically significant. The mean age at the onset of the diabetes was about 7, in those without it was about 8. In 6 cases the neuropathy was mixed sensory-motor distal symmetrical, while in two cases it was only sensory, distal symmetrical.

TABLE 1

DISTRIBUTION OF NEUROPATHY ACCORDING TO THE AGE

P = n.s. (Chi square)

| AGE (Years) | NEUROPATHY | | | MEAN DURATION of DIABETES (months) |
	ABSENT	MILD	MODERATE SEVERE	
12 No. cases 16	12 (75 %)	2 (12.5 %)	2 (12.5 %)	26
13 - 16 No. cases 14	10 (71.5 %)	1 (7.1 %)	3 (21.4 %)	56
3 - 16 Total cases 30	22 (73.3 %)	3 (10 %)	5 (16.7 %)	41

There was no significant relationship between sex and duration with neuropathy. On the basis of the duration of the diabetes (Fig.1) the patients were divided into three groups: those with the same diabetic duration or lower than 24 months, those with a duration of from 25 to 59 months and those over 60 months. In these groups neuropathy was present in 16.6%, in 28.6% and in 36.3% respectively. There is no significant relationship with the duration even if we divide the patients into 2 groups: 12 years or under and from 13 to 16 years.

A high significance (P < 0.005 Chi square) was found for neuropathy with glyco-metabolic control of diabetes (Fig.2).

One limitation in our date derives from the fact that there were only a few cases with fair and poor glyco-metabolic controls. (In our cases there was no significant relationship between the degree of glyco-metabolic control and the duration of the diabetes).

Particular attention was given to the study of the C.V. of nerves to confirm the clinical diagnosis of neuropathy as well as to detect initial electrophysiological abnormalities, that is, subclinical neuropathy.

We observed that with an increase in the duration of the diabetes there is a statistically significant decrease in the C.V. of the left peroneal nerve (M.C.V.) (from 50.6 $\pm$ 1.7 to 43 + 2.2) and in the right median (S.C.V.) from 61.1 + 1.3 to 55.6 + 2) while the decrease was not significant in other nerves.

As seen in clinical neuropathy, the degree of glyco-metabolic control is also very important in determining a decrease in the C.V. (Fig.2). In fact, concerning the peroneal and tibial nerves, there is a significant decrease in M.C.V. between the group with excellent and good glyco-metabolic controls and the group with fair and poor controls.

DISTRIBUTION OF NEUROPATHY ACCORDING
TO THE GLYCO-METABOLIC CONTROL

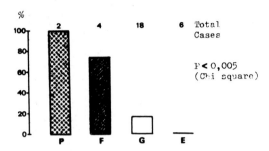

MOTOR CONDUCTION VELOCITY IN PATIENTS WITH DIFFERENT METABOLIC CONTROL (MEAN ± SEM)

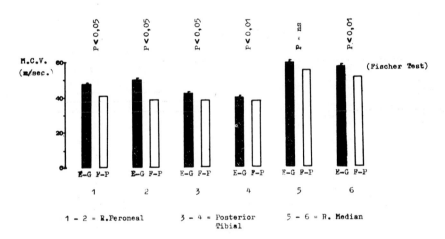

1 - 2 = R.Peroneal   3 - 4 = Posterior   5 - 6 = R. Median
                                Tibial

The C.V. of nerves was pathological in a higher number of patients than those having clinical neuropathy. (subclinical neuropathy).

The nerves most affected seemed to be the left (43.3%) and right (40%) median (S.C.V.), while the right and left posterior tibials of the lower limbs were affected in 36.6 % and 33.3 % of cases respectively, and the right and left peroneal nerve in 30% and 33% of cases respectively.

CONCLUSIONS

The findings of our study are in agreement with Lawrence et al. [2] and Gamstorp et al. [3] that neuropathy is a complication of diabetes in infancy as well as childhood. There is a 26% incidence if only the clinical form is considered and about 35% considering the sub-clinical form as well.

Unlike in adults, in children the clinical onset of diabetes coincides with its real onset so that one may affirm that there is not statistically significant relationship between the duration of diabetes and the appearance of neurological complications. This data dissociates diabetic neuropathy from the vascular complications of diabetes which are in significant relationship to its duration. Furthermore, the presence of diabetic neuropathy in infancy-childhood, toghether with other data,[4,5,6] is contrary to a vascular pathogenetic hypothesis, while a metabolic hypothesis assumes greater importance[7,8]. On the other hand, it is more difficult to control diabetes in children than in adults, so that even in children with a very low real duration there is the appearance of neuropathy. Our study, therefore, stresses the need for careful control of diabetes in order to avoid its possible neurological complications.

REFERENCES

1. White, P., Joslin, E.P., Root, H.F., Marble, A. (1959) The treatment of diabetes mellitus Ed. by Febiget, Philadelphia, pp., 47

2. Lawrence, D.G., Loche, S. (1963) Br.Med.J., 5333, 784.

3. Gamstorp, I., Shelburne, S.A.Jr., Engelson, G., Redond, D., Traisman, H.S. (1966) Diabetes, 15, 411.

4. Pirart, J. (1965) Diabetes 14, 1.

5. Chopra, J.S., Hurwitz, L.J., Montgomery, D.A.D. (1969) Brain 92, 391.

6. Ward, J.D. (1974) Diabetes Proc. 8th Congr.Inter.Fedn., Bruxelles 1973, Excerpta Medica, Amsterdam, pp.419

7. Gabbay, K.H., (1966) Science, 51, 209.

8. Gabbay, K.H., Tze, W.J. (1972) Proc.Nat.Acad.Sci.USA, 69, 1435.

Peripheral Neuropathies
N. Canal and G. Pozza, eds.
© 1978 Elsevier/North-Holland Biomedical Press

F AND H RESPONSES IN THE EVALUATION OF CONDUCTION VELOCITY IN THE PROXIMAL
TRACTS OF PERIPHERAL NERVES IN DIABETIC AND ALCOHOLIC PATIENTS

W. TRONI, L. BERGAMINI and F. LACQUANITI
Neurological Clinic, University of Turin, Turin (Italy)

ABSTRACT

The F and H responses were used for the evaluation of the conduction velocity
in the more proximal districts of peripheral nerves in normal subjects, in diabetic and alcoholic patients without clinical signs of peripheral neuropathy.
The results obtained in pathological conditions suggest the doubtful reliability of the use of F wave in clinical practice, particularly in recording from
EDB. The conduction velocity in the H pathway is early reduced especially in
alcoholics. This finding may indicate an earlier involvement of the afferent
pathway than of the efferent one in the monosynaptic circuit in subclinical
patients.

INTRODUCTION

The traditional methods for determining the motor and sensory conduction velocity do not allow the exploration of the most proximal segments of the peripheral nerves. The H and F responses, that could be helpful to this aim, have
not been much exploited for conduction studies because clear, univocal methods
providing results directly comparable with those obtained from the distal segments are not yet available.

Kimura[1] in 1974 first used the F wave in the measurement of the motor conduction velocity in the proximal tracts of the upper limbs. More recently (1977)
Panayiotopoulos et al[2] have proposed a similar method for the lower limbs.

The present work has two main goals : first, we want to consider some unclear
and questionable methodological aspects related to the use of F wave in conduction studies ; second, on the basis of the obtained data, we apply F and H responses to the study of subclinical peripheral neuropathies to evaluate their
real usefulness in the clinical practice in the measure of the C.V. in the proximal segments of the lower limbs.

MATERIALS AND METHODS

This study was carried out in 30 normal subjects (21-63 Yr.; mean : 36.2),
26 diabetic patients (14-64 Yr.; mean : 39.1) and 22 alcoholic patients (31-
58 Yr.; mean : 42.6), all of them without clinical signs of peripheral neuro-

thy. We determined in both lower limbs, the "distal" maximal motor conduction velocity (dMMCV) in the knee-ankle tract and the "proximal" maximal motor conduction velocity (pMMCV) in the knee-cord tract by using M and F responses recorded from the extensor digitorum brevis muscle (EDB) with surface electrodes by supramaximal stimulation of the deep peroneal nerve at the knee. We calculated the pMMCV following the formula (Panayiotopoulos et al.)[2] :

$$\frac{(\text{ Distance between L1 and the stim. point at knee x 2) cm.}}{(\text{ shortest } F_k - M_k \text{ latency} - 1 \text{) msec.}}$$

For each determination a hundred of serial stimuli at the frequency of 0.5/sec. were delivered. In order to avoid contamination by randomly occurring voluntary potentials, we chose for pMMCV estimate only the minimum-latency F waves recurring more than once with the same latency and morphology (see results).

Similarly we determined dMMCV in the poples-ankle tract and pMMCV in the poples-cord tract by using M and F responses recorded from the abductor digiti minimi muscle (ADM) with a coaxial needle electrode by supramaximal stimulation of the posterior tibial nerve at the poples.

Furthermore the conduction velocity in the monosynaptic pathway (HCV) was bilaterally valued by employing the M and H responses recorded from soleus muscle with a coaxial needle electrode by stimulating the posterior tibial nerve at the poples. The following formula was used :

$$\frac{(\text{ Distance between L1 and the stimulus point at poples x 2) cm}}{(\text{ H latency} - M_p \text{ latency} - 1 \text{) msec.}}$$

It must be stressed that this HCV represents no more than an "H index" because it is a mean between a fast afferent pathway and a much slower efferent one.

RESULTS

Normal subjects. Recording from EDB, we observed in all subjects F responses but with a high variability of frequency (in some cases more than 90 % of stimuli elicited F waves, in others only 5-10 % of stimuli did so). It must be noted that, as shown in fig. 1 (where a brief sequence of responses is presented), the large pool of the recorded F waves is composed actually by a limited number of well recognizable potentials of simple morphology which occur at random but with constant shape and latency throughout the recording session (the same potentials are identified with the same letter in fig. 1).

Recording from ADM, the antidromic responses appear, on the contrary, in nearly all stimulations and very often show a composed and polyphasic morphology.

In table I all the results are summarized ; note that the pMMCV is higher

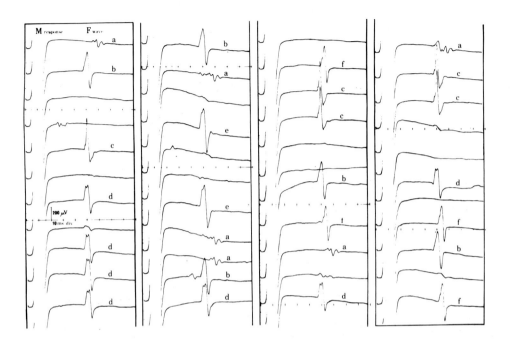

Fig. 1 F responses from EDB. For explanations see text.

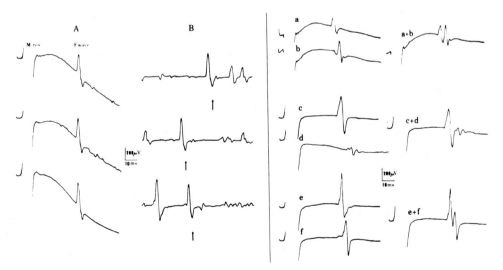

Fig. 2 For explanations see text

than dMMCV in both deep peroneal and posterior tibial nerve in good agreement with the well accepted[3] proximal-distal .gradient of motor C.V. The highest values were observed for the HCV and this is not surprising if we consider the contribution of the fast Ia afferent fibres.

Diabetic and alcoholic patients. On EMG examination, in many diabetic and alcoholic patients we often found an evident reduction of the pattern of voluntary recruitment in EDB that was clinically unsuspicious. In these cases, although a quantitative estimate has not been made, a marked reduction of the number of the single antidromic potentials was observed.

Recording from ADM, no significant differences with controls were noted in the features and frequency of the antidromic discharge.

Recording from EDB, in both diabetic and alcoholic patients pMMCV is significantly more reduced than dMMCV (- 8 m/s and -4.5 m/s respectively for diabetics; - 4.5 m/s and - 1.9 m/s respectively for alcoholics below the normal values).

Recording from ADM, on the contrary, the decrease of pMMCV and dMMCV is homogeneous and does not corroborate the previous results obtained from EDB. (- 4.8 m/s and - 4.3 m/s respectively for diabetics ; - 1.9 m/s and - 0.9 m/s respectively for alcoholics below normal values ; note that in the last the decreases are not significant).

The HCV values in both diabetic and alcoholic patients are more reduced than the dMMCV of the posterior tibial nerve. For diabetics however the difference between the reduction of HCV and that of dMMCV is not significant (- 6.9 m/s for the HCV and - 4.3 m/s for the dMMCV below normal values).
In alcoholics instead the same difference is significant (- 4.5 m/s for the HCV and - 0.9 for the dMMCV below normal values).

DISCUSSION

The features of the antidromic responses from EDB, consisting in several types of low amplitude potentials randomly occurring with constant latency and morphology, seem to suggest that most F waves, at least in the case of EDB recording, represent actually the antidromic discharge of single spinal motor neurones as proposed by Feasby and Brown as well[4]. We could indeed record, during voluntary contraction of EDB, rare potentials that proved to be identical with particular F waves (fig. 2, left) thus providing a further clue supporting our hypothesis about the nature of the F wave. Sometimes the simultaneous discharge of two motor neurones was observed : in these cases two simple potentials were recorded paired in a combined morphology in which the single components were still distinguishable (fig. 2,right). Within each subject a great variability of recurrence exists among different types of F waves indicating a parallel variability in the likelihood of antidromic discharge among different motor neurones.

These features of the antidromic discharge clearly indicate that, recording from EDB, the evaluation of the pMMCV is actually based on the conduction velocity of a single motor fibre.

TABLE I

		E D B		A D M		
		dMMCV	pMMCV	dMMCV	pMMCV	HCV
Controls	Range	42.8 - 55.3	49.4 - 58.2	40.1 - 48.7	45.4 - 54	53.6 - 59
	Mean ± SD	49 ± 2.6	54.4 ± 1.9	45.9 ± 1.7	50.9 ± 1.8	55.9 ± 1.5
Alcoholics	Range	40.3 - 52.3	43.6 - 55	35.6 - 49.4	37 - 53.4	43.9 - 58.3
	Mean ± SD	47.1" ± 2.9	49.9" ± 2.8	45 ' ± 3.2	49 ' ± 3.6	51.4" ± 3.3
Diabetics	Range	33.2 - 54.6	35.6 - 56	36.6 - 47.5	40.6 - 53.4	43 - 57.7
	Mean ± SD	44.5"' ± 4.1	46.4"' ± 3.7	41.6"' ± 2.7	46.1"' ± 2.6	49"' ± 3.2

*= not significant with Student t test. ' = P<0.05 with Student t test.
'' = P<0.01 with Student t test.   ''' = P<0.001 with Student t test.

It is evident that the correct determination of the pMMCV requires therefore the recording of the antidromic discharge of the motor neurones with maximal conduction velocity. Of course the larger is the sample size of the F waves recorded, the higher is the likelihood of a reliable estimate of pMMCV. Thus it is clear that the margin of safety of the method can decrease in clinical states characterized by a loss of motor fibres and this is particularly true if large size motor neurones are prominently involved. Therefore, even on a mere theoretical ground, this method from EDB is burdened, in our opinion, with heavy and unavoidable limits. On the contrary, the higher frequency of the antidromic responses from ADM can make the use of this derivation site a more reliable one.

The greater involvement of pMMCV in both diabetic and alcoholic patients represents a striking result if we consider the general agreement of pathologists about the prevalent distal damage and about the scanty abnormalities of the anterior roots (afferent and efferent pathway of the F response) in diabetic and [5-6] alcoholic[7] neuropathies. Moreover the results obtained from ADM, not confirming the prevalent proximal involvement, seem to invalidate the reliability of the results obtained from EDB. A possible reason for this fact can be found in the subclinical denervation of EDB seen on EMG examination in a lot of our patients. Also recent quantitative studies[8] have pointed out a marked loss of motor units in EDB of diabetics without clinical signs of neuropathy. Probably a similar situation is present in alcoholics. It is not amazing that, in these cases, a marked decrease in the number of distinct F waves recorded was observed. This finding, probably expression of a reduced number of functioning motor fibres, may be a factor of unreliability of this method applied to EDB because, as previously remarked, the likelihood of recording the F wave at minumum latency is grossly reduced. In three diabetics and in two alcoholics indeed, we were compelled to estimate the pMMCV on the basis of a single recorded F wave.

The early fall of C.V. along the H pathway is the most interesting datum emerged from our study, particularly in alcoholics. Also Blackstock et al.[9] in asymptomatic alcoholics, reported a clear increase in the mean latency of the H reflex (+ 3.3 ms) above controls with a near normal dMMCV of the deep peroneal nerve. Since we have no data for suspecting a prominent involvement of the motor fibres of soleus, the increase in the latency of the H response seems to suggest an early lesion in the afferent pathway. This comes out also from the results of Guiheneuc and Bathien[10] who found in alcoholics a severe decrease in the H max./ M max. ratio, indicating a prominent loss of Ia afferent fibres. Moreover there are several pathological reports on the severe degeneration of nerve cells of the spinal ganglia and on the pronounced segmental demyelination of the posterior roots in diabetic[5,6] and alcoholic[7] neuropathy. However it must be noted that pathological studies performed post-mortem in patients with advanced neuropathy provide poor informations about the time occurrence of these lesions which, from our results, seem to be an early finding in subclinical patients. The early involvement of the spinal ganglia cells can furthermore explain the equally early fall of the sensory potential amplitude : a well known finding in alcoholic patients.[11]

Although further data are needed, the evaluation of the conduction velocity in the H pathway seems to be, in our opinion, a method useful for the early diagnosis of peripheral neuropathy especially in the alcoholic one. This fact may be justified by an early demyelination of the posterior roots in these pathological conditions.

REFERENCES

1. Kimura,J. (1974) F-wave velocity in the central segment of median and ulnar

nerves., Neurology, 24, 539-546.

2. Panayiotopoulos, C.P., Scarpalezos, S. and Nastas, P.E. (1977) F-wave studies on the deep peroneal nerve. Part 1. Control Subjects., J. neurol. Sci., 31, 319-329.

3. Kaeser, H.E. (1970) Nerve conduction velocity measurement. In: P. J. Vinken and G. W. Bruyn (Eds), Handbook of Clinical Neurology, Vol 7, North-Holland, Amsterdam, pp. 116-196.

4. Feasby, T.E. and Brown, W.F. (1974) Variation of motor unit size in the human extensor digitorum brevis and thenar muscles., J. Neurol. Neurosurg. Psychiat., 37, 916-926.

5. Dolman, C.L. (1963) The morbid anatomy of diabetic neuropathy., Neurology, 13, 135-142

6. Thomas, P.K. and Lascelles, R.G. (1966) The pathology of diabetic neuropathy. Quart. J. Med., 35, 489-509.

7. Vignon, G.M., Megard, M. and Marin, A. (1956) Une observation anatomo-clinique d'acropathie ulcèro-mutilente., Presse Méd., 64, 1954-1956.

8. Hansen, S. and Ballantine, J.P. (1977) Axonal dysfunction in the neuropathy of diabetes mellitus. A quantitative electrophysiological study., J. Neurol. Neurosurg. Psychiat., 40, 555-564

9. Blackstock, E., Rushwort, G. and Gath, D. (1972) Electrophysiological studies in alcoholism., J. Neurol. Neurosurg. Psychiat., 35, 326-334.

10. Guiheneuc, P. and Bathien, N. (1976) Two patterns of results in polyneuropathies investigated with the H reflex., J. neurol. Sci., 30, 83-94

11. Bergamini, L., Gandiglio, G., Fra, L., Bergamasco, B., Bram., S. and Mombelli, A.M. (1965) Alterazioni della conduzione nervosa sensitiva e motoria in alcoolisti cronici privi di segni di neuropatia periferica., Riv. Pat. nerv. ment., 86, 31-49.

COMPRESSION NEUROPATHIES

Peripheral Neuropathies
N. Canal and G. Pozza, eds.
© 1978 Elsevier/North-Holland Biomedical Press

CONDUCTION BLOCK IN ACUTE COMPRESSION

ROGER W. GILLIATT

Institute of Neurology, Queen Square, London, WC1N 3BG

This review begins with the classical studies of
Dr. Denny-Brown and his colleagues at the end of World War II,
as these were the first to indicate the presence of a
characteristic anatomical change caused by acute compression.
Although for many years neurologists had been aware that
compression could produce a conduction block lasting for days
or weeks, the nature of the anatomical change was quite obscure.
One hundred years ago Erb himself referred to "a change in the
molecular constitution of the motor nerves so as to abolish
their power of conduction"[1]. Seventy years later, the
situation was no better; Seddon[2] gave a good clinical
description of these cases, for which he coined the term
"neurapraxia", but was forced to admit "neurapraxia is as yet
insecure morphologically".

The papers of Denny-Brown, Brenner and others[3-7] are therefore
extremely important ones. In peripheral nerves damaged by
compression, percussion, stretching or cooling, it was noted
that the injury resulted in selective myelin damage,
longitudinal sections showing gaps in the myelin sheaths
without degeneration of the axons. These myelin defects were
identified with the type of change described by Gombault in
1880[8], which we now know as segmental demyelination.

In the years before Denny-Brown's papers the concept of
segmental demyelination had become rather neglected, and our
present realisation of its great importance in both the
peripheral and the central nervous system really stems from
this work on mechanical lesions of peripheral nerves and the
later work in Denny-Brown's unit by Fisher and Adams[9] on
demyelination in the roots of autopsied patients with
diphtheritic polyneuropathy. This led to the experimental

study by Waksman, Adams and Mansmann[10] of diphtheritic neuritis
in rabbits and guinea-pigs, and to the first electrophysiological
studies of diphtheritic animals, those of Kaeser and Lambert[11]
in America and of McDonald[12,13] in New Zealand.

Our understanding of conduction delay and conduction block
in demyelinated fibres has been greatly clarified by the work
of Sears, Rasminsky and Bostock. In their first paper
Rasminsky and Sears[14] showed that conduction in partially
demyelinated rat nerves remained saltatory until it was
blocked completely, the slow velocity being accounted for by
greatly increased nodal delays at individual nodes of Ranvier.
Conduction delay could easily be converted into conduction
block by a small change in the physical state of the
preparation, such as a slight rise in temperature[15].
Subsequently, continuous conduction over demyelinated internodes has been demonstrated[16,17] but the factors which determine in a damaged fibre whether conduction becomes continuous
or is blocked completely still require to be elucidated.

In acute nerve compression conduction is of course blocked
or delayed from the time of the injury, whereas degeneration
of the paranodal myelin takes several days. The conduction
defect during the first 24 hours cannot therefore be due to
paranodal demyelination. To what then is it due? The answer
came from the beautiful electron microscope preparations made
by my colleague Dr. Ochoa, which showed that compression in the
experimental animal causes movement of the nodes of Ranvier,
with distortion and invagination of paranodal myelin[18].
It as also shown that the movement is in opposite directions
at each edge of a compressed zone (Fig. 1), from which it may
be assumed that the force which moves the axoplasm and
invaginates the myelin is the pressure difference between
one point and another along the course of the axon. As there
is no pressure gradient in the centre of the compressed
region the nodes in the centre remain normal.

site of compression

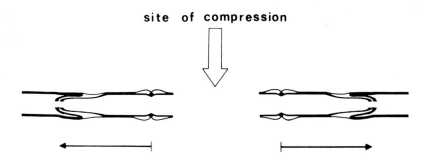

Figure 1

The postulated sequence of events at each node is therefore
as follows. First of all, nodal displacement with stretching
and invagination of paranodal myelin. The Schwann-cell junction
retains its original position, marking the old site of the node
by a slight indentation, from which the node may be displaced
for a distance of more than 100 µm. The part of the myelin
sheath between the two degenerates, giving rise to a comparable
length of paranodal demyelination. Remyelination subsequently
occurs in the usual way. In severe cases there is obvious
mechanical damage to the distorted myelin, with rupture of
lamellae at the time of compression, so that the transverse
resistance of the myelin may be reduced sufficiently to block
saltatory conduction from the time of injury. In mild cases,
however, the distorted paranodal myelin does not appear to
have been grossly damaged, although the nodal gap is occluded,
and it is possible that in such cases the buried nodes behave
like the locally anaesthetised nodes in Tasaki's classical
experiments on saltatory conduction[19].

Once paranodal demyelination has occurred, we have a
situation similar to that studied by Rasminsky and Sears in
their diphtheritic rat nerves, and we can assume that the
same physiological considerations would apply. By stimulating
and recording from the exposed nerve a few days after
compression it is possible to show that the conduction delay

and conduction block is limited to regions near the edges of
the cuff, and that the same nerve fibres in the centre of the
compressed zone have a normal excitability and conduction
velocity[20].

The duration of the conduction block which can be produced
by compression varies greatly from one example to another. In
both man and animals severe lesions may show a block which does
not begin to recover for 8 - 10 weeks, and in which some fibres
are still blocked after 4 - 6 months[21,22,23]. The factors
upon which the duration of block depends are still not fully
understood but the magnitude of the compressive force and its
duration are of obvious importance[21]. The length of the
lesion is also important, suggesting that a long lesion is
more likely than a short one to contain a few nodes at which
repair is delayed[24].

The cause of the delayed repair after compression injury is
itself an interesting problem; there is the possibility that
reactive swelling of Schwann cell cytoplasm within the compact
myelin (ad-axonal Schwann-cell oedema) may be a relevant factor,
as this persists for many weeks after injury, leading to
delayed demyelination of the distended myelin sheath[18].

Regardless of its cause, the persistence of conduction
block for many weeks after acute compression injury has
important clinical implications. For the electromyographer
it means that if a local block can be identified by nerve
stimulation, even in the presence of Wallerian degeneration
in other fibres of the same nerve, surgical exploration should
not be undertaken as the block is likely to recover with the
passage of time[25]. This interpretation is only justified when
a single episode of compression has occurred; in chronic or
recurrent compression other considerations may apply.

The effects of prolonged conduction block on the function
of the distal part of the axon and on the paretic muscle which
it innervates are of some theoretical and practical interest.
The authors of the 'double crush syndrome'[26] have postulated
that proximal compression might impair axonal transport and
make the distal part of the axon more susceptible to further

injury. For acute compression blocks there is no evidence that this occurs, since regeneration following distal nerve crush has been shown to be normal in fibres in which impulse traffic has been abolished by a proximal compression block[27].

There are, however, changes in the extrajunctional muscle membrane during acute compression block[28], including a rise in sensitivity to applied ACh[29], which raise the possibility that the conduction block can itself cause spontaneous fibrillation in the inactive muscle[28,30]. The issue is not fully decided but recent experiments on subhuman primates suggest that a conduction block produces no more than a minimal rise in insertion activity in an affected muscle and that spontaneous fibrillation does not occur in the absence of Wallerian degeneration[31].

The histological and physiological features of acute compressive lesions emphasise the direct mechanical nature of the injury; nerve ischaemia due to occlusion of the vasa nervorum seems a less important factor[32]. Whether ischaemia plays any role in causing or exaggerating the nerve damage is still debated[33,34] but recent evidence from subhuman primates suggests that ischaemia of the compressed tissues does not contribute to the nerve damage provided that the duration of the ischaemia is short[35]. In these experiments ischaemia of the hind limb from a cuff round the thigh for three or four hours was sometimes sufficient to cause transient skin and muscle oedema under and distal to the cuff. However, ischaemia of this duration did not affect the outcome of local compression of the anterior tibial nerve at the ankle, when this was carried out during the period of total limb ischaemia.

This result is in agreement with the fact that a pressure block is most likely to be caused by a compressing force which is large, acting over an area which is small[24], conditions which favour direct mechanical damage without ischaemia. Thus tourniquet paralysis in patients was frequently seen when narrow rubber tourniquets or Esmarch bandages were used in orthopaedic surgery but became relatively rare after pneumatic tourniquets had been generally adopted[21,36,37,38].

310

1. Erb, W.H. (1876) in von Ziemssen, H.W., Cyclopaedia of the Practice of Medicine, New York, William Wood & Co., 11.

2. Seddon, H.J. (1943) Brain, 66, 237-288.

3. Denny-Brown, D. and Brenner, C. (1944) Arch. Neurol. Psychiat., 51, 1-26.

4. Denny-Brown, D. and Brenner, C. (1944) Arch. Neurol. Psychiat., 52, 1-19.

5. Denny-Brown, D. and Brenner, C. (1944) J. Neurol. Neurosurg. Psychiat., 7, 76-95.

6. Denny-Brown, D. Doherty, M.M. (1945) Arch. Neurol. Psychiat., 54, 116-129.

7. Denny-Brown, D., Adams, R.D., Brenner, C. and Doherty, M.M. J. Neuropath. exp. Neurol., 4, 305-323.

8. Gombault, A. (1880) Arch. Neurol. (Paris), 1, 11-38.

9. Fisher, C.M. and Adams, R.D. (1956) J. Neuropath. exp. Neurol., 15, 243-268.

10. Waksman, B.H., Adams, R.D. and Mansmann, H.C. (1957) J. exp. Med., 105, 591-614.

11. Kaeser, H.E. and Lambert, E.H. (1962) Electroenceph. clin. Neurophysiol. Suppl., 22, 29-35.

12. McDonald, W.I. (1963) Brain, 86, 481-500.

13. McDonald, W.I. (1963) Brain, 86, 501-524.

14. Rasminsky, M. and Sears, T.A. (1972) J. Physiol., 227, pp 323-350.

15. Rasminsky, M. (1973) Arch. Neurol., 28, 287-292.

16. Rasminsky, M., Kearney, R.E., Aguayo, A.J. and Bray, G.M. (1978) Brain Res., 143, 71-85.

17. Bostock, H. and Sears, T.A. (1976) Nature, 263, 786-787.

18. Ochoa, J., Fowler, T.J. and Gilliatt, R.W. (1972) J. Anat., 113, 433-455.

19. Tasaki, I. (1953) Nervous Transmissions. Charles C. Thomas, Springfield, Illinois.

20. Gilliatt, R.W., McDonald, W.I. and Rudge, P. (1973) J. Physiol., 238, 31-32P.

21. Fowler, T.J., Danta, G. and Gilliatt, R.W. (1972) J. Neurol. Neurosurg. Psychiat., 35, 638-647.

22. Rudge, P. (1974) J. Bone Jt. Surg., 56B, 716-720.

23. Trojaborg, W. (1977) J. Neurol. Neurosurg. Psychiat., 40, 50-57.

24. Rudge, P., Ochoa, J. and Gilliatt, R.W. (1974) J. neurol. Sci., 23, 403-420.

25. Payan, J. (1970) J. Neurol. Neurosurg. Psychiat., 33, 157-165.

26. McComas, A.J., Jorgensen, P.B. and Upton, A.R.M. (1974)
    Canad. J. neurol. Sci., 1, 170-179.

27. Williams, I.R. and Gilliatt, R.W. (1977) J. neurol. Sci.,
    33, 267-273.

28. Cangiano, A., Lutzemberger, L. and Nicotra, L. (1977)
    J. Physiol., 273, 691-706.

29. Gilliatt, R.W., Westgaard, R.H. and Williams, I.R. (1977)
    J. Physiol., 271, 21-22P.

30. Trojaborg, W. (1978) Muscle and Nerve, in press.

31. Gilliatt, R.W., Westgaard, R.H. and Williams, I.R. (1978)
    J. Physiol., in press.

32. Gilliatt, R.W. (1975) in Eleventh Symposium on Advanced
    Medicine, Lant, A.F. ed. Pitman Medical, London, 144-163.

33. Lundborg, G. (1975) J. Bone Jt. Surg., 57A, 938-948.

34. Mäkitie, J. and Teräväinen, H. (1977) Acta neuropath.
    (Berl.), 37, 55-63.

35. Williams, I.R., Gilliatt, R.W. and Jefferson, D. (1977)
    Electroenceph. clin. Neurophysiol., 43, 592.

36. Bruner, J.M. (1951) J. Bone Jt. Surg., 33A, 221-224.

37. Bruner, J.M. (1970) Hand, 2, 39-42.

38. Klenerman, L. (1962) J. Bone Jt. Surg., 44B, 937-943.

Peripheral Neuropathies
N. Canal and G. Pozza, eds.
© 1978 Elsevier/North-Holland Biomedical Press

PATHOLOGY AND PATHOGENESIS OF TRAUMATIC NERVE LESIONS IN ANIMALS AND MAN, WITH
SPECIAL REFERENCE TO CHRONIC ENTRAPMENT

JOSE OCHOA

Department of Neurology, Dartmouth Medical School, Hanover, New Hampshire,

03755 USA

ABSTRACT

There exist well defined pathological situations related to local nerve

trauma where the effects of mechanical injury dissociate from those of anoxia.

Motor and sensory paralysis follow acute local compression of a limb above

systolic pressure. Such disorder of nerve function is immediately reversible

upon reestablishing blood flow. Lewis et al[1] showed this is caused by ischemia

and not by direct mechanical injury to the nerve. No structural changes can be

detected. More severe acute compression may cause paralysis and sensory loss,

from local conduction block, lasting weeks or a few months. Myelinated and

unmyelinated axons remain largely intact but demyelination is prominent (Denny-

Brown and Brenner[2]). The primary lesion which leads to demyelination is

obviously mechanical in origin and involves invagination of the extremities

(paranodes) of myelin segments - like an intussusception - in opposite direct-

ions under each edge of the compressed region (Ochoa et al[3,4]; Gilliatt, this

volume).

Myelinated fibres underlying chronic entrapment also suffer displacement of

structural components of myelin segments, again in opposite directions on either

side of the entrapped region, but there is no obliteration of the nodes of

Ranvier. Slippage of myelin lamellae explains progressive exposure of the axon

at the paranodes which point towards the area of entrapment, and buckling of the

opposite paranodes. Active demyelination, axonal degeneration and fibrosis

follow (Ochoa and Marotte[5]; Neary et al[6]).

Violent local nerve injury interrupts axons and may open breaches in peri-neurium. Attempts at repair by terminal axonal regeneration follow inevitably. Axonal outgrowths which escape beyond the perineurial continent overproliferate and fail to mature from lack of reconnection: dissident perineurial cells enclose them in miniature fascicles. In experimental neuromas these sprouts are abnormally excitable (Wall and Gutnick[7]): perhaps they explain spontaneous pain in human neuromas (Ochoa[8]).

INTRODUCTION

Local nerve lesions are no longer the dull chapter in nerve pathology. Indeed, some aspects of the pathology and pathogenesis of local nerve lesions caused by compression and entrapment have proven to be unexpectedly interesting. This is partly due to the fact that the nerve pathology at the single fibre level is quite spectacular, but mostly, it is due to the fact that the fine structural changes of the nerve fibres literally portray the mechanism of their causation.

It is difficult to envisage why relatively banale conditions, such as those resulting from nerve compression and entrapment, excite so much controversy regarding their pathogenesis. Both the advocates of direct mechanical injury and those of nerve ischemia have come up with apparently incontrovertible arguments and nobody would dare contradict the evidence that both ischemia and mechanical compression per se are quite capable of damaging nerves; however, when it comes to the specific cause of the primary pathology of nerve fibres in explicit conditions such as "Neurapraxia" or such as the "Carpal Tunnel Syndrome", then there must be discrete causative agents susceptible of investigation. Whether such pathological changes are responsible for all the clinical and electrophysiological manifestations is entirely another matter which deserves separate analysis.

In the following we will endeavor to produce convincing evidence to support that the common causative agent which explains the primary nerve fibre pathologies underlying both neurapraxia and chronic nerve entrapment is mechanical and not ischemic. For those who react instinctively against such dictum it may be worth a brief critical analysis of some pieces of information which appear to support the contrary. First, the experiments of Lewis, Pickering and Rothschild[1] demonstrating with classic elegance that local compression of an arm, above systolic pressure, leads to ascending paralysis and anesthesia from ischemia and not from direct mechanical nerve damage. The key experiment involved installing a sphigmomanometer cuff above systolic pressure in the upper arm, which was regularly followed by ascending paralysis and anesthesia of the limb. On release of the cuff, there was regular recovery of function almost immediately. Having installed the cuff and having awaited the usual 20-30 minutes until sensory-motor paralysis, a second cuff was installed at similar pressure proximal to the first one. Upon release of the first cuff there was no recovery, indicating that sustained ischemia and not local compression over a discrete area of nerve was responsible for the functional nerve defect. But here, paralysis and anesthesia are immediately reversible on restoring circulation and there is no demonstrable structural lesion. Obviously, such condition is quite independent from the relatively longstanding local nerve block which may occur following more prolonged and severe local compression (neurapraxia), and where Denny-Brown and Brenner[2] first demonstrated underlying demyelination. Although Denny-Brown and Brenner construed their acute demyelinating block as due to ischemia, modern microscopy has disclosed an early lesion of myelinated fibres which leads to demyelination and can only be explained through the action of mechanical forces (Ochoa et al[3]; Ochoa et al[4]). Such lesion is reviewed in Professor Gilliatt's chapter in this volume and will not distract us any further. Second, the famous experiment of Grundfest[9] on the effects of compression upon nerve conduction in vitro. This experiment was strategically quoted by Denny-Brown and Brenner[2] in support of nerve ischemia as the cause of neurapraxia; the argument may appear to be invulnerable, but probably is not. Grundfest, who was not interested in nerve pathology, observed that excised stretches of nerve within a pressure chamber would withstand tremendous pressures without conduction failure, provided there was oxygen in the chamber. A natural though falacious interpretation of this experiment is the following: anoxia is the cause of damage in nerve compression. A particular feature of the primary lesion of myelinated fibres underlying neurapraxia renders invalid the above interpretation: such lesion only occurs at the sites of pressure gradients between compressed and uncompressed nerve, and therefore could not be expected to occur in fragments of nerves compressed equally throughout their length within pressure chambers. Third, there is the common observation that nocturnal acroparesthesiae in carpal tunnel syndrome are promptly relieved by shaking the hand, "as though reestablishing circulation in an ischemic nerve". Indeed, it is perfectly possible that rapidly reversible paresthesiae of this kind are due to nerve fibre dysfunction caused by ischemic anoxia. But, is there a causal relationship between anoxia and the characteristic nerve fibre pathology found underlying chronic entrapment? Hopefully the evidence to be produced below will be convincing in a negative direction. The explanation for nocturnal acroparesthesiae in the carpal tunnel syndrome is probably found in the human experiments by Gilliatt and Wilson[10]: damaged nerves are more susceptible to ischemia and may generate paresthesiae earlier and more intensely than the normal.

In summary, to prelude this presentation, we have identified and questioned the pertinence of some pieces of information which form the basis for the common belief that ischemia is behind the pathogenesis of all forms of compression and entrapment neuropathies.

What follows is largely an account of collaborative work done at Queen Square
in London and at Dartmouth in the U.S.A. with my colleagues Drs. R. W. Gilliatt,
T. J. Fowler, P. Rudge, D. Neary, and Lauren Marotte. The findings in acute
compression leading to neurapraxia are reviewed in Gilliatt's chapter in this
volume. Here we concentrate on chronic entrapment.

After the peculiar lesion of myelinated fibres was identified underlying
tourniquet paralysis (Ochoa et al[3]) and also underlying an experimental form
of "Saturday Night Paralysis" (Rudge et al[11]), it seemed desirable to find out
whether a similar lesion was present underlying chronic entrapment. In other
words, there was an immediate question to explore: is _chronic_ entrapment just
the result of cummulative subclinical _acute_ compressions? The answer is no and
emerges from the application of plain histopathology. If only to dispel pessi-
mistic statements in the literature regarding the potential of histopathology in
this area, we will indulge in a heavily illustrated chapter and allow morphology
to speak for itself.

MATERIAL AND METHODS

Conventional histological methods applied to the median nerve at the carpal
tunnel in guinea pig were the initial basis of the studies to be described. The
application of improved fixation methods and, particularly, the use of ultrathin
longitudinal sections of myelinated fibres for electronmicroscopy, allowed
definitive insight into the nature of the primary lesion of myelinated fibres
underlying chronic entrapment[12]. Fresh postmortem human material was subsequently studied by Neary et al[13]: among twelve median nerves at the wrist
and twelve ulnar nerves at the elbow, obtained from random autopsies, there was
a surprisingly high incidence of local abnormalities, entirely similar to those
found in guinea pigs. Some of the fine structural features of abnormal single

human myelinated fibres obtained from that exclusive collection have been reported by Ochoa and Neary[14], as well as other general ultrastructural features in a proven post mortem case of ulnar entrapment at the elbow, studied by Neary and Eames[15].

Biopsy material from entrapped nerves in man, worked with a range of modern techniques, is exceptionally rare and probably limited to a few personal examples of lateral cutaneous of the thigh nerve from patients with meralgia paresthetica. Such material has yielded additional information on quantitative electronmicroscopy of unmyelinated fibres in human nerve entrapment.

RESULTS

It was Pierre Marie and Foix[16] who discovered that a cause for thenar muscle atrophy is an anatomical lesion of the median nerve at the wrist. Using their vintage histological stains they noticed that myelin tended to disappear at the level of the carpal tunnel in their patient. However, they did not examine the nerve distal to the wrist. Fifty years later, Thomas and Fullerton[17] studied another post mortem specimen of median nerve from a case of carpal tunnel syndrome proven electrophysiologically. Again myelin stains showed paucity of myelin at the level of the tunnel but cross sections of the nerve trunk at the palm showed reappearance of myelinated fibres. Clearly then, the local nerve lesion was not one that led necessarily to local axonal interruption: there must have been an element of local demyelination. Then came the discovery from Queen Square that guinea pigs aged 2 and over suffer from carpal tunnels..., and Gilliatt and his associates[18,19] confirmed local demyelination in the median nerve under the wrist in guinea pigs. They also described a peculiar distortion of the myelin segments proximal to the wrist: unlike the normal more or less symmetrical segments, these had a bulbous end and a tapered end, like long thin tadpoles. Consistently, the bulbous ends were directed away from the wrist, towards the axilla, fading away progressively up the forearm.

While working at Queen Square in Gilliatt's department, Ochoa and Marotte[4] adopted the guinea pig model of chronic nerve entrapment, primarily to check for the presence of indications of acute compression injury, i.e., "intussusception" of myelin segments. No suggestion of such change was ever found, even in young animals. This, in addition to the distinct changes found, indicated that the nerve fibre lesion underlying chronic entrapment is basically different from that underlying neurapraxia and not its relentless accummulation. Interestingly, however, when single microdissected nerve fibres were followed along the median nerve into the palm, it was found that distal to the carpal tunnel, the rigorous polarity of the distorted myelin segments (internodes), described by Gilliatt and collaborators[18] became reversed (Figure 1).

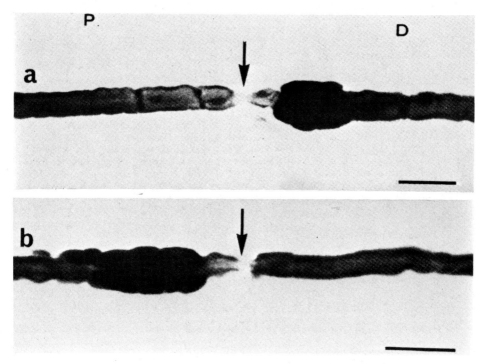

Fig. 1. Paranodal regions of deformed internodes; a was taken from above and b from below the wrist. The nodal gap is arrowed; P: proximal; D: distal. Bars: 20 µm.
From: Ochoa, J. and Marotte, L., in J. Neurol. Sci., 1973, 19:491-495.
Reproduced by permission of Elsevier, Amsterdam.

320

Tracing the lesion back, chronologically, in young animals showing mild
distortion of myelin segments but no local demyelination, a turning point could
often be demonstrated under the region of the tunnel (Figure 2a). With age,
the lesions become more grotesque, the nodal gaps become widened, and local
demyelination and remyelination follow (Figure 2b). Eventually, axons get
interrupted and their distal portions degenerate (Figure 2c).

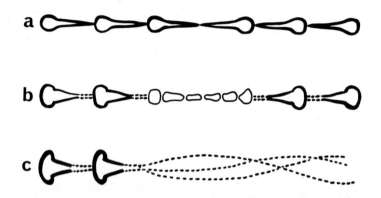

Fig. 2. Progression of the primary lesion of myelinated fibres underlying
chronic entrapment. a) Distorted myelin segments from median nerve of young
guinea pig. Polarity is reversed at the wrist. b) Increased deformity of the
myelin segments with partial exposure of axon towards the tapered ends of internodes. Thinly remyelinated segments repair local demyelination at the wrist.
c) Grotesque bulbous ends of distorted internodes and signs of Wallerian degeneration and regeneration at the wrist. Modified from Figure 5.5, Ochoa, in
Management of Peripheral Nerve Problems edited by Omer and Spinner, Saunders,
1978.

The fine structure of distorted myelin segments, as displayed in ultrathin
longitudinal sections is revealing of their pathogenesis. In brief, at the
tapered paranodes, groups of internal myelin lamellae appear to have slipped
away and buckle at the bulbous paranodes, where they are often found abnormally
inturned (Figure 3).

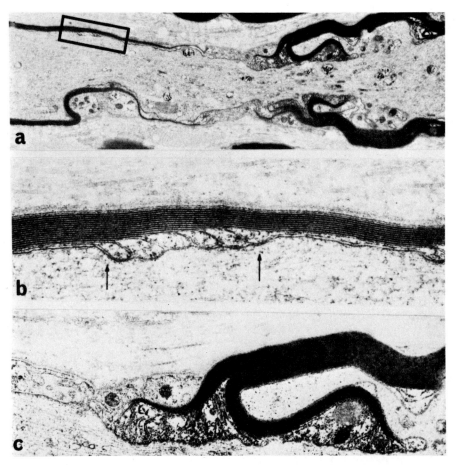

Fig. 3. a: low power electron micrograph of a moderately abnormal fibre taken
from above the wrist. The paranode on the left is tapered. The bulbous paranode on the right shows inturning of a group of inner lamellae. R: node of
Ranvier x 7000.
 b: enlargement of the area enclosed in the rectangle in a. Six myelin lamellae end in cytoplasmic loops between the arrows. x 48,000.
 c: detail of the bulbous paranodes. x 20,000
From: Ochoa, J. and Marotte, L., in J. Neurol. Sci., 1973, 19:491-495.
Reproduced by permission of Elsevier, Amsterdam.

The bulbous paranodes grow progressively larger from convolution of redundant

myelin which progressively deserts the paranodes closer to the site of entrap-

ment, as in Figure 4, illustrating human post mortem single fibre pathology.

322

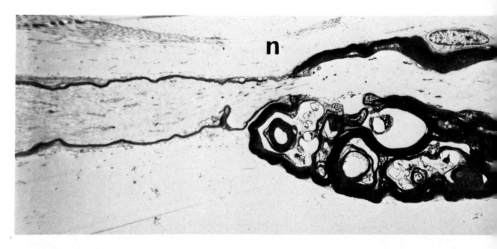

Fig. 4.   Low-power electron micrograph of single distorted fibre cut longitud-
inally (n=node of Ranvier).
From: Ochoa, J. and Neary, D., in Lancet, 1975, page 632.
Reproduced by permission of the Editors.

Loss of myelin (and remyelination) are, at least initially, confined to the

tapered ends of the myelin segments, thus providing good evidence that "demye-

lination" starts as simple slippage of myelin lamellae.   Active demyelination

seems to proceed at the level of the bulbs, where contorted myelin, perhaps

upset molecularly, may be invaded by mononuclear cells.   There is no reason why

ischemia should selectively damage the distal paranodes above the wrist and the

proximal paranodes below the wrist.

Figure 5 illustrates polarized demyelination affecting progressively the

tapered paranodes as the wrist is approached.

Although essentially different from acute "intussusception" underlying

neurapraxia, the peculiar telescoping of myelinated segments described above is

highly reminiscent of the former in the sense that there has been displacement

of structural components in opposite directions on either side of the entrapped

region.   In the acute lesion, however, the prime mover is probably squeezed

axoplasm which, finding an obstacle at the normally narrowed nodes of large

diameter fibres, dislocates axolemma while tethered myelin follows passively.

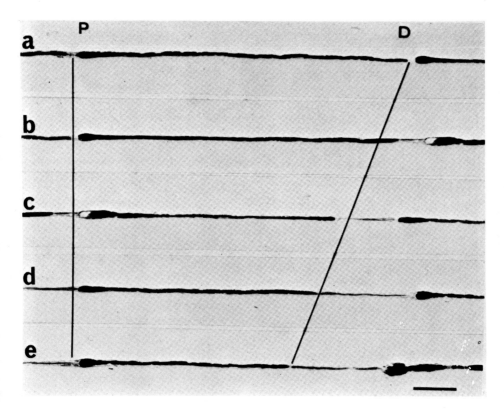

Fig. 5. Five consecutive internodes (a–e) taken from above the wrist, displayed to emphasize the asymmetry of the internodes and progressive demyelination of the tapered ends. P: proximal; D: distal. Bar: 100 μm.
From: Ochoa, J. and Marotte, L., in J. Neurol. Sci., 1973, 19:491–495.
Reproduced by permission of Elsevier, Amsterdam.

In chronic telescoping the mechanism remains obscure. A tenable interpretation is the following: repeated minor trauma, or perhaps repeated stretching or friction against flexor tendons or bone, might elicit pressure waves which propagate in opposite directions along axons, shattering the innermost myelin lamellae which would detach and slip away. Since outer lamellae remain attached to axolemma, the redundant inner lamellae can only inturn and contort into bulbous paranodes. Under these circumstances if the myelin sheath were to be unrolled, it would appear skewed rather than symmetrical as in the normal (Figure 6).

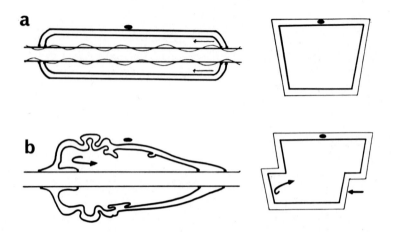

Fig. 6. a) Normal myelin segment and unrolled myelin sheath (right).
Hypothetical pressure waves along axon.
b) Distorted segment with tapered end due to myelin slippage and
bulbous end containing inturned redundant myelin lamellae.
Skewed unrolled myelin (right).
From: Ochoa, Chapter 5, in "Management of Peripheral Nerve Problems", edited by
Omer and Spinner, 1978.
Reproduced by permission of the Editors and W. B. Saunders Company.

As reported by Marotte in median nerves from affected guinea pigs, unmyelinated fibres are relatively spared in entrapped nerves from patients with meralgia
paresthetica, emphasizing the separate vulnerability of axon as opposed to
myelin. The cause of eventual loss of axons remains unclear, and it is anybody's
guess whether direct mechanical injury, impaired axoplasmic flow or even
ischemia might be responsible.

REFERENCES

1. Lewis, T., Pickering, G.W., and Rothschild, P. (1931) Heart, 16, 2.

2. Denny-Brown, D., and Brenner, C. (1944a) Arch. Neurol. Psych., 51, 1.

3. Ochoa, J., Danta, G., Fowler, T.J., and Gilliatt, R.W. (1971) Nature, 233,
    265.

4. Ochoa, J., Fowler, T.J., and Gilliatt, R.W. (1972) J. Anat., 113, 433.

5. Ochoa, J., and Marotte, L. (1973) J. Neurol. Sci., 19, 491.

6. Neary, D., Ochoa, J., and Gilliatt, R.W. (1975) J. Neurol. Sci., 24, 283.

7. Wall, P.D. and Gutnick, M. (1974b) Nature, 248, 740.

8. Ochoa, J. (1977) Electroenceph. and Clin. Neurophysiol., 43, 597.

9. Grundfest, H. (1936) Cold Spring Harbor Symposia on Quantitative Biology, 4, 179.

10. Gilliatt, R.W., and Wilson, T.G. (1954) J. Neurol., Neurosurg. and Psychiat., 17, 104.

11. Rudge, P., Ochoa, J. and Gilliatt, R.W. (1974) J. Neurol. Sci., 23, 403.

12. Ochoa, J. (1972) J. Neurol. Sci., 17, 103.

13. Neary, D., Ochoa, J., and Gilliatt, R.W. (1975) J. Neurol. Sci., 24, 283.

14. Ochoa, J., and Neary, D. (1975) Lancet, March 15.

15. Neary, D., and Eames, R.A. (1975) Neuropath. and Appl. Neurobiol., 1, 69.

16. Marie, P., and Foix, C. (1913) Revue Neurologique, 26, 647.

17. Thomas, P.K., and Fullerton, P.M. (1963) J. Neurol. Neurosurg. Psychiat., 26, 520.

18. Fullerton, P.M., and Gilliatt, R.W. (1967) J. Neurol. Neurosurg. Psychiat., 30, 1967.

19. Anderson, M.H., Fullerton, P.M., Gilliatt, R.W., and Hern, J.E.C. (1970) J. Neurol., 33, 70.

Peripheral Neuropathies
N. Canal and G. Pozza, eds.
© 1978 Elsevier/North-Holland Biomedical Press

RECOVERY OF SENSORY POTENTIALS AFTER ISCHAEMIC BLOCK BY PNEUMATIC COMPRESSION OF VARYING DURATION.

GIUSEPPE CARUSO, LUCIO SANTORO, ANNA PERRETTI, and BRUNO AMANTEA.

Department of Clinical Neurophysiology, Neurologic Clinic, and Department of Anaesthesia and Rehanimation. 2nd Fac. of Medicine, "Nuovo Policlinico", University of Naples, 80131 Naples, Italy.

ABSTRACT

In 34 normal volunteers from 19-32 years of age the forearm was compressed for periods of 15, 30, 45 and 60 minutes by a 8 cm wide pneumatic cuff rapidly inflated to a pressure of 320 mm Hg.

The sensory responses to supramaximal stimulation of median nerve on digit III were recorded distally (at wrist) and proximally (at elbow and axilla) to the compression.

During forearm compression, maximum conduction velocity gradually decreased from digit III to wrist and from wrist to elbow, whereas it did not change significantly from elbow to axilla, thus confirming the assumption that ischaemia simultaneously affects all classes of axons contained in the nerve trunk.

During an observation of one hour after cuff release, a significant correlation between the duration of compression and the time needed to reach pre-compression values of potential amplitude and conduction velocity was observed at all the three recording sites. On the other hand, improvement was clearly delayed along the compressed nerve segment when compared to the recovery observed at the wrist, thus emphasizing the role of local pressure.

The oxygen requirement of mammalian peripheral nerves is rather low, even during increased activity [1,2]. However, when the blood supply to a limb is arrested, conduction velocity is progressively reduced until the complete block along the nerves subjected to ischaemia [3-12]. Evoked action potentials gradually disappear in a distal-ward direction from the site of blood occlusion, and after 1O to 3O minutes, according to the distance from the point of stimulation, they are no longer detectable. The older the subjects, the longer the persistence of the evoked responses and the less marked the slowing in conduction velocity [12].

In experimental short-lasting ischaemia, on removing the occlusion and restoring the blood flow to the limb, no structural changes occur and nerve functions rapidly normalize. In animals, a pressure of 1,OOO mm Hg for a period of 3 hours is necessary to give an effect that will last as long as five months [11].

To produce experimental ischaemia in man, a pneumatic cuff, rapidly inflated to a pressure above the systolic blood pressure, is maintained around the limbs for a suitable period of time. Serial nerve conduction is then measured distally to the occlusion and values compared to those observed before ischaemia.

By such a procedure, however, it is difficult to differentiate whether ischaemia primarily affects one of the different classes of axons contained in the nerve trunk, or contemporaneously impairs all fibres. Moreover, as there is no distinction between the effects of direct local nerve compression and those depending on blood occlusion, it is not possible to say whether it is the ischaemia or the compression that causes the conduction block.

Thus, to verify whether there is a selective "resistance" to ischaemia between fast and slow conducting fibres, and to control to what extend nerve fibres could be damaged by the pressure itself, we decided to use a small pneumatic cuff inflated to a constant pressure, and to record action potentials proximally and distally to it (Fig. 1).

We therefore, under general anaesthesia by a mixture of O.5 - 1.5 per cent Fluothane and 4O per cent nitrous oxide, occluded the blood flow to the upper limb by means of a 8 cm wide pneumatic cuff inflated to a pressure of 32O mm Hg and maintained it around the forearm for periods of 15, 3O,

45 and 6O minutes. Our subjects were 34 normal informed consent volunteers from 19 to 32 years of age (the average 24. 7), 19 males and 15 females.

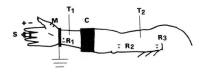

Fig. 1. Drawing of the positioning of the electrodes and of the pneumatic cuff. S-stimulating electrode on digit III; R1, R2 and R3 - stigmatic leading - off and remote electrodes; M-concentric needle electrode inserted in abductor pollicis brevis muscle; T1 and T2 - thermoneedles connected to electrical thermometer; C-cuff.

Sensory potentials evoked by supramaximal stimuli to digit III at 1 per second frequency were recorded from median nerve at the wrist, elbow and axilla as described by Buchthal and Rosenfalck [13]. Control estimates of maximum orthodromic sensory conduction velocity from digit III to wrist, from wrist to elbow and from elbow to axilla, and sensory response amplitude at the three different sites of recording were taken both before anaesthesia and inflation of the cuff, and then every five minutes, or less, during compression. After the release of the blood-pressure-cuff, recordings were taken at intervals of one minute for the first ten minutes, and then every five minutes for the remaining 5O minutes.

Surface temperature of the arm was kept at 36-37°C by an automatically controlled infra-red heat source, and near-nerve temperature was measured by two thermo-needles previously inserted in the limb proximal and distal to the cuff and connected to an electrical thermometer. Thus, the deep temperature did not vary by more than 1-1°, 5 C before circulatory arrest, or during and after occlusion.

In this preliminary report attention is focused on the investigation of the recovery time-course; it is worth mentioning, however, that the time and the rate of amplitude-decrease of the recorded sensory action potentials at the elbow and the axilla during blood occlusion was the same. Moreover, maximum conduction velocity along this most proximal nerve segment (that is, elbow - axilla) did not change significantly up to the first 1O to 15 minutes of ischaemia.

These results agree with previous observations by Behse and Buchthal [14] and with the assumption of Kamp-Nielsen and Kardel [15], that ischaemia results in a gradual and progressive attenuation of impulse propagation along all nerve fibres rather than in a selective block primarily affecting the fastest conducting axons. Should this not be so, a slowing in maximum conduction velocity proximal to compression would certainly be expected from a higher susceptibility and conse quent conduction block of the largest fibres.

Regarding to the recovery phase of the nerve conduction parameters, we refer here to the preliminary results obtained from three groups of subjects in whom compression was maintained for periods o f 15, 45 and 60 minutes. A more detailed statistical analysis of the data is at present being carried out, however even from this rough study, some significant differences among the groups are evident.

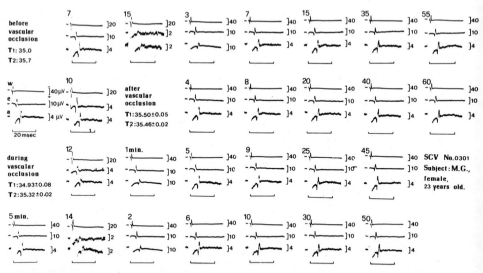

Fig. 2. From top to bottom. Sensory nerve action potentials evoked by supra-maximal stimulation of digit III and recorded from wrist (w), elbow (e) and axilla (a) before, during (15 minutes) and after vascular occlusion. See text for details.

Fig. 2 illustrates the course of changes in potential amplitude and sensory conduction time occurring in a 23 year old girl over a 15 minute period of

blood occlusion, and during one hour of post-ischaemic observation. From
top to bottom, it can be seen that already one minute after the cuff was
deflated, potential amplitude improves almost to pre-ischaemic values both
in the distal and proximal sites of recording. At the same time, latencies
to wrist and axilla are 9 to 12 per cent above pre-compression figures, while
conduction time from digit to elbow is still increased by 19 per cent. Four
minutes later, however, the nerve fibres appear to conduct normally both
distally and proximally to the site of cuff compression.

These figures are in contrast with the results obtained in the experiment
carried out on a 27 year old girl, and illustrated in Fig. 3. This shows the

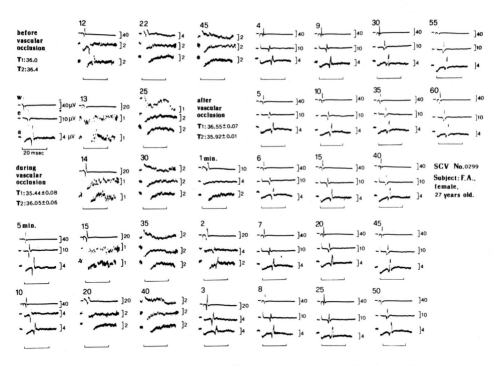

Fig. 3. Sensory nerve action potentials evoked and recorded as in Fig. 2.
Duration of complete vascular occlusion: 45 minutes. See text for details.

changes occurring in sensory nerve conduction parameters during and after
45 minutes of blood occlusion. It can be seen that one minute after removing
the cuff, no potential can be observed in either of the recording sites situated
proximal to compression, and that the potential amplitude at the wrist appears

more than 85 per cent below the pre-ischaemic value. After 5 minutes, about 65 per cent of pre-compression amplitude is regained at the wrist, whereas sensory response amplitudes at the elbow and axilla are still 60 per cent below previous figures. After one hour, amplitude is about "normal" at the wrist, but it is still 30 per cent below pre-compression values at the elbow and axilla. The serial latencies to action potentials recorded along the nerve at the three different levels during one hour of post-compression observations fit in with amplitude values.

Further information on the relationship between the length of cuff compression at 320 mm Hg and recovery time of nerve conduction parameters is shown in Figures 4-8, where, in two groups of subjects comparative changes in sensory potential amplitude and in maximum conduction velocity after relief of the blood occlusion are expressed as per cent deviation figures from pre-ischaemic stimulation.

In figures 4-8, the curves refer to mean values of 15 subjects: 7 with a 15 minute blood occlusion (broken lines), and 8 in whom cuff compression was

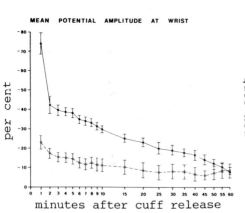

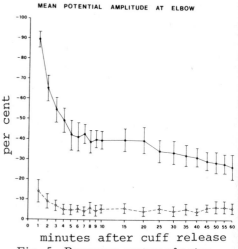

Fig. 4. Recovery curves of potential amplitude at the wrist. On ordinate the percentage deviation from pre-ischaemic figures; on abscissa, on logarithmic scale, the minutes after cuff release. Continuous line: 8 subjects with a 45 minute blood occlusion; broken line: 7 subjects with a 15 minute lasting compression. See text for details.

Fig. 5. Recovery curves of potential amplitude at the elbow. Ordinate, abscissa and subject groups as in Fig. 4. See text for details.

maintained for 45 minutes (continous lines). On ordinate, the deviation from pre-ischaemic value, in per cent; on abscissa, on logarithmic scale, the time from removing compression, in minutes.

Differences between recovery curves are evident. However, as far as potential amplitude at the wrist is concerned (Fig. 4), no significant difference can be seen after 55-60 minutes. At this point, in fact, both groups regain 90 per cent of pre-compression amplitude.

On the contrary, mean response amplitude at the elbow (Fig. 5) and at the axilla (Fig. 6) even 60 minutes after cuff release are below 20 to 30 per cent of previous figures.

On comparing the two groups of subjects, recovery curves are significantly different also in maximum conduction velocity in the segments from digit to wrist (Fig. 7), and from wrist to elbow (Fig. 8). Moreover, through the nerve segment, compressed for 45 minutes, mean value of velocity after one hour observation is still about 10 per cent below the figures obtained from digit to wrist.

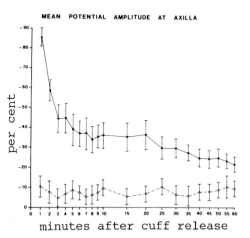

Fig. 6. Recovery curves of potential amplitude at the axilla. Ordinate, abscissa and subject groups as in Fig. 4. See text for details.

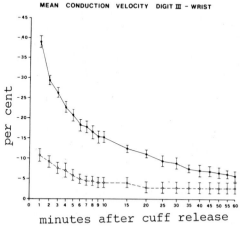

Fig. 7. Recovery curves of maximum sensory conduction velocity from digit III to wrist. Ordinate, abscissa and subject groups as in Fig. 4. See text for details.

334

When some of these data were presented during September 1977 in Amsterdam [16], our conclusions suggested that the recovery difference between the
nerve functions through the nerve segment subjected to only ischaemia (that
is, from digit to wrist) and the ischaemic and compressed nerve segment
(that is, from wrist to elbow), would probably be greater if compression
duration was longer.

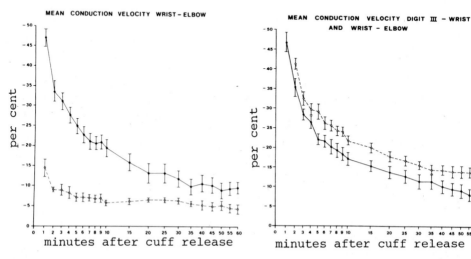

Fig. 8. Recovery curves of maximum sensory conduction velocity
from wrist to elbow. Ordinate,
abscissa and subject groups as in
Fig. 4. See text for details.

Fig. 9. Recovery curves of maximum
sensory conduction velocity from digit
III to wrist (continuous line) and from
wrist to elbow (broken line) in 9 subjected with a 60 minute lasting blood occlusion. Ordinate and abscissa as in Fig. 4.
See text for details.

With reference to this point we have investigated a further 9 volunteers
and compressed the nerve up to as much as an hour at 320 mm Hg. Fig. 9
shows some preliminary comparisons of the time-course of conduction velocity recovery along these two nerve segments. As in figures 4-8, on ordinate
the percentage deviation from pre-ischaemic figures, and on abscissa the
minutes after cuff release. In this Figure, however, the continuous line
refer to the maximum velocity from digit to wrist, and the broken one to
that from wrist to elbow. The two curves are rather similar, although the
broken line remains systematically higher than the other, and it, during the

last 15 minutes of observation, is almost parallel to the abscissa. It is to be stressed, moreover, that one minute after the removal of compression, conduction velocity from wrist to elbow could be estimated in only one subject out of nine, while velocity from digit to wrist could be measured in 8.

CONCLUSIONS

Perhaps, it should not be excluded that the earlier improvement occurring in the most distal nerve portion is, at least in part, related to the shorter length of the nerve between stimulating cathode and recording electrodes. Statistical treatment of our data is still in progress. Nevertheless, these preliminary results agree with those obtained by Gilliatt and co-workers[17] in the baboon, and suggest: 1. that there is a significant relation between the duration of blood occlusion and the recovery time of nerve conduction parameters, and 2. that improvement through the nerve segment subjected to local pressure appears delayed.

REFERENCES

1. Gerard, R.W. (1927) Studies on nerve metabolism. II. Respiration in oxygen and nitrogen. Am.J. Physiol., 82, 381.

2. Gerard, R.W. (1932) Nerve metabolism. Physiol. Rev., 12, 469.

3. Clark, D., Hughes, J. and Gasser, H.S. (1935) Afferent function in the groups of nerve fibers of slowest conduction velocity. Am. J. Physiol., 114, 69.

4. Buelbring, E. and Burn, J.H. (1939) Vascular changes affecting the transmission of nervous impulses. J. Physiol. (Lond.), 97, 250.

5. Bentley, F.H. and Schlapp, W. (1943) Experiments on the blood supply of nerves. J. Physiol. (Lond.), 102, 62.

6. Magladery, J.W., McDougal, D.B., jr. and Stoll, J. (1950) Electrophysiological studies of nerve and reflex activity in normal man. II. Effects of ischaemia. Johns Hopkins Hosp. Bull., 86, 291.

7. Cathala, H.-P. and Scherrer, J. (1963) Modifications du potentiel de nerf, sous l'influence d'un brassard ischémisant chez l'homme. Rev. Neurol., 108, 201.

8. Abramson, D.I., Hlavova, A., Rickert, B.L., Talso, J., Schwab, C., Feldman, J. and Chu, L.S.W. (1970) Effect of ischemia on median and ulnar motor nerve conduction velocities at various temperatures. Arch. Phys. Med. Rehabil., 51, 463.

336

9. Abramson, D.I., Hlavova, A., Rickert, B.L., Talso, J., Schwab, C., Feldman, J. and Chu, L.S.W. (1970) Effect of ischemia on latencies of median nerve in the hand at various temperatures. Arch. Phys. Med. Rehabil., 51, 471.

10. Abramson, D.I., Rickert, B.L., Alexis, J.T., Hlavova, A., Schwab, C. and Tandoc, J. (1971) Effect of repeated periods of ischemia on motor nerve conduction velocity in forearm. J. Appl. Physiol., 30, 636.

11. Fowler, T.J., Danta, G. and Gilliatt, R.W. (1972) Recovery of nerve conduction after a pneumatic tourniquet: observations on the hind-limb of the baboon. J. Neurol. Neurosurg. Psychiat., 35, 638.

12. Caruso, G., Labianca, O. and Ferrannini, E. (1973) Effect of ischaemia on sensory potentials of normal subjects of different ages. J. Neurol. Neurosurg. Psychiat., 36, 455.

13. Buchthal, F. and Rosenfalck, A. (1966) Evoked action potentials and conduction velocity in human sensory nerves. Brain Research, 3, 1-122.

14. Behse, F. and Buchthal, F. (1975) Slowing in maximum nerve conduction velocity during acute hypoxia due to block of large fibres or to slowing along all fibres? Nodiska Neurologkongressen, Stockholm, 11-14 June, 1975.

15. Kamp Nielsen, V. and Kardel, T. (1974) Decremental conduction in normal human nerves subjected to ischemia? Acta Physiol. Scand., 92, 249.

16. Caruso, G., Santoro, L., Perretti, A. and Amantea, B. (1977) Recovery of sensory nerve conduction after "ischaemic" block by pneumatic compression. Preliminary observations on median nerve in normal subjects. 9th Internat. Congress of Electroencephal. and Clin. Neurophysiol., Amsterdam, 4-9 September, 1977.

17. Gilliatt, R.W., Fowler, T.J., Ochoa, J. and Rudge, P. (1975) The effect of acute compression on nerve conduction. A quantitative study. Studies on Neuromuscular Diseases. Proc. Internat. Symp., Giessen, 1973. Eds. Karger, Basel, 1975.

Peripheral Neuropathies
N. Canal and G. Pozza, eds.
© 1978 Elsevier/North-Holland Biomedical Press

IDIOPATHIC CARPAL TUNNEL SYNDROME: A CLINICAL AND ELECTROPHYSIOLO-
GICAL STUDY OF 50 PATIENTS

COMI G. (°), GUALTIERI G. (°°) , RODOCANACHI M. (°), and LOZZA L.(°)
(°) Clinic of Nervous Diseases, University of Milan Medical School
(°°) Department of Orthopedic, "G. Pini" Institute, Milan

Carpal tunnel syndrome is the commonest type of entrapment disease in the upper limbs.

In most cases the clinical features are sufficiently characteristic to allow a confident diagnosis to be made.

Electrophysiological studies are of the most value when they
provide clear evidence for a local injury to the median nerve in
the carpal tunnel region especially in patients whose symptoms and
signs are unusual or indefinite.

Simpson [1] first reported a prolongued motor terminal delay at
wrist in carpal tunnel syndrome. Results of nerve conduction studies on large series of patients have been reported [2,3,4,5].
Gilliatt and Sears [6] first demonstrated that sensory conduction
may be abnormal while motor latency remains within the normal
range. In subsequent studies [7] it has been shown that slowing of
sensory conduction along the median nerve from palm to wrist
could be demonstrated when conduction from digit to wrist and motor latency were normal. Other authors [8] suggested that border
line cases of entrapment to wrist could be recognized comparing
amplitude of sensory action potentials in median and ulnar nerves
in the same subject.

In the present study results of median and ulnar nerve conduction and needle EMG examination of thenar and ipothenar muscles
in patients with idiopathic carpal tunnel syndrome (I.C.T.S.)
are reported.

Electrophysiological abnormalities are related to duration of
symptoms, involvement of right or left hand, and recovery after
surgery.

MATERIALS AND METHODS

All patients with clinical evidence of a generalized peripheral neuropathy, with lesions involving other nerves or with
disorders such as diabetes, alchoolism, uremia or pernicious
anemia which predispose to peripheral nerve disease or in which
involvement of median nerve was suspected to be related to job
were excluded. 50 patients were studied: 49 females and one man.
The mean age of the patients was 52 years with an range between
33 and 73 years. The mean age of onset of the disease coincided
in one case with the use of the pill and in two cases with pregnancy. The mean duration of the disease was quite elevated: 3.4
years, with a range between 1 month and 1 year.

Sensory conduction was determined along the median nerve (digit
II° - wrist) and ulnar nerve (digit V° - wrist). Sensory action
potential (S.A.P.) amplitude, peak to peak, and latency, to negative peak, were considered. Motor conduction velocity (elbow -
wrist) and distal motor latency (D.M.L.) in median and ulnar nerves
were also measured. For conduction studies surfaces electrodes
were employed. Parameters were compared to values in 50 healthy
subjects matched for age.

For needle EMG mean duration and number of phases of motor
unit potentials, pattern a full effort and fibrillation or positive sharp waves were evaluated.

Tests were performed in a room at a constant temperature (24° -
26° C.).

RESULTS

18 patients had monolateral I.C.T.S., 16 interesting the dominant and 2 the non dominant hand. 32 patients had a bilateral
involvement: in 20 of them the dominant hand was more severely
affected, in 11 both hands were equally severelly affected and
only one had the non dominant hand more severelly affected.

Opponens pollicis muscle showed fibrillation potentials and/or
positive shwrp waves in 67 % of cases, signs of loss of motor
units in 80 %, increased duration of motor units potentials in 50 %
and more than 12 % of poliphasic potentials in 52 % of cases.

Signs of denervation were found only in 7 % of cases in abductor digiti minimi muscle. In 2 patients abnormalities were bilateral

The results of median nerve conduction studies are summarized in Table 1.

MEDIAN NERVE CONDUCTION STUDIES IN CONTROL SUBJECTS AND PATIENTS WITH I.C.T.S.

		I.C.T.S.	CONTROL	SIGNIFICANCE
D.M.L. (msec)	mean[a]	6.3±2.6	3.2±0.5	p 0.001
	range	3.2-12.5	2.6-4.7	
M.C.V. (m/sec)	mean	53.3±5.8	58.4±2.5	p 0.001
	range	45-64	52-65	
S.A.P.ampl. (micronvolt)	mean	5.0±5.7	21±8.8	p 0.001
	range	0-22	9-40	
S.A.P.lat. (msec)	mean	4.9±1.1	2.8±0.3	p 0.001
	range	3.0-6.1	2.3-3.5	

[a]Mean ± S.D.

Ulnar nerve motor and sensory conduction mean values in I.C.T.S. patients and controls were not statistically different. Nevertheless abnormalities were found in small number of cases of I.C.T.S.
Frequency of electrophysiological abnormalities - Table II.
An abnormal latency of S.A.P. was the most sensitive finding of involvement of median nerve at wrist. Only one case showed a normal S.A.P. latency with an abnormal D.M.L.
Determination of sensory conduction from digit to palm and from palm to wrist made possible to find abnormalities in the segment of nerve underneath the flexor retinaculum in three cases in which S.A.P. latency and amplitude were normal.
Concerning ulnar nerve in one case an abnormal D.M.L., in another

case an abnormal S.A.P. latency and in another one a slowed maximum motor conduction velocity in the elbow-wrist tract were found. A reduced S.A.P. amplitude was found in 10 % of cases.

The ratio of median to ulnar nerve S.A.P. amplitude was consistenly greater than one in our group of normal subjects. This ratio was found to be less than one in 76 out of 82 cases. So this test, recommended by Long and Seah [8], confirme its sensibility in the diagnosis of I.C.T.S.

TABLE II
FREQUENCY OF ELECTROPHYSIOLOGICAL ABNORMALITIES IN 82 CASES OF I.C.T.S.

	Criterion of abnormalities	Frequency (%)
Median nerve		
D.M.L.	4.7 msec	76
M.C.V.	50 m/sec	26
S.A.P. amplitude	9 micronV.	70
S.A.P. latency	3.6 msec	95
Ulnar nerve		
D.M.L.	3.7 msec	1
M.C.V.	50 m/sec	1
S.A.P. amplitude	8.1 micronV.	10
S.A.P. latency	3.1 msec	1

Motor conduction velocity related to distal motor latency in median nerve (Figure 1). Median nerve M.C.V. was slowed in the elbow-wrist tract in 26 % of cases. M.C.V. was plotted against D.M.L. The entity of slowing in the forearm is related to the degree of slowing at wrist.

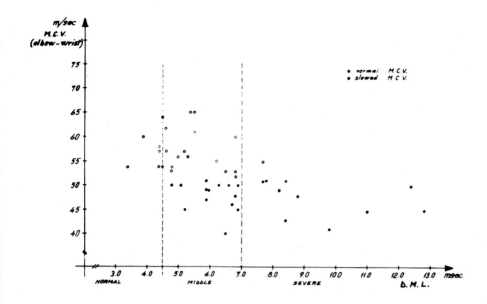

Fig. 1. Relationship between median nerve M.C.V. in the forearm
and D.M.L. The open circles represent normal values of M.C.V., the
filled circles the abnormal values. The vertical lines devide the
patients in three groups with normal, middle and severe involvement
of D.M.L.

Electrophysiological abnormalities related to duration of disease. (Figure 2-3). D.M.L. and S.A.P. amplitude were related by
correlation coefficients to the duration of symptoms in years. No
statistically significative relationship was demonstrated. S.A.P.
was allready absent in some cases in the first few months of disease. D.M.L. was also very augmented in the same period.

Post-operative findings. Table III. 15 patients were re-examined
3-5 months after surgical decompression. Mean values of median nerve
S.A.P. amplitude and latency and D.M.L. were improved. The signifi-
cativity of the difference between pre and post-operative data was
demonstrated using the paired t test. D.M.L. had returned to normal range in 53 % of cases, S.A.P. amplitude in 47 % of cases and
S.A.P. latency in 33 % of cases. In all cases one or more parameters were ameliorated.

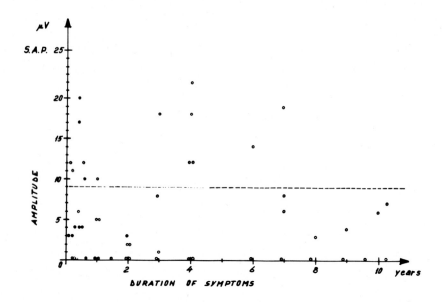

Fig. 2. Median nerve S.A.P. amplitude at wrist related to duration of symptoms in I.C.T.S.

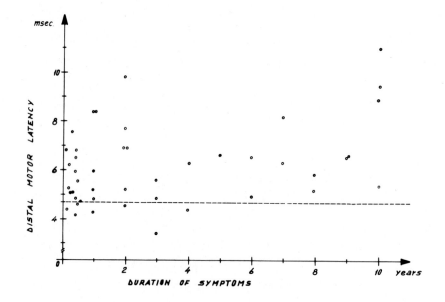

Fig. 3. Median nerve D.M.L. at wrist related to duration of
symptoms in I.C.T.S.

TABLE III

MEDIAN NERVE ELECTROPHYSIOLOGICAL FINDINGS PRE AND POST-OPERATIVELY
IN 15 CASES OF I.C.T.S.

	D.M.L. (msec)	S.A.P. lat. (msec)	S.A.P. ampl. (micronV.)
Pre-operative	7.3±2.84	4.45±0.53	4.4±0.53
Post-operative	4.5±1.03	3.57±0.57	9.27±0.66
Significance	0.005 p 0.001	p 0.001	0.005 p 0.001

CONCLUSIONS

In our study the distribution for sex and age, the modality of
involvement of the hands and the frequency of electrophysiological
abnormalities are in agreement with data reported by other authors.
It was also confirmed that an alteration of median nerve sensory
conduction at wrist is the most peculiar electrophysiological finding for I.C.T.S.

However a lack of correlation between the severity of the disease - as determined with electrophysiological examination -
and its duration has to be pointed out. This finding is in disagreement with the study carried out by Kemble [3] in which a statistically significative relationship between D.M.L. and duration
of the disease is found. Nerve conduction abnormalities do not
usually correspond to the onset of clinical symptomatology, as it
is shown by finding of abnormalities of sensory and/or motor velocity conduction in asymptomatic hands. This fact can in part
explain the lack of correlation. Furthermore it is possible that
conservative treatments previously carried out by some of the
patients had modified the course of the disease. Our data suggest
that nerve involvement is rapidly worsening in the first few months
since the onset of disturbances, afterwards it remains fairly im-
modified or in any case it progresses very slowly. The good

functional recovery of nerve conduction and the regression of disturbances after surgical decompression advise an early operation in cases in which severe signs of denervation are detected.

The finding of a very small number of cases with lesions of the ulnar nerve in our group of I.C.T.S. is in contrast with the high incidence of ulnar nerve lesions found by Sedal et al.[4]. Our results therefore do not agree with the hypotesis of the presence of a more generalized subclinical neuropathy in a significative number of patients with I.C.T.S.

At last the age of onset of the disease and its temporal relationship with pregnancy and the use of pill - as found in our cases - suggest to carrie out deeper endocrinological studies in these patients.

REFERENCES

1. Simpson, J.A. (1956) Electrical signs in the diagnosis of carpal tunnel and related syndromes. J. Neurol. Neurosurg. Psychiat., 19, 275-280.

2. Kaeser, H.E. (1963) Diagnostische probleme beim karpal tunnel syndrom. Dtsch. Z. Nervenheilk., 185, 453-460.

3. Kemble, F. (1968) Clinical manifestations related to electro-physiological abnormalities measurement in the carpal tunnel syndrome. Electromyography, 8, 19-26.

4. Sedal, L., McLeod, J.G., Walsh, J.C. (1973) Ulnar nerve lesions associated with the carpal tunnel syndrome. J. Neurol. Neurosurg. Psychiat., 36, 118-123.

5. Thomas, P.K. (1960) Motor nerve conduction in the carpal tunnel syndrome. Neurology, 10, 1045-1050.

6. Gilliat, R.W., Sears, T.A. (1958) Sensory nerve action potentials in patients with peripheral nerve lesions. J. Neurol. Psychiat., 21, 109-118.

7. Buchthal, F., Rosenfalk, A. (1971) Sensory conduction from digit to palm and from palm to wrist in the carpal tunnel syndrome. J. Neurol. Neurosurg. Psychiat., 34, 243-252.

8. Loong, S.C., Seah, C.S. (1971) Comparison of median and ulnar sensory nerve action potentials in the diagnosis of the carpal tunnel syndrome. J. Neurol. Neurosurg. Psychiat., 34, 750-754.

Peripheral Neuropathies
N. Canal and G. Pozza, eds.
© 1978 Elsevier/North-Holland Biomedical Press

RELATIONSHIP BETWEEN ARM PARAESTHESIAS AND ENTRAPMENT SYNDROMES IN
397 PATIENTS:ELECTROMYOGRAPHIC FINDINGS.

RUDI SCHOENHUBER,CARLO PAGANI and FILOMENA PRATTICHIZZO
Neurological Department,University of Modena,Via del Pozzo 71,
Modena (Italy)

ABSTRACT

397 unselected patients suffering from paraesthesias of the upper
limb were examined by electromyography.Only 7% had signs pointing
to a radicular lesion,while 57% had an entrapment neuropathy,mostly
at the carpal tunnel.22% showed no pathological findings.

INTRODUCTION

Paraesthesias and pain in the hands and arms are common as isolated complaint.The patient usually describes numbness,tingling or
pain of the entire hand and,at least at early stages,abnormal signs
are frequently absent or unreliable at the clinical examination.It
is therefore not surprising that the approach to these patients varies with the specialisation and training of the consulted physi-
cian.The management of this clinical problem has been changing repeatedly in the last century in concomitance with reports of new
syndromes,which from time to time have enjoyed popularity and gained wide,though transient acceptance by the medical audience[1].

Early in our century attention was directed to the neurovascular
bundle at its entry in the arm.The cervical rib was soon recognized
to be a possible cause of compression of the brachial plexus and
the subclavian vessels.Then it was thought that similar symptoms
could occur also in the absence of the rib and various causes were
found of what now is usually called the thoracic outlet syndrome[2].

Later the role of the prolapsed intervertebral disc,known to produce sciatica,was also applicated to the upper limb.Semmes and Mur-

phey[3] in 1943 suggested that laterally protruded cervical discs
could account for many cases precedently ascribed to the thoracic
outlet syndrome.Frykholm[4] stressed that radicular pain could occur
also in the absence of disc protrusion,simply due to compression by
osteoarthrosic spurs,and concluded that "most cases of brachialgia
are probably of radicular origin".This view prompted neurosurgeons
to operate on the cervical spine,when prolapsed disc tissue was
found or suspected or X-rays showed spondyloarthrosis.

About at the same time attention was shifted to the entrapment
neuropathies,particularly to the carpal tunnel syndrome,by the papers of Cannon (1946)[5] and Brain (1947)[6].

It is possible that so many different types of lesion are capable of producing pain and paraesthesias in the hand and arm,but it
is unlikely that they are all equally important and frequent.Becau-
se of the difficulty of a correct diagnosis based on anamnestic and
clinical data,most patients seen in general practice are treated as
if they were suffering from cervical disc protrusion or spondylosis
and only rarely the possibility of an entrapment neuropathy is considered.

For proper management of these patients it is important to know
what and how frequent are the different causes of brachialgias.In
order to assess this we studied 397 patients presenting this symptom using neurophysiological techniques.

MATERIALS AND METHODS

From 1975 to 1977 397 patients with the presenting diagnosis of
arm and hand paraesthesias were studied electromyographically in
the Neurological Department of the University of Modena.The age of
the patients ranged from 10 to 76 years,with a mean age of 41.5
years.The males were 176,the females 221.

In all patients the sensory action potential of the median and
ulnar nerve was recorded at the wrist after digital stimulation.The
motor conduction velocity was studied in the median nerve stimula-

ting at the wrist,the elbow and at the clavicular fossa,and in the ulnar nerve stimulating at the wrist,below and above the elbow and at the clavicular fossa.The radial and the proximal nerves were studied only when there were clinical indications.All electroneuro-graphic recordings were done with surface electrodes and compared with the normal values[7].

In all patients the opponens pollicis and the abductor digiti quinti were examined with concentric needle electrodes.In selected cases also other muscles were examined.

RESULTS

Table 1 shows the electromyographic findings of the patients.The various causes of paraesthesias found in the 35 patient with multiple aetiology are shown in table 2.

TABLE 1

EMG DATA IN 397 PATIENTS WITH ARM AND HAND PARAESTHESIAS

Entrapment neuropathies			229	57.4%
Carpal tunnel	93	23.3%		
Ulnar-elbow	68	17.1%		
Outlet	30	7.5%		
Ulnar-wrist	24	6.0%		
Radial	12	3.0%		
Pronator	2	0.5%		
Radicular lesion			27	6.8%
Polyneuropathy			17	4.3%
Multiple aetiology			35	8.8%
Normal			89	22.7%

DISCUSSION

Our data do not confirm the general belief that most brachial-gias are of radicular origin.Only 7% of our patients showed signs denervation with radicular distribution.This is in contrast with

TABLE 2

EMG DATA IN 35 CASES WITH PARAESTHESIAS OF MULTIPLE AETIOLOGY

Carpal tunnel + ulnar-elbow	12
Polyneuropathy + carpal tunnel	7
Polyneuropathy + ulnar-elbow	6
Outlet + ulnar-elbow	6
Radicular + ulnar-elbow	2
Radicular + outlet	1
Radicular + carpal tunnel	1
Outlet + carpal tunnel	1

the data of Mayfield[8] who found clinical and/or radiological eviden ce of cervical disc or spondylosis in 513 out of a series of 961 patients for whom a cause of brachialgia could be found (Fig.1).

Clinical diagnosis,n=961,Mayfield,1971

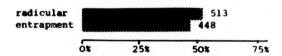

EMG diagnosis,n=308,present study

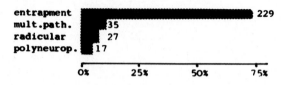

Fig.1.Causes of hand and arm paraesthesias.Upper part:clinical dia-
gosis (Mayfield,1971[8]).Lower part:EMG diagnosis (present study).

The diagnosis of Mayfield rested on clinical and radiographic elements only,which may explain the high incidence of radicular le -
sions.It must be said that neurophysiological techniques tend
to underestimate radicular lesions and to overestimate entrapment
neuropathies.The first are detectable only when they produce neu-
rotmesis and result in denervation,while the second become apparent
already at the stage of local demyelination,being brought out by
local slowing of conduction velocity.This caveat notwithstanding,
the predominance of entrapment aetiology in our series is worth-
stressing.

The carpal tunnel syndrome heads the list of the entrapment neuropathies in our material,a finding in agreement with previous reports[8](Fig.2).The incidence of ulnar nerve compression at the el-

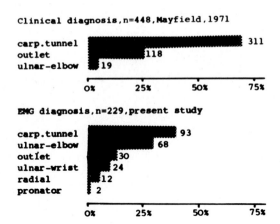

Fig.2.Relative incidence of entrapment neuropathies.Upper part:
clinical diagnosis (Mayfield,1971[8]).Lower part:EMG diagnosis (present study).

bow (68 cases) and at the wrist (24 cases) is higher than it would be expected from the clinical literature.This is probably due to the difficulty to diagnose this syndrome on mere clinical grounds.

The thoracic outlet syndrome is certainly less frequent that it used to be thought,but it still deserves consideration by the clinician concerned with arm and hand paraesthesias.

Polyneuropathy,multiple entrapments and the association of entrapment neuropathies with radicular lesions represent 13% of our case material and could be hardly diagnosed without the aid of neurophysiological techniques,which are indispensable for detecting curable causes of paraesthesias in the upper limb.

REFERENCES

1. Lishman,W.A. and Russel,W.R.(1961)Lancet,ii,941-947.

2. Urschel,H.C. and Razzuk,M.A.(1972) New Engl.J.Med.,286,1140-43.

3. Semmes,R.E. and Murphey F.(1943) J.Amer.Med.Ass.,121,1209-1214.

4. Frykholm,R.(1951) Acta Chir.Scand.,Suppl.160,1-149.

5. Cannon,B.W. and Love,J.G.(1946) Surgery,20,210-216.

6. Brain,W.R.,Wright,A.D. and Wilkinson,M.(1947) Lancet,i,277-282.

7. Pagani,C.,Schoenhuber,R. and Tuscano,G.(1977) Il Policlinico - Sez.Chir.,84,423-428.

8. Mayfield,F.H.(1971) in Handbook of Clinical Neurology,Vinken, P.J. and Bruyn,G.W. eds.,Elsevier,Amsterdam,pp 430-446

Peripheral Neuropathies
N. Canal and G. Pozza, eds.
© 1978 Elsevier/North-Holland Biomedical Press

COMPARISON OF ORTHODROMIC AND ANTIDROMIC SENSORY NERVE
CONDUCTION IN POLYNEUROPATHIES AND IN CARPAL TUNNEL SYNDROME

HANS-PETER LUDIN, JUERG LUETSCHG and FIAMMETTA VALSANGIACOMO
Neurological Clinic, University of Berne, Inselspital,
CH-3010 Berne (Switzerland)

INTRODUCTION

It was the aim of the present study to compare the diagnostic
value of orthodromic and antidromic sensory nerve conduction
measurements. In patients with a polyneuropathy or a carpal
tunnel syndrome, the results of measurements from the median
nerve employing both methods were compared.

MATERIALS AND METHODS (for details see Ludin[1])

30 patients (age 16 to 77 years) with minimal or beginning
polyneuropathies of different etiologies and 26 patients (age 22
to 65 years) with a mild carpal tunnel syndrome were examined.
The diagnosis was confirmed in all cases by additional clinical
and laboratory findings and by the further course of the disease.

The following parameters were considered and compared with the
normal values which have been published previously[1]. In the antidromic method the nerve action potentials were recorded from the
index finger with ring electrodes after stimulating with surface
electrodes at the wrist and at the elbow. In most instances stimulation was submaximal. The latency was measured to the negative
onset of the averaged nerve action potential. From these latencies
the conduction velocities between elbow and wrist and between
wrist and digit II were calculated. In agreement with previous
experience with normal subjects, it was not considered to be
definitely abnormal if no antidromic nerve action potential could
be recorded or if it could not be clearly distinguished from a
volume conducted muscle potential[2]. For the orthodromic measurements supramaximal stimulation (50 to 70 mA) was applied at the
index finger with ring electrodes. The nerve action potentials

were recorded with unipolar needle electrodes at wrist and
elbow. Each potential was averaged 500 times. The latencies were
measured to the first positive peak. The maximum conduction
velocity was calculated from index finger to wrist and from
wrist to elbow. The amplitude was measured from the highest
positive to the highest negative peak. In addition the number of
potential components were counted. All components reaching at
least 10 per cent of the maximal amplitude were included. The
duration of the nerve action potential was measured from the
beginning of the first to the end of the last component which
had been counted.

RESULTS

  Polyneuropathies. The antidromic conduction velocity (Fig.1)
was slightly decreased in one or both segments in only 8 cases.
In 14 patients a definite antidromic potential could be recorded
by stimulating neither at the wrist nor at the elbow. In two
cases there was no potential only when stimulating in the elbow.
In all but one patient orthodromic sensory nerve action potentials could be recorded at both wrist and elbow. In a 32 year-old
woman suffering from a hereditary sensory neuropathy type II no
definite nerve action potential could be detected at all. Eleven
patients had a slowed conduction velocity (Fig. 2) in one or
both segments. The slowing was borderline to discrete in most
instances. Many of the remaining values were situated in the
lower normal range. The amplitude of orthodromic nerve action
potentials (Fig. 3) was not an especially sensitive parameter in
the present material. Most values lay in the lower normal range.
Only 7 patients exhibited pathological values, some of which
were still at the borderline. In 21 cases the duration of an
evoked potential (Fig. 4) was longer than normal at one or both
of the 2 recording sites. A potential with an increased number of
components was found in 19 cases. In 9 patients these 2 parameters represented the only pathological findings.

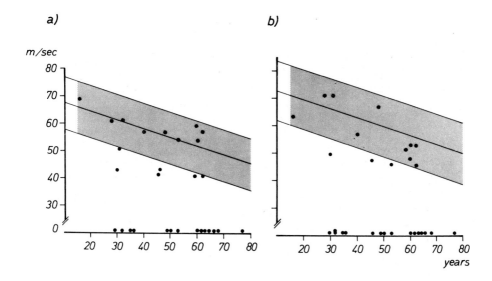

Fig. 1. Antidromic sensory nerve conduction velocity in the median nerve between elbow and wrist (a) and between wrist and digit II in 30 patients with polyneuropathies.

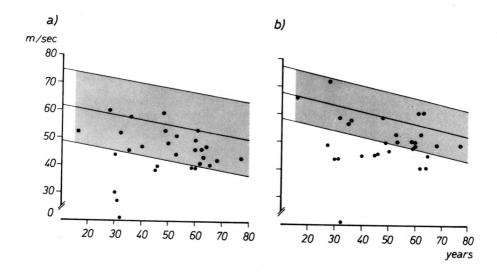

Fig. 2. Orthodromic sensory nerve conduction velocity in the median nerve between digit II and wrist (a) and between wrist and elbow (b) in 30 patients with polyneuropathies.

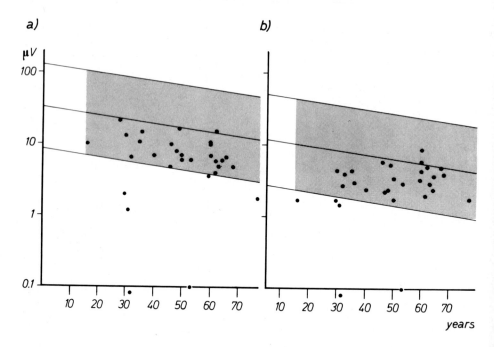

Fig. 3. Amplitude of orthodromic sensory nerve action potentials recorded from the median nerve at wrist (a) and at elbow (b) in 30 patients with polyneuropathies.

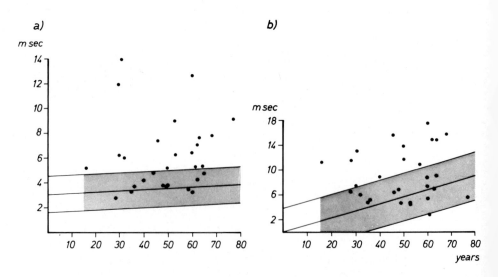

Fig. 4. Duration of orthodromic sensory nerve action potentials from the median nerve recorded at wrist (a) and at elbow (b) in 30 patients with polyneuropathies.

Carpal tunnel syndrome. With the antidromic method 12 patients
had definite nerve action potentials. In all these cases conduction velocity was decreased between wrist and digit II (Fig. 5a).
Orthodromic potentials could be recorded in all cases; 22 had
conduction velocities lower than normal between index finger and
wrist (Fig. 5b). In 4 cases the values were in the lowest range of
the normal. With both methods, all conduction velocities between
wrist and elbow were normal. In only 5 cases did orthodromic

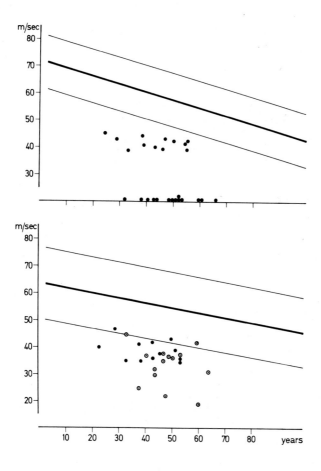

Fig. 5. Antidromic (top) and orthodromic (bottom) sensory nerve
conduction velocity in the median nerve between digit II and
wrist in 26 patients with a carpal tunnel syndrome. Open circles
with dot indicate patients having no definite antidromic potential.

action potentials have a low amplitude; in all these cases the distal conduction velocity was reduced. Potential duration and number of components were abnormal in 10 and 11 cases respectively. Two of these patients had normal conduction velocities between index finger and wrist.

If distal motor latency is taken into consideration, it can be said that 11 of the 14 patients having no definite antidromic potential, had an increased distal motor latency. Of the remaining three cases, 2 had abnormal orthodromic conduction velocity between digit II and wrist and one only had pathological orthodromic nerve action potentials.

CONCLUSIONS

28 of 30 patients with polyneuropathies had abnormal findings when recording sensory nerve action potentials from a median nerve with the orthodromic method. Potential duration and number of components were the most useful individual parameters. They were abnormal in 21 and 19 cases respectively. Antidromic sensory nerve conduction measurement from a median nerve proved to be of little value for the detection of mild or beginning polyneuropathies - the results being clearly abnormal in only 8 of 30 cases. If this diagnosis is considered, orthodromic nerve action potential recording is indicated. For the diagnosis of the carpal tunnel syndrome, however, antidromic sensory combined with motor conduction velocity is a very helpful and reliable screening method. Only in exceptional cases will the additional recording of orthodromic potentials be necessary.

REFERENCES

1. Ludin, H.P. (1976) Praktische Elektromyographie, Enke, Stuttgart, pp. 1 - 181.
2. Ludin, H.P., Lütschg, J. and Valsangiacomo, F. (1977) Z. EEG - EMG, 8, 173 - 179.

TABLE 2
CPT-SYNDROME UNDER PSYCHOPHARMACOTHERAPY

Patients	sex	age	drugs		latency from onset therapy to first symptoms of CPT (months)
E.H.	f	67	amitriptylin oxacepam Hydergin(R)	AD T	36
H.S.	f	62	amitriptylin promethacin Stutgeron(R)	AD N	18
H.K.	m	57	amitriptylin di-K-cloraceptat	AD T	18
E.G.	f	55	amitriptylin clordiacepoxid Hydergin(R) Optalidon(R) Modenol(R)	AD T	13
J.B.	f	46	amitriptylin DHE	AD	6
A.D.	f	54	amitriptylin clordiazepoxid	AD T	5
K.F.	f	71	oxacepam pracepam sulpirid	T T N	3

AD = antidepressant
T = tranquillizer
N = neuroleptic

A reverse time relationship between CPT syndrome and depression could not be observed in our patients: None of the patients seeing the doctor because of a CPT syndrome developed a depression later on (mean observation period 10 months). This should be the case at least in some patients if the co-incidence of CPT and involution-depression would be due to the fact that both have the same age distribution or are due to the same hormonal deficit syndrome. At least the possibility that certain drugs used in the therapy of depression could cause a CPT syndrome in predisposed patients should be discussed. Possible causative mechanism could be: Increase in bodyweight, edema and impairment of peripheral nerve function.

SUMMERY

Until now, ulnar nerve lesion is regarded as the most frequent type of peripheral nerve compression lesion[2]. In a neurological practice, however, CPT syndrome was found about 5 times as often as ulnar nerve lesion. An interesting observation was made in seven patients under long-term psychopharmacotherapy who later on developed a CPT syndrome.

REFERENCES

1. Jantz, D.
   Über das Karpaltunnelsyndrom als Grundlage von Schwangerschafts-
   paraesthesien.
   Dt.med.Wschr. **87**, 1457 (1962)

2. Mummenthaler, M.
   Die Ulnarislähmungen. Über 314 "nichttraumatische" eigene
   Beobachtungen.
   Schweiz.med.Wschr. **90**, 815 (1960)

Peripheral Neuropathies
N. Canal and G. Pozza, eds.
© 1978 Elsevier/North-Holland Biomedical Press

MICROELECTROPHYSIOLOGIC STUDIES ON THE NATURE OF NEUROMUSCULAR TRANSMISSION
BLOCK CAUSED BY PERIPHERAL NERVE INJURY

NORITOSHI SHIBUYA, M.D., KAZUTAKE MORI, M.D., YOSHIO NAKAZAWA, M.D. and
MITSUHIRO TSUJIHATA, M.D.
Department of Neurology, National Kawatana Hospital, Kawatanamachi,
Higashisonogigun, Nagasaki, 859-36 Japan

ABSTRACT

Neuromuscular transmission block due to an injury of the peripheral nerve
appears in the early stages of reinnervation. In microelectrode methods,
miniature end-plate potentials (MEPPs) were of normal amplitude but of decreased
frequency. The quantum content of the end-plate potential (EPP) decreased
significantly, while the quantum size of the EPP was within normal limit.
The time course of the EPPs was remarkably prolonged despite the normal time
course of MEPPs. Abnormal end-plate responses returned to normal after day
40. Neuromuscular transmission block in the early stages of reinnervation
could best be explained by a failure of impulse to invade the axon terminal
and by the decreased number of acetylcholine (ACh) quanta readily available
for release from the nerve terminals. It is likely that the metabolism of
ACh and calcium ions is not appropriate in immature nerve terminals.

INTRODUCTION

Neuromuscular transmission block has been found occasionally in the course
of motor neuron diseases and anticholinesterase drugs are of benefit to these
patients. We have reported that edrophonium responsive waning appears during
the period of reinnervation after mechanical injury of the peripheral nerve.[1]
In order to elucidate this nature, we studied microelectrophysiologically
the changes of the neuromuscular transmission during the period of reinnervation
after the nerve crush.

MATERIALS AND METHODS

Female Sprague-Dawley rats (initial body weight 100 gm) were used. The
sciatic nerve was exposed at the central region of the thigh and was crushed
for 30 seconds each at two levels with a 3mm wide Pean's forceps. Following
the nerve crush, changes at the neuromuscular transmission were observed till
day 60.

The extensor digitorum longus muscle and deep peroneal nerve were removed

under sodium pentobarbital anesthesia for in vitro recordings of resting
membrane potential (RP), spontaneous MEPP and EPP. The muscle was immersed
in the bathing fluid at a temperature of 29 to 30°C and stretched to its physiologic length. The bathing fluid was composed of 135 mM NaCl, 15 mM $NaHCO_3$,
10 mM Na_2HPO_4, 5.0 mM KCl, 2.0 mM $CaCl_2$, 1.0 mM $MgCl_2$, 11.0 mM glucose and
choline chloride 10^{-5}M, and was bubbled with 5 percent carbon dioxide and 95
percent oxygen with a resulting pH of 7.4. MEPPs and EPPs were detected by
conventional microelectrode techniques,[2] displayed on a cathode ray oscillo-
scope and recorded on an oscillofilm for measurements. The glass microelectrodes were filled with 2 M potassium acetate. Tip resistance was between
7 and 15 megohms. Fibers were used for measurements if the rise time of MEPPs
was less than 0.7 msec. Excluding "giant" potentials, 100 to 200 potentials
in a single fiber were measured to determine the mean amplitude and frequency
of spontaneous MEPPs. For recordings of EPPs evoked by nerve stimulation,
d-tubocurarine (3 x 10^{-7}gm/ml) was added to the bathing fluid in order to
eliminate muscle twitching. Sixty EPPs evoked by repetitive nerve stimulation
of 1 per second were recorded. Estimates were made from measurements of 50
EPPs after discarding the first ten EPPs. The amplitudes of MEPPs and EPPs
were corrected for non-lineality of the end-plate response assuming a transmitter equilibrium potential to be -15 mV and for the standard RP of 90 mV.[3]
Quantum size (q) and quantum content (m) were calculated from amplitude distributions of trains of EPPs, on the assumption that the number of quanta in
the EPPs fluctuated according to a Poisson distribution.[4] q and m were obtained
from the relation   q = variance of EPP/mean EPP, m = mean EPP/q.

RESULTS

Resumption of synaptic transmission first occurred 20 days after the nerve
crush when MEPPs appeared. RP showed no difference from the control on day
20 and thereafter when reinnervation took place. As shown in Figure 1 and
Table 1, MEPP frequency during day 20 to 35 decreased significantly ($p < 0.001$),
but it returned to normal after day 40. MEPP amplitude during this period
also decreased against values in normal control and showed variation in size
(Figure 1). However, there was no statistically significant difference (Table
1). The half decay time of MEPPs was 1.53 $\pm$ 0.03 msec (mean ± s.e., n = 57,
number of fibers) in normal muscles, and 1.67 $\pm$ 0.08 msec (n = 8) in reinnervated muscles on day 20 after the nerve crush. No significant difference in
the time course of MEPPs was found between normal muscle fibers and reinnervated muscle fibers. EPP evoked by a single nerve stimulus showed remarkable
prolongation of the distal latency and time course, and a decrease of amplitude

TABLE 1

END-PLATE RESPONSES FROM THE REINNERVATED MUSCLE

	RP	MEPP		EPP	
		Amplitude	Frequency	Quantum size (q)	Quantum content (m)
	(mV)	(mV)	(per second)	(mV)	
Control	77.3±0.5 (n=107)	0.94±0.02 (n=107)	1.36±0.04 (n=107)	2.16±0.44 (n=14)	99.62±7.79 (n=14)
Crushed, day 25	75.8±1.7 (n=8)	0.72±0.07 (n=8)	0.48±0.07* (n=8)	1.93±0.16 (n=14)	50.46±6.53* (n=14)
day 40	77.7±1.5 (n=3)	0.92±0.07 (n=3)	0.85±0.23 (n=3)	4.01±0.57 (n=5)	35.37±5.60* (n=5)
day 60	84.4±1.9 (n=5)	0.75±0.05 (n=5)	1.56±0.29 (n=5)	1.71±0.34 (n=8)	101.79±18.93 (n=8)

* Significantly different from control (p < 0.001)
 n = number of fibers   The values are the mean±s.e.

as shown in Figure 2. The half decay time of EPPs on day 20 after the nerve
crush was significantly prolonged to 2.53 ± 0.08 msec (n = 70, number of
potentials from different fibers) in contrast to the control value of 1.47 ±
0.03 msec (n = 45)(p < 0.001). When the motor nerve was stimulated repetitively
with high frequency, the amplitude of the EPPs in some end-plates increased
by twofold to threefold at the beginning of stimulation (Figure 3). In the
analysis of the quantal composition of the EPP (Table 1), the quantum content
of the EPP showed a significant decrease by student's t-test during day 20 to
40 compared with the value in the control, but it returned to a normal value
on day 60. The quantum size showed no significant difference.

DISCUSSION

In the early stages of reinnervation, the end-plates showed the following
electrophysiologic characteristics: 1. RP was normal; 2. MEPP frequency was
markedly reduced, while MEPP amplitude was in the low-normal range; 3. EPPs
had a small amplitude and their time course was greatly prolonged; 4. A progressive increase in the amplitude of EPPs was seen at some end-plates during
repetitive nerve stimulation with high frequencies; 5. The quantum content
of the EPP was abnormally small, but the quantum size of EPP was within normal
limit. These findings indicate that neuromuscular block in the early stages
of reinnervation is probably caused by presynaptic impairment.

The number of ACh quanta released by nerve impulse is affected by the
number of quanta readily available for release from the nerve terminal and

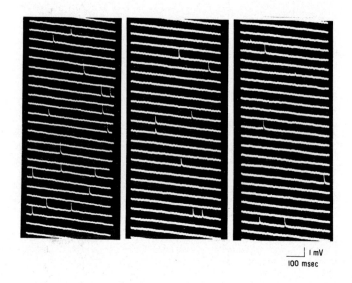

Fig. 1. Intracellular recordings of miniature end-plate potentials from the extensor digitorum longus muscle. Left: Recording from a normal muscle fiber. Center: Recording from a reinnervated muscle fiber 20 days after the nerve crush. Right: Recording 30 days after the nerve crush. Note that MEPP frequency shows a marked decrease after the nerve crush.

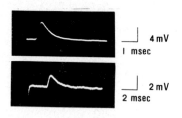

Fig. 2. End-plate potential evoked by a single nerve stimulus

Upper: EPP recorded intracellularly from a normal muscle fiber
Lower: EPP recorded from a reinnervated muscle fiber on day 20 after the nerve crush

Note the remarkably prolonged distal latency and time course of EPP on day 20 after the nerve crush.

by the probability of release. We have estimated the number of quanta assuming that quantum content of the EPP is distributed according to Poisson's law. However, Bennett and Florin[5] reported that statistical probability of release (P) was high ($P > 0.5$) at newly formed synapses and suggested that transmitter release could not be described by Poisson statistics but by binomial statistics when synapses are forming in reinnervated mammalian muscle. If their assumptions are correct, it might not be proper to compare the quantum content

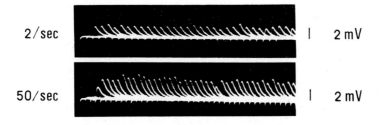

Fig. 3. Intracellular recording in vitro of end-plate potentials evoked by repetitive nerve stimulation. Note the progressive increase in amplitude of EPPs evoked by 50/sec nerve stimulation. RP = 80 mV d-tubocurarine 3x10^{-7} g/ml

in immature synapses with that in normal ones. Kuno and associates[6] observed that the quantum content of the EPP was positively correlated with the size of the nerve terminal. Tsujihata and Engel[7] observed electron microscopically, in the early stages of reinnervation, a significant decrease of the nerve terminal area and the number of synaptic vesicles per unit nerve terminal area, but no changes over the post-synaptic regions. In our experiment on repetitive nerve stimulation with high frequencies, the amplitude of EPPs increased by nearly twofold to threefold. This waxing is seen when the depolarization of the nerve terminal is suppressed by magnesium ions and low calcium ion concentration. Thus, a decreased number of ACh quanta released by nerve impulse is suggested. Moreover, if spontaneous release of transmitter reflects the resting level of calcium ions within nerve terminal,[8] calcium ions in immature nerve terminals may also be reduced, and changes in the calcium ion concentration in the nerve terminal may produce large alterations in the number of ACh quanta released.

In the early stages of reinnervation, the distal latency and time course of EPPs were remarkably prolonged. Despite the prolonged time course of EPPs, the time course of MEPPs was within normal limit and the MEPP amplitude showed no significant difference from the normal control. This may suggest that the prolonged time course of EPPs may be the delayed conduction time of impulse which results in a delay of depolarization in the synaptic boutons.

It has been well known that the conduction of nerve impulse is blocked at the nerve terminals in the early stages of reinnervation owing to the fact that motor axon re-establish synaptic connections through collateral sprouting with denervated muscle fibers, and newly formed axon terminals are initially unmyelinated and small in size. Dennis and Miledi[9] found that the 'non-

transmitting' synapses are present during early stages of end-plate reinnervation and concluded that transmission failure is caused by a block of impulse
conduction in the distal motor axon. Stålberg and Thiele[10] reported with their
method of single fiber EMG that conduction of impulse is probably blocked at
the branching points of axonal sprouting and considered that this neurogenic
blocking may contribute to the fatigue clinically experienced in patients with
motor neuron diseases.

Consequently, it is most likely that the fundamental defect of neuromuscular
transmission appearing in the early stages of reinnervation consists of the
impairment of impulse invasion and the decreased number of ACh quanta at the
nerve terminals. It is also likely that the metabolism of ACh and calcium
ions is not appropriate in immature nerve terminals.

REFERENCES

1. Shibuya, N., Hazama, R., et al. (1975) J. Neurol. Sci., 25, 463-471.
2. Fatt, P. and Katz, B. (1951) J. Physiol. (Lond.), 115, 320-370.
3. Katz, B. and Thesleff, S. (1957) J. Physiol. (Lond.), 137, 267-278.
4. Elmqvist, O., Hoffmann, W.W., et al. (1964) J. Physiol. (Lond.), 174, 417-434.
5. Bennett, H.R. and Florin, T. (1974) J. Physiol. (Lond.), 238, 93-107.
6. Kuno, M., Turkanis, S. A., et al. (1971) J. Physiol. (Lond.), 213, 545-556.
7. Tsujihata, M. and Engel, A. G. unpublished data.
8. Alnaes, E. and Rahamimoff, R. (1975) J. Physiol. (Lond,), 248, 285-306
9. Dennis, M. J. and Miledi, R. (1974) J. Physiol. (Lond.), 239, 553-570.
10. Stålberg, E. and Thiele, B. (1972) J. Neurol. Neurosurg. and Psychiat., 35, 52-59.

Peripheral Neuropathies
N. Canal and G. Pozza, eds.
© 1978 Elsevier/North-Holland Biomedical Press

PRESSURE NEUROPATHIES - THE NEED FOR MICROSURGICAL APPROACH

V. DOLENC and J.V. TRONTELJ

V.D.: University Hospital for Neurosurgery, University Medical Centre, Zaloška 7, 61105 Ljubljana, Yugoslavia

J.V.T.: Institute of Clinical Neurophysiology, University Medical Centre, Zaloška 7, 61105 Ljubljana, Yugoslavia

ABSTRACT

Due to improved diagnostics, increasing numbers of patients with various pressure neuropathies are referred for surgical treatment. Classical surgery usually provides excellent results in mild cases, but tends to fail in advanced cases, with pronounced neurological deficit. On operation, the latter cases usually show extensive intraneural fibrosis and atrophy of the nerve distal to the site of compression. It is postulated that removal of intraneural fibrotic tissue while sparing the vascular bed is essential for restoration of neural function.

The paper reports on a series of 233 patients (88 with carpal tunnel syndrome, 42 with cubital syndrome of the ulnar nerve, 33 with thoracic outlet syndrome, and 70 patients with other peripheral pressure neuropathies). The results were evaluated clinically and neurophysiologically and were rated good in a majority of the cases.

The results prove that microsurgery is the method of choice in the treatment of pressure neuropathies.

INTRODUCTION

Various pressure neuropathies represent an increasing proportion of patients treated for peripheral nerve problems in neurosurgical hospitals. This proportion is even higher if one includes cervical and particularly lumbar root lesions, which are certainly nothing but entrapment neuropathy. However these will not be discussed in the present paper.

Diagnostic possibilities have improved in the recent years as a result of the excellent scientific work of many of the honorary members of this meeting. As a neurosurgeon I feel strongly that these possibilities have to be used to achieve early diagnosis, particularly since entrapment neuropathy is one of the relatively few treatable neurological diseases.

PATIENTS

I should like to report on our experience with the neurosurgical treatment of entrapment neuropathies since 1972, when we introduced the microsurgical techniques in Ljubljana. In these 6 years we operated on 233 patients with various types of compression neuropathies (Table 1).

TABLE 1

Compression neuropathies treated microsurgically since 1972.

Carpal tunnel syndrome	88
Cubital syndrome of ulnar nerve	42
Thoracic outlet syndrome	33
Other compression neuropathies	70
T o t a l	233

As can be seen, carpal tunnel syndrome was much more common than other types of nerve entrapment.

The category "other compression neuropathies" comprises of entrapment of various nerves in scar tissue due to rather recent injury, except for a few non-traumatic cases (Table 2).

Among the patients with carpal tunnel syndrome, as many as one third turned out to be related to some old injury at the wrist (Table 3). Among the remaining patients, one third had an additional entrapment of the same nerve fibres at a more proximal site, i.e. double entrapment. As is also seen in the table, the incidence of carpal tunnel syndrome of non-traumatic aetiology is, in our material, six times higher in females. It is also of interest that nearly one half of the non-traumatic cases showed evidence of bilateral involvement.

TABLE 2

"Other compression neuropathies" of Table 1.

Entrapment of	No. of cases
Radial nerve	20
Median nerve	6
Ulnar nerve	3
Sciatic nerve	10
Peroneal nerve	22
Tibial nerve	9
Total	70

TABLE 3

88 cases operated for carpal tunnel syndrome.

	Post traumatic	Non-traumatic	Bilateral	Double entrapment
Males	19	9	4	1
Females	10	50	20	13
Total	29	59	24	14

In contrast to the carpal tunnel syndrome, traumatic aetiology seems to predominate in cubital syndrome of the ulnar nerve (Table 4). Here too we had cases of double entrapment, with an additional compression at the thoracic outlet or at the root level.

From 33 cases operated for thoracic outlet syndrome only 3 were males (Table 5). 12 cases had a rudimentary cervical rib, and the remaining 21 cases had a large transverse process of C7 vertebra associated with the so-called scalenus medius band (Bonney, 1965), with a hard fibrotic medial margin.

The diagnosis of the particular entrapment was made in each case according to the current neurological and neurophysiological criteria and was proved on operation. In none of the cases was there a negative finding on operation.

TABLE 4

42 cases operated for cubital syndrome of the ulnar nerve.

	Posttraumatic	Non-traumatic	Bilateral	Double entrapment
Males	19	5	0	3
Females	13	5	1	2
Total	32	10	1	5

TABLE 5

33 patients operated for thoracic outlet syndrome.

	Cervical Rib	Scalenus muscles	Bilateral	Double entrapment
Males	2	1	1	0
Females	10	20	4	2
Total	12	21	5	2

SURGERY

Classical approach was used in each of the entrapment syndromes. Conventional neurolysis was performed as the first stage of operation. In the second stage, when removing the thickened epineurium and the accumulated fibrotic tissue between the individual nerve bundles, magnification was always used. Intraneural fibrotic tissue was accumulated not only in the compressed length of the nerve trunk but extended up to 1 centimetre both in the proximal and distal direction, where it could be even more increased than in the compressed segment, thus contributing to a bulging appearance of the pre- and poststenotic segments. Naturally the prestenotic bulging is also due to the stop, or slowing, of the axoplasmic flow.

In the third stage of the operation, a higher magnification was used (up to 40x) to separate the individual funiculi, special attention being paid to sparing the vascular bed and interfunicular bridges.

Being aware of vulnerability of the already damaged nerve fibres, we did not use tourniquet ischaemia or regional anaesthesia in any of the patients.

RESULTS

Results of the treatment were evaluated both clinically and neurophysiologically. Pain and paraesthesiae disappeared within a few hours of operation in all carpal tunnel patients and in a majority of other patients. In the remaining patients, pain and paraesthesiae disappeared in less than 3 months.

Muscle atrophy, when present, recovered gradually, improving sometimes for as long as one year, particularly in cubital syndrome of the ulnar nerve and thoracic outlet syndrome. Patients with longstanding extreme atrophy and almost complete loss of motor units in affected muscles did generally not show much motor recovery. Most of other patients, i.e. 80%, recovered practically completely according to clinical criteria, while neurophysiological parameters, particularly sensory and motor conduction and amplitude of the M-wave and sensory nerve potentials, showed marked improvement, and in a proportion of patients (25%) even complete normalization. All patients regained ability to perform previously hindered motor actions within less than one year.

DISCUSSION

In comparison to the results obtained by the classical surgical methods (e.g. Lascelles et al., 1977; Benini 1975; Gilliatt et al., 1970), the results in our series of patients, which is completely nonselected, are considerably better. Having visual experience of the appearance of the intraneural structures in the entrapped nerve we cannot imagine any significant recovery following simple neurolysis without epineurectomy and removal of interfunicular fibrotic tissue, except for mild cases or cases of relatively short duration.

In other cases, axonal compression persists after neurolysis. The thickened epineurium represents a rigid tube with decreased inner diameter; the thickened epineural septa reaching between the individual funiculi further reduce the vital space for the axons. In other words, there is an additional inner entrapment, as we call it, which has to be relieved if any degree of functional improvement is to be achieved. In suppport to this view we can quote 5 patients operated upon in the classical way (1 - 3 times) without any improvement; when reoperated with the microsurgical method they showed good or fair recovery.

Therefore we are convinced that there is no substitute for microsurgical approach in the treatment of chronic entrapment neuropathies.

REFERENCES

1. Benini, B. (1975) Das Karpaltunnel Syndrom und die übrigen Kompessionssyndrome des Nervus medianus, Georg Thieme Verlag, Stuttgart, pp. 125-129.

2. Bonney, G. (1965) The scalenus medius band, a contribution of the study of the thoracic outlet syndrome. Journal of Bone and Joint Surgery (British) 47, 268-277.

3. Gilliatt, R.W., Le Quesne, P.M., Logue, V. and Sumner, A.J. (1970) Wasting of the hand associated with a cervical rib or band. Journal of Neurology, Neurosurgery and Psychiatry 33, 615-624.

4. Lascelles, R.G., Mohr, P.D., Neary, D. and Bloor, K. (1977) The thoracic outlet syndrome, Brain 100, 601-612.

Peripheral Neuropathies
N. Canal and G. Pozza, eds.
© 1978 Elsevier/North-Holland Biomedical Press

MICRONEUROSURGICAL TREATMENT OF THE ENTRAPMENT NEUROPATHIES OF THE UPPER LIMB

F.CASTELLANOS,R.GUILLEN,J.M.CASTILLA and J.JIMENEZ-CASTELLANOS
Service of Neurosurgery.University Hospital.Seville (Spain)

ABSTRACT

The purpose of this paper is to review our personal experience in the surgical treatment of the entrapment neuropathies of the upper limb followed during the last three years.
We performed in all the cases the interfascicular or perineural fascicular neurolysis with microneurosurgical technique.

INTRODUCTION

The place of neurolysis in the treatment of peripheral nerve injuries has received great attention in the literature.It
is a known fact,that since the introduction of the operating
microscope in 1964,there has been a tremendous change in the
operative treatment of peripheral nerve surgery.The extent of
nerve lesions can be more accurately estimated,with minimal
trauma to the area of the nerve damage[1].

The entrapment neuropathies are specific form of pressure
neuropathy in which nerve injury results from compression by
neighboring anatomical structures and developed by a variety
of conditions[2,3].Their diagnosis is clinical and must be done
in the early stages since the impairment of motor and sensory
nerve functions is usually reversible.The aid of the electrophysiological conduction velocity test of the nerve action
potentials is of a great importance[4].

Failure to improve following medical and postural treatment
suggest as necessary the surgical liberation of the nerve.

In addition,there is no doubt that of the three surgical techniques in entrapment neuropathies: conventional decompression,
decompression and epineural neurolysis and decompression and
perineural fascicular or interfascicular neurolysis,the microsurgical techniques are superior to conventional methods of
surgery[5],because individual fascicles can be exposed and libe-
rated from scar strangulation,removing the external sheet of
the epineurium.In fact with the perineural fascicular neurolysis
even the perineurium of each and every fascicle should remain
intact and not be traumatized.

However we must acknowledge that discussions still continue
about these methods of treatment,so that in the present work
we express our personal experience during the last three years.

CLINICAL MATERIAL AND METHODS

We have studied 13 cases of entrapment neuropathies of the
upper limb in 12 patients which had to be admitted to the Neurosurgical Service (Prof.Jimenez-Castellanos),during the years 1975
to 1977,for surgical treatment.

The evaluation of clinical features was realized from three
points of view: Motor functions (**paralysis and atrphy**),Sensory
functions (paresthesia,hypo or anaesthesia an pain) and Electro-
neurophysiological methods (electromyographycal abnormalities
as fibrillation potentials,motor and sensory conduction velocity
and motor distal latency).The system of grading used was from
0.- normal function, 1.- minimal disturbance,to 2.- severe disturbance, so we can provided the basis for judging the efficacy
of our treatment[6].We performed in all the cases the perineural
fascicular neurolysis with the microneurosurgical technique of
SAMII.Seven of our cases need also anterior transposition (super-
fitial way) of the ulnar nerve in the elbow,and in one case
we make a bilateral carpal tunnel approach.

Clinical data,localization,treatment effected on each one of the patients and evolutionary control of the results after three to six months of surgery,appear reflected in the Tables I and II.

TABLE I

ENTRAPMENT NEUROPATHIES OF THE UPPER LIMB

Operative results in 13 cases treated by interfascicular neurolysis.

Cases Nº	Localization	Symptoms	Treatment	Results
1 46,M	Left ulnar n. Cubital T.	M2,S2,A2 EMG.2	If.neurolys. Ant.transp.	Mo,S1,A1 EMG.o
2 64,M	Left ulnar n. Cubital T.	M2,S2,A2 EMG.2	If.neurolys. Ant.transp.	Mo,S1,A1 EMG.o
3 54,M	Left median n. Int.bicip.T.	M1,S1,A1 EMG.1	If.neurolys. Decompression	Mo,So,Ao EMG.o
4 24,M	Right median n. Int.bicip.T.	M2,S1,A2 EMG.2	If.neurolys. Decompression	M1,So,A1 EMG.1
5 53,M	Right ulnar n. Cubital T.	M2,S2,A2 EMG.2	If.neurolys. Ant.transp.	M1,S1,A1 EMG.1
6 29,M	Right ulnar n. Cubital T.	M1,S1,A1 EMG.1	If.neurolys. Ant.transp.	Mo,So,Ao EMG.o
7 24,M	Right ulnar n. Cubital T.	M2,S2,A2 EMG.2	If.neurolys. Ant.transp.	Mo,So,Ao EMG.o
8 34,M	Left ulnar n. Cubital T.	M1,S1,A1 EMG.1	If.neurolys. Ant.transp.	M1,So,A1 EMG.1
9 43,M	Right median n. Carpal T.	M1,S1,Ao EMG.1	If.neurolys. Decompression	Mo,So,Ao EMG.1
10 45,F	Left ulnar n. Cubital T.	M2,S2,A2 EMG.2	If.neurolys. Ant.transp.	M1,S1,A2 EMG.1
11 43,M	Right median n. Carpal T.	Mo,S2,Ao EMG.1	If.neurolys. Decompression	Mo,So,Ao EMG.o
12 43,M	Left ulnar n. Guyon's T.	M1,S2,Ao EMG.2	If.neurolys. Decompression	Mo,So,Ao EMG.o
13 43,M	Left median n. Carpal T.	M1,S1,Ao EMG.1	If.neurolys. Decompression	Mo,So,Ao EMG.o

DISCUSSION

The surgical attitude towards entrapment neuropathies has oscillated,since the first experience of LEARMONTH in 1933, from the very interventionist posture[7,8,1],that recommended surgical intervention as soon as possible with decompression at the entrapment level and adequate exposure of the nerve,to the most moderate posture of waiting a demostrable improvement in nerve functions with medical and postural treatment[9,10].

As regards the surgical approach,we think that it is the only satisfactory form of treatment,and also,it is only during operation with the aid of the operating microscope,that one can distinguish with certainty between normal and fibrotically changed epineurium,with a magnification rate of from 10 to 25 powers.

TABLE II

ENTRAPMENT NEUROPATHIES OF THE UPPER LIMB

Results of clinical controls (3 - 6 months)

Nerve	Localization		Good	Fair	Poor
Ulnar	Guyon's Tunnel	1	1	–	–
	Cubital Tunnel	7	5	2	–
Median	Carpal Tunnel	3	3	–	–
	Bicip. Tunnel	2	1	1	–
Total		13	10	3	–
		100%	77%	23%	–

Our study present the results of a short series of 13 cases of entrapment neuropathies of the upper limb.Eight patients with entrapment of the ulnar nerve,seven of them at the elbow, in the "cubital tunnel" of Feindel and Stratford,and the remain-

der case at the wrist in the Guyon's tunnel.The median nerve
was affected in five cases: three carpal tunnel syndromes and
two at the level of the elbow in the internal bicipital tunnel,
one by compression of the Struther's ligament,and the other
case showed the whole median nerve involved at the level of
the pronator teres muscle in the upper forearm,with motor and
sensory disorders.

The patients'ages were ranging from 24 to 64 years with an
average of 42 years.As far as the sex is concerned was observed
a great predominance of male in 11 cases,that could be in relation with occupational or microtraumatic etiology.Surgical
approach was realized after medical and postural treatment
proving to be unsuccessfull,with failure to improve the nerve
functions and increase of abnormal electrophysiological signs.
We do not consider advisable to use local steroid therapy.

When considering surgical treatment for entrapment neuropathies,one must take into account the operatory instructions
and techniques to be used.Conventional decompression and microsurgical approach for perineural fascicular neurolysis was
always realizes.The diagonally placed small fascicles must be
preserved and the use of bipolar coagulation avoid the damage
of neural blood supply and postoperative ischemic injuries.

The clinical and electrophysiological evolutionary control
of our cases was performed by the same observer three to six
months after surgery,with an average time of 4.5 months.The
results were good in ten cases (77%) and fair in three cases.
The improvement was excellent as regards pain,subjective sensory disorders and muscular weakness,but in contrast the muscle atrophy was little improved.The results of comparative
electrophysiological measurement were improved except in the
cases where there were important preoperative signs of denervation.

Finally,in order to the surgical classification of neural compression,[1] the first type of injury only needs conventional decompression,but in the other two types,with thickening and neural atrophy,we feel obliged to do the perineural fascicular neurolysis because most failure or bad results with conventional techniques are probably caused by scar tissue from epineurium.

REFERENCES

1. Samii,M.(1975) Moderns aspects of peripheral and cranial nerve surgery. Advances and Tech.Stand.in Neurosurgery. Vol.2,3-84.Springer Verlag.Wien.

2. Staal,A.(1970) The entrapment neuropathies. In Handbook of Clinical Neurology.Elsevier.Amsterdam.vol 7,part I,285-325.

3. Marenghi,P.and Soncini,G.(1976) La sindrome del canali di Guyon. L'Ateneo Parmense.Act.Bio.Med.47, 177-184.

4. Zilch,H.and Buck-Gramcko,D. (1975) Ergebnisse der Nerven-wiederherstellungen an der oberen Extremität durch Mikro-chirurgie. Handchirurgie 7, 21-31.

5. Gassmann,N and Segmüller,G. (1976) Das Karpaltunnelsyndrom. Helv.chir.Acta, 43, 699-702.

6. Castellanos,F. (1978) Lesiones traumaticas neurales del miembro superior:Experiencia personal.Rev.Quir.Esp.(in press)

7. Curtis,R.and Eversman,W.(1973) Internal neurolysis as an adjunt to the treatment of the carpal tunnel syndrom. J.Bone Jt.Surg. 55A, 733-740.

8. Noterman,J.et al.(1975) La pathologie chirurgicale du nerf peripherique. Acta Chir.Belg. Suppl.I, 1-192.

9. Seddon,H.J.(1972) Surgical disorders of the peripheral nerves. Churchill Livings.London.

10. Kenesi,C.and Scheffer,J.C. (1977) Le debridement chirurgicale du canal carpien. Rev.du Rhumatisme. 44 (1), 35-40.

METABOLIC, GENETIC
AND INFLAMMATORY NEUROPATHIES

Peripheral Neuropathies
N. Canal and G. Pozza, eds.
© 1978 Elsevier/North-Holland Biomedical Press

ELECTROMYOGRAPHY AND NERVE CONDUCTION VELOCITY MEASUREMENTS
IN GENETIC NEUROPATHIES

F. ISCH

Service d'Electromyographie, Clinique Neurologique, Hospices
Civils, 67005 STRASBOURG CEDEX (France)

ABSTRACT

Our knowledge on the electrophysiological aspects and anatomo-
pathological correlations in genetic neuropathies has expanded
during recent years. The object of this paper is to assess the
significance of routine electromyography and nerve conduction measurements in a large series of patients presenting clinical signs
of hereditary neuropathy or heredodegenerative syndroms.

INTRODUCTION

Lambert, (1962[1]), Kaeser, (1965[2]) and Isch et al (1966[3]) reported
the contribution of nerve conduction velocity measurements in the
delimitation of atrophies resulting from soma or peripheral nerve
lesions in chronic or progressive neurogenic atrophies. Hence, a
participation of the peripheral nervous system in heredodegenerative syndroms was clearly shown. Ultrastructural studies (Dyck,
(1973[4]), P.K. Thomas, (1973[5]) and correlations between conduction
velocity and the ultrastructure of nerves (Isch-Stoebner et al,
(1973[6]), Mc Leod et al, (1973[7]) demonstrated the predominance of
segmental demyelination in the slowing of conduction velocity and
the frequency of "onion bulbs" in peripheral nerve fibres in degenerative syndroms. However, these correlations do not allow any
physiopathological or etiological classification ; real progress
came from biochemical studies showing a metabolic disorder resulting in abnormalities of nerve fibers : autosomal recessive metabolic disorder in phytol metabolisme with accumulation of Phytanic
Acid in Refsum's Disease (Alexander, (1966[8]), Rake and Saunders,
(1966[9]) primary deficiency of Arylsulphatase A in Metachromatic
Leukodystrophy (Austin et al, (1966[10]). Unfortunately, in the majority of cases biochemical tests are negative and it seems that

clinical definition, EMG and conduction velocity measurements are still essential in the diagnosis of a degenerative syndrom of peripheral nerve fibers.

MATERIALS AND METHODS

171 records of patients examined in the Service d'Electromyographie du Centre Hospitalier et Universitaire de Strasbourg were studied. Reasons of referral varied from progressive distal amyotrophies in the lower limbs, foot deformations (principally pes cavus), gait disturbances or clinical pictures of spinocerebellar heredodegeneration. All age groups were represented but we were more selective for patients over 50 years of age, excluding cases where suspicion of such disorders as alcoholism or diabetes mellitus, complicating a neurological picture of heredodegeneration, was legitimate.

Routine electromyography was performed in the distal muscles of the upper and lower limbs, using Broncks coaxial needle electrode, followed by motor nerve conduction measurements. Muscles of the forearm and legs were tested, according to clinical data, in search of subacute denervation (fibrillation potentials and positive sharp waves) or signs of progressive or chronic neurogenic atrophy (reduction in number of motor unit potentials with high frequencies on vigorous voluntary contraction). Motor conduction velocities were determined along the Common Peroneal and Tibial nerves (normal values over 45 m/sec) and the Median and Ulnar nerves (normally over 50 m/sec). In cases of marked distal peripheral lesions in the lower limbs, conduction measurements may not be obtainable ; in the upper limbs they often give valuable information even in the absence of clinical signs (Isch et al, (1966[3-6]).

Conduction velocity of afferent fibers was measured on the reflex potentials in the Abductor Digiti Minimi, in some cases. Sensory conduction measurements were not performed, for technical reasons.

30 % of the patients were followed up for several years with clinical examination, EMG, conduction measurements and biological tests. Unfortunately we do not dispose of complete records for each patient because of the mode of recruitement in our Unit.

However, some correlations between conduction velocity measurements and ultrastructural aspects were carried out, and, to a limited extent, biochemical studies.

Two cases of Amyloïd neuropathy without clear evidence of genetic factor involved, and ten patients presenting "mal perforants" where the role of other metabolic factors (diabetes mellitus...) could not be differenciated, were excluded.

RESULTS

1° Routine electromyogramm rarely shows signs of subacute denervation (fibrillation potentials, positive sharp waves). These were present only in one case of Refsum's disease (18 years old male) in the distal muscles of the lower limbs conveying possible aggravating phases in the course of the disease.

On vigorous voluntary contraction, tracings of chronic or progressive neurogenic atrophy, frequently obtained, are undistinguishable from these seen in spinal atrophies (fig IB, 2B and C). On the other hand, the presence of an interference pattern without signs of denervation does not exclude anomalies in conduction (fig IC, 2A and C).

2° Motor nerve conduction velocity measurements have always conceded valuable information : slowing of conduction velocity has always been significant : inferior to 35 m/sec in median and ulnar nerves, 30 m/sec in the Common Peroneal and Tibial nerves.

DISCUSSION

In neuropathies with innate metabolic disorder (Table I) our results (slowing of conduction velocity) are in agreement with the related literature. In metachromatic leukodystrophy, slowing is prominent in the afferent and efferent fibers of large diameter (fig IA). In Refsum's disease slowing is marked in the upper limbs contrasting with a rich interference pattern of voluntary activity (fig 2D).

In spinocerebellar heredodegenerations (Table II) numerous works reported the frequency of associated peripheral nerve fibers lesions to such a degree that frontiers with peripheral heredodegenerative diseases of the Charcot-Marie-Tooth type may be less rigorous (De Recondo, 1977[11]). In table II, Friedreich syndroms

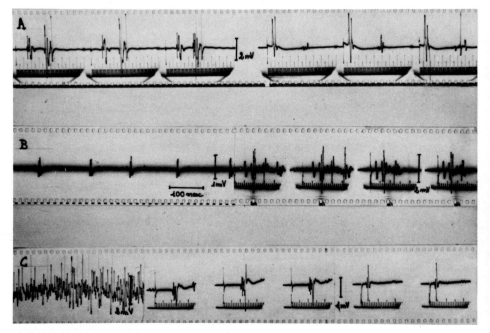

Fig. I.

A : Metachromatic leukodystrophy : 9 years old boy ; Conduction velocity of
Tibial nerve. Motor and reflex responses. C.V. of motor and afferent fibers :
17-19 m/sec.

B : 2 years old girl : family disease with pyramidal syndrom in the lower
limbs and signs of chronic neurogenic atrophy. No etiology found. Voluntary
activity in left extensor digitarum brevis. C.V. of Common Peroneal
37-25 m/sec.

C : 9 years old boy : pes cavus, bilateral Babinski sign and impairment of
deep sensibility. In lower limbs C.V. 20 m/sec. Rich activity in Abductor
Digiti Minimi. C.V. of Ulnar n. 16-17 m/sec. No clinical signs in upper limbs.

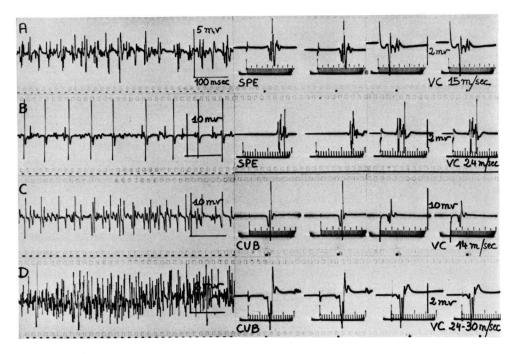

Fig. 2.

A : 18 years old female : pes cavus without other neurological signs. Family
incidence. m. Extensor Digitorum Brevis : intermediate activity without signs of
denervation. C.V. in Common Peroneal : 15 m/sec.

B : 22 years old male : pes cavus (no family incidence), pyramidal syndrom
in lower limbs. m. Extensor Digitorum Brevis : simple tracing with high frequencies (chronic neurogenic atrophy). C.V. of Common Peroneal : 24 m/sec.

C : 58 years old male : Ataxia with tremor in upper limbs (Roussy-Levy ?)
m. Abductor Digiti Minimi : Intermediate activity with high amplitude potentials and some high frequencies (chronic neurogenic atrophy). C.V. Ulnar :
16 m/sec.

D : 18 years old male : progressive distal polyneuritis-Refsum's disease.
Inexcitability of nerves in lower limbs. m. Abductor Digiti Minimi : Rich
activity without signs of denervation. C.V. Ulnar : 24-30 m/sec.

with the classical signs (ataxia predominating in the lower limbs
loss of deep reflexes, impairment of deep sensibility, pes cavus,
cyphoscoliosis, bilateral Babinski sign, impairment of coordination
in the upper limbs) were grouped. In comparison with our first
series (3) the proportion of cases without conduction impairment
is important and some of them are in an advanced stage of the
disease. Therefore, the absence of slowing of conduction velocity
cannot be considered as a sign of good prognosis in the course of
the disease.

TABLE 1

Metabolic Neuropathies	C.V. ↓	N.C.V.
Refsum's disease	1	–
Metachromatic Leukodystrophy	2	–
Niemann-Pick disease	1	–

TABLE II

Spinocerebellar degeneration	C.V. ↓	N.C.V.
Friedreich's type	17 (5 fam.)	14
P. Marie	2 (1 fam.)	–
Roussy-Levy	3	–

   The presence of a progressive distal amyotrophy associated or
not with bilateral pes cavus in the lower limbs constitutes a difficult nosological problem in the absence of biochemical criteria
(Table III). These progressive distal amyotrophies may resemble
some chronic polyneuritis i.e Refsum's disease or hereditary amy-
losis. Appreciation of foot deformation may be perplexing : pes
cavus with distal amyotrophy of varying degree or distal amyotrophy with foot deformation of varying degrees. Furthemore, sensory
impairment may be of different degrees not allowing clear clinical

TABLE III

Peripheral Motor Heredodegenerations	C.V.⊥	N.C.V.
Progressive distal amyotrophy (Charcot-Marie-Tooth?)	20 (3fam.)	12 (1 fam.)
Dejerine-Sottas polyneuropathy	1	-
Pes Cavus	16 (5fam.)	47 (2 fam)
Progressive distal amyotrophy + pyramidal syndrom	14 (3fam.)	5
Pes Cavus + pyram. syndrom	5	11

TABLE IV

Pes Cavus with normal C.V.	
- isolated	31 (2 fam.)
+ neurogenic atrophy (with normal C.V.)	8
+ degenerative stigure	8
+ pyramidal syndrom	11

limits between the Charcot-Marie-Tooth disease and the Dejerine-Sottas hypertrophic polyneuropathy. Palpable thickening of the peripheral nerves in the latter, though a valuable diagnostic sign is not invariably present. Detection of "onion bulbs" in nerve biopsy should be appreciated quantitatively due to their unspecified character (Dyck P.J., (1975[12]) - Said G. (1978[13]). The association of a distal amyotrophy, with or without pes cavus, with a pyramidal syndrom approaches the clinical picture of meta-chromatic leukodystrophy ; but to what degree the Pyramidal syn-drom becomes a prere quisite of a spasmodic family paraplegia of Strumpell Lorrain...

A family incidence was found in some cases of each of these syndroms. In their majority, they occur sporadically within a family.

The proportion of bilateral pes cavus (Table IV) accompanied or not by other symptoms (amyotrophy, pyramidal signs...), is augmented in the absence of lesions of peripheral nerve fibers.

Hence, motor nerve conduction velocity measurements appear as an important semeiologic element for the dissociation of the various syndroms where peripheral nerve fiber lesion are suspected.

SUMMARY

The contribution of detection electromyography and, prominently, of conduction velocity measurements is essential in the delimitation of genetic neuropathies. Conduction impairment may be found in the absence of signs of neurogenic atrophy. Routine electromyography is helpful in following up the evolution of the peripheral nerve lesion. Slowing of motor nerve conduction velocity is significant except in cases of advanced stages where all fibers are inexcitable. Our series of 171 patients shows various clinical pictures : chronic polyneuritis, progressive spastic paraplegia, syndroms resembling Friedreich's ataxia, isolated familial pes cavus. In some cases the etiology may be defined : innate metabolic disorder in Refsum's disease or metachromatic leukodystrophy. The majority of cases consist of heredodegenerations of peripheral nerve fibers : Charcot-Marie-Tooth disease, hypertrophic Dejerine-Sottas polyneuropathy are the most representative entities. Spinocerebellar degenerations comprising more clinical signs constitute even more complexe entities.

Conduction velocity measurements are valuable in defining the presence of a degenerative syndrom of peripheral nerve fibers in a complex clinical picture.

ACKNOWLEDGEMENTS

I wish to thank Dr. Cécile ISCH-TREUDDARD and Dr. L. MIDDLETON for their help in the preparation and translation of this paper.

REFERENCES

1. Lambert, E.H. (1962) Diagnostic value of electrical stimulation of motor nerves, Electroencephal. Clin. Neurophysiol., suppl. 122, pp. 9-16

2. Kaeser, H.E. (1965) Veränderungen der Leitungsgeschwindigkeit bei Neuropathies und Neuritiden, Fortschr. Neurol. Psych, 33, pp. 221-250

3. Isch, F., Isch-Treussard, C. and Jesel, M.(1966) La mesure de la vitesse de conduction des fibres nerveuses dans les atrophies neurogènes chroniques ou progressives, Rev. Neurol., 115, pp. 122-129.

4. Dyck, P.J., (1973) Ultrastructural Alterations in Myelinated Fibers, New Developments in Electromyography and Clinical Neurophysiology édit. by J.E. Desmedt, 2, pp192-226 Karger Basel.

5. Thomas, P.K. The Ultrastructural Pathology of unmyelinated nerve Fibers, Ibid, pp 227-239.

6. Isch, F., Stoebner, P., Jesel, M. and Isch-Treussard, C. Conduction Velocity and Ultrastructure of Nerves, Ibid, pp 240-247.

7. Mc Leod, J.G., Prineas, J.W. and Walsh, J.C. The relations hip of Conduction Velocity to Pathology in peripheral nerves, Ibid, pp 248-258.

8. Alexander, W.S. (1966) Phytanic Acid in Refsum's Syndrom, J. of Neurol. Neurosurg. Psychiat., 29, pp 412-416.

9. Rake, M, and Saunders, M. Refsum's Disease a disorder of lipid metabolism. Ibid, pp 417-422.

10. Austin, J., Armstrong, D., Shearer, L. and Mc Afee, D (1966) Metachromatic form of diffuse cerebral sclerosis. VI. A rapid test for the sulfatase A deficiency in metachromatic leukodystrophy (MLD) urine, Arch. Neurol. (Chic), 14, pp 259.

11. Recondo, J. (de) (1977) Hérédo-dégénérescences spino-cérébelleuses. Encycl. Méd. Chir. Paris Neurologie 17079 B[10], 7

12. Dyck, P.J. (1975) Inherited neuronal degeneration and atrophy affecting peripheral motor, sensory and autonomic neurons in Dyck Thomas Lambert : Peripheral Neuropathy. W. Saunders Philadelphia, pp 825-867.

13. Said, G. (1978) Névrites hypertrophiques primitives, Encycl. Méd. Chir. Paris Neurologie. Fasc. 17080 B[10], 3.

Peripheral Neuropathies
N. Canal and G. Pozza, eds.
© 1978 Elsevier/North-Holland Biomedical Press

THE LONG TERM ISSUE OF ACUTE IDIOPATHIC POLYNEURITIS (LANDRY-
GUILLAIN-BARRE SYNDROME)

MARCO MUMENTHALER, HANS-PETER LUDIN, LIVIA N. ROSSI,
NIKLAUS B. LOEFFEL
Department of Neurology, Inselspital, CH - 3olo Berne

INTRODUCTION

When they first described the disease - which was later named
after them - Guillain, Barré and Strohl (1916) considered it
to have a very good prognosis. Professor Georges Guillain, one of
the authors (M.M.) first teacher in Neurology, used to speak of
"une maladie bénigne et spontanément curable". As a matter of fact
they had to admit later, that fatal outcome due to ascending paralysis with respiratory insufficiency was possible[2]. Such cases
therefore did not differ from what Landry had described in 1859
as "paralysie ascendante aiguë", which in 4 out of his 5 original
cases wasn't fatal. We therefore fully agree, that if an eponym
has to be used, one should talk about the Landry-Guillain-Barré
syndrome (LGBS)[13,25].

The respiratory and infectious complications of LGBS are quite
well mastered by modern intensive care medicine. One therefore
expects mortality to become lower and lower. Our purpose was to
give an account of the course and the mortality in 154 personal
cases and to analyse the long term issue of the so-called "cured"
cases. We base this paper on two former publications[11,21] and on
additional 31 cases observed since.

MATERIAL AND METHODS

During a period of 15 years, from 1963 to 1977, the diagnosis
of LGBS was made in 198 in-patients of the Berne University
Hospital. 44 of these were children less than 16 years old at the
acute disease stage. After elimination of insufficiently documented or misdiagnosed cases, the data of 154 patients could be
analysed, 97 of which were re-examined after a period between

o.9 and 12.3 years, in average 5.o3 years. The age at follow up
was between 7 and 78 years.

RESULTS

The clinical picture in the acute phase

To be included in this study the cases had to fulfill the
following definition, i.e. an acute or subacute illness with
flaccid, mainly motor paralysis, which had reached its maximum
in 8 weeks or less, which shows an increased protein content in
the cerebrospinal fluid (CSF), with or without cranial nerve and
central nervous system participation[5]. A few cases with normal CSF
protein values, but otherwise fulfilling these criteria were included. After elimination of insufficiently documented cases and
following the criteria just mentioned 154 cases were retained and
analysed. 87 were males and 67 females; 44 were younger than
16 years in the acute phase; the age at the beginning varied from
1.6 to 88 years. In 78 cases an other disease or particular event
preceded the LGBS, in general a non-specific infection of upper
respiratory tract or a gastrointestinal disorder. 3 adults had
been bitten by an insect in the weeks preceding the acute illness,
but none by a tick. One had had a zoster in the first trigeminal
division, one a paratyphus B, one an epidemic hepatitis, one an
acrodermatitis chronica atrophicans (Herxheimer) (without indication for a tick-infection), one an infectious mononucleosis and
one a variola-vaccination two weeks earlier.

Initial symptoms consisted of paresthesias in half the cases
(in 3 followed first by cranial nerve weakness), paresthesiae
together with motor weakness of the limbs in 1/4 of the cases and
only motor weakness initially in the remainder. Even in those cases beginning with paresthesiae, motor weakness was soon prominent.

The progression was from distal to proximal in 3/4 of our cases
and in nearly all of them it spread from the legs to the arms.
All the cases presented here had reached maximal motor weakness
within 4 weeks with the only exception of 3 cases where progression lasted up to 8 weeks. The average time from beginning of weakness to its maximum was 12 days.

TABLE 1

CLINICAL SIGNS IN THE ACUTE PHASE OF 154 PATIENTS WITH LANDRY-GUILLAIN-BARRE SYNDROME

	N	%
Motor weakness	148	96
Sensory impairment	lol	66
Cranial nerve signs	68	44
CNS involvement	17	11

The signs at the maximum of the acute phase are summarized in TABLE 1. Flaccid motor paralysis was always prominent. In 125 out of 148 cases the arms as well as the legs were affected, in 21 cases only the legs and as a rarity in 2 adults only the arms. In 2 cases fasciculations were observed. The tendon reflexes were abolished in all cases. Sensory loss was present in 66 % of all patients, but could in general be demonstrated less frequently in children. In 17 % of adults there was no history of paresthesiae and no sensory loss at the examination. In several cases, where no sensory loss could be demonstrated clinically, pathological sensory nerve action potentials however could be recorded. Cranial nerve paralysis was present in 68 of the 154 cases, somewhat more frequently in adults (51 %) than in children (32 %). In nearly 2/3 of the cases the facial nerve was affected, in most cases bilaterally. TABLE 2 gives the figures for all cranial nerves.

Important respiratory insufficiency was present in 23 patients, all adults, which had to be treated by intubation or tracheostomy and artificial respiration for a period up to 4 weeks. Disturbance of sphincter functions was rare and was observed in only 14 of our cases, always in the form of urinary retention or incontinence, never as a loss of bowel control. Obstipation however was the rule. Tachycardia and hypertension were quite frequent in severely paralysed patients, also outside of infectious pulmonary or other secundary complications. In 16 of the patients neck-stiffness and in

TABLE 2

CRANIAL NERVE SIGNS IN 154 PATIENTS WITH LANDRY-GUILLAIN-BARRE
SYNDROME

Eye motility disorders	12
Vth nerve involvement	1
Facial palsy	45
IXth + Xth nerve involvement	3o
XIth nerve involvement	6
XIIth nerve involvement	7
Total	1o1 cranial nerve involvement in 68 cases (44 %)

several (not examined systematically) a positive Lasègue sign was
present. There was no relation to the cell count in the CSF. Quite
a number of patients mentioned aching pains, mainly in the legs
and hands in the course of the disease, but in 3 patients pain was
a very early and very prominent symptom.

TABLE 3

CNS SIGNS IN 154 PATIENTS WITH LANDRY-GUILLAIN-BARRE SYNDROME

Pyramidal tract involvement	9
Ataxia	6
Dystonic features	2
Action myoclonus	1
Gaze paralysis	1
Disturbed consciousness	1
Total	2o symptoms in 17 cases (11 %)

Central nervous symptoms were rare, may however be part of a
"polyradiculitis". 17 of the 154 patients had symptoms, which indicated participation of the central nervous system in the disease

process (TABLE 3). The prevalence in children was noteworthy: 9 out of 41 (22 %) had central nervous symptoms. These were, however, not very striking and consisted mainly of slight cerebellar ataxia, which was not just paretic ataxia. 5 of the 113 adults had pyramidal tract signs, which were accompanied in 2 cases by choreoathetotic movements of the arms and dystonic oral movements, in a third case by an action myoclonus of both arms and in one patient by a gaze paralysis. One adult patient was disoriented and one had an ataxia.

The cerebrospinal fluid could be examined in 141 cases. In 122 (87 %) the typical increase of protein with normal cell count, the "dissociation albumino-cytologique" was found. Total protein in one case was 795, in another even 16oo mg %. 19 of the patients had normal protein values, 6 in a single sample before the end of the second week. In 13 adults however with otherwise typical clinical signs and course, protein was normal 3 weeks ore more after onset of the disease process. 2 of these cases had a slight increase in cell count, which was present in 13 further cases, i.e. in a total of 15 of the 141 cases (1.4 %). 3 of these, however, showed in a second sample taken 2 or more weeks later, the typical albumino-cytological dissociation.

In addition to the respiratory insufficiency mentioned above in 23 patients we observed the following neurological complications: a 14-year-old girl had papilloedema and an increase of the CSF pressure to 5o cm water. A Rickham reservoir had to be applied. 5 patients had a recurrence of their polyneuritis after 4 - 5 months and after 1, 2, 8 and 13 years respectively after an initial complete recovery. One young woman had a neuralgic shoulder amyotrophy (paralytic brachial neuritis) with local pain and a paralysis persisting for several months after the clearing of the weakness due to the LGBS.

Amongst the 154 patients only 4 deaths were observed which bore an immediate or indirect relationship to the Guillain-Barré syndrome. All 4 patients were adults: a 7o-year-old man died 56 days after the beginning of his symptoms because of pneumonia with respiratory insufficiency; a 66-year-old man died after 4 days

from pulmonary embolism; a 61-year-old man with diabetes mellitus, hypertonia and cardiac insufficiency died after 3 weeks of respiratory treatment with pneumonia and a 22-year-old woman after 6 days because of sepsis, probably due to a pre-existing ulcerative colitis and proctocolectomy. The overall mortality was therefore 2.9 %.

Follow up study

TABLE 4
RESIDUAL SIGNS IN 97 PATIENTS WITH LANDRY-GUILLAIN-BARRE SYNDROME

	N	%
Motor weakness	2o	21
Absent reflexes	24	25
Sensory signs	14	14
Cranial nerve signs	3	3
CNS signs	6	6
Total	67 signs in 43 patients == (44 %)	

Only in 97 of the 154 patients was follow up possible. We saw them again after a period of between o,9 and 12,3 years, an average of 5,o3 years. Their ages at the follow up examination was between 7 and 77 years. Of these 97 patients, 54 (56 %) were completely cured on re-examination. 43 patients showed residual symptoms (TABLE 4). Motor weakness, present in 2o cases (21 %), was mainly distal in the lower extremities. In 24 cases one or more tendon reflexes were missing, mainly the ankle jerks. 7 of these, however, had no motor weakness or other signs or symptoms. Sensory loss was present in 14 adults, but in none of the children, not even in the older and co-operative ones. These 14 adults had a "stocking" distribution of sensory loss, 11 only for vibration and 3 in addition also for touch. Cranial nerve paralysis at follow up was not found in the children, twice was a minimal facial weakness observed in 2 adults and once a bilateral very marked peripheral facial palsy was present 2 years after the acute

illness in a 53-year-old woman. Amongst the CNS signs present in
6 cases at follow up were ataxia in 5, 4 of which were children.
In the adult with ataxia there was also a positive Babinski sign.
Another adult showed a dissociated nystagmus. All signs had already been present during the acute phase.

Electrophysiological examinations were done at follow up in
55 patients, 36 children and 19 adults. The results have been
described earlier[11, 21]. In summary 11 showed abnormal findings
on needle electromyography (EMG) of the extensor digitorum brevis muscle, including fibrillations and a reduced interference
pattern or single oscillations on maximal active innervation. All
these patients also had clinical residual signs. There were, however, patients with clear-cut sensory loss or loss of reflexes
who had a normal EMG in the above-mentioned muscle. All patients
without any clinical signs had a normal EMG. The conduction velocity measurements, motor and sensory, did not show a constant relationship to the residual clinical signs. In 11 of the 36 children[21] and in a similar proportion of the adults a disturbance of
conduction velocity mostly in the carpal tunnel was found without
any residual clinical signs.

It was our impression, that during the acute phase of the
disease, only 2 clinical features seemed to be of prognostic
value for the amount of recovery: patients who had a particularly
pronounced tetraparesis seemed most frequently to have residual
signs at follow up. In addition a particularly long time span between the moment at which the initial signs reached their maximum
and the moment when recovery started seemed to be correlated with
frequent residual signs at follow up. It was not our impression,
that corticosteroid treatment had any real benefic influence on
the course of the disease or on the degree of recovery[11,21].

DISCUSSION AND CONCLUSIONS

The comparison of our personal observations with the data from
the literature in the large material presented here does not differ
essentially from the conclusions we published earlier[11,21]. We
like therefore only to stress a few points, which in our opinion
may complete the classical picture of LGBS and facilitate the

diagnosis:

- The disease can present in every age group: small children [1,3,5,9,12,21], but also in very old people. Our youngest patient was 1,6 years, our oldest 88 years old.

- The disease presents in about 5o % of cases only with motor symptoms and always were motor symptoms soon prominent even in the presence of sensory symptoms or signs[14,2o,25].

- Cranial nerve signs are frequent and were present in 44 % of our patients. Most prominent was a facial palsy in 2/3 of these cases. The Fisher syndrome[4] in his classical form however seems rare.

- Central nervous system participated in 17 of the 154 cases (11 %) to the disease process. This confirms the data of the literature[5] and stresses, that in the presence of CNS signs in an otherwise typical case, one should not hesitate to make the diagnosis of LGBS.

- The typical "dissociation albumino-cytologique" was present in 87 % of the CSF examined. The presence of increased cell count in a few cases had no bearing on the clinical aspect or the prognosis[8]. The normal CSF in the very beginning may become typically altered after 3 weeks[7].

- The mortality of 4 out of 154 cases (2.9 %) is very low. All the cases had additional severe diseases or handicaps. Prognosis quo ad vitam is therefore better in children. Similar figures are given in the literature[14,15,19].

- At follow up the presence of residual signs is frequent: we found 67 signs in 43 of the 97 cases (44 %) we reviewed after o.9 and 12.3 years. In accordance with others absent tendon reflexes and motor weakness are the most frequent residual signs[8,9,16,19]. Residual facial weakness is rare. These signs were never a real handicap in children and rarely in adults.

- Of probable negative prognostic value for the amount of residual signs were a profound paralysis[9,18,19] and a long duration of maximal motor weakness before the beginning of recovery[3,17].

- The treatment with corticosteroid had also in our experience no positive influence on the disease course[13,18,19,22,23,24,25].

SUMMARY

154 cases of Landry-Guillain-Barré syndrome are analysed following age range, presenting symptoms, signs and complications in the acute disease phase. 4 patients died. At follow up after o.9 and 12.3 years 97 cases were seen. 44 % showed some residual signs, mainly motor weakness and absent tendon reflexes. They were very rarely handicapped.

REFERENCES

1. Banerji, N.K. and Millar, J.H.D. (1972) Develop. Med. Child. Neurol. 14, 56-63

2. Barré, J.A. (1938) J. belge Neurol. Psychiat. 38, 314-322

3. Eberle, E., Brink, J., Azen, S. et al. (1975) J. Pediat. 86, 356-359

4. Fisher, M. (1956) New Engl. J. Med. 255, 57-65

5. Gamstorp, I. (1974) Develop. Med. Child Neurol. 16, 654-658

6. Guillain, G., Barré, J.A. and Strohl, A. (1916) Bull. Soc. Méd. Hôp. Paris 4o, 1462-147o

7. Haymaker, W. and Kernohan, J.W. (1949) Medicine (Baltimore) 28, 59-141

8. Kaeser, H.E. (1964) Schweiz. Arch. Neurol. Psychiat. 94, 278-286

9. Kotlarek, F., Lenard, H.G. and Schulte, F.J. (1974) Mschr. Kinderheilk. 122, 198-2o2

lo. Landry, O. (1859) Gaz. hebd. méd. Chir. 6, 472-474

11. Löffel, N.B., Rossi, Livia N., Mumenthaler, M. et al. (1977) J.Neurol.Sci. 33, 71-79

12. Low, N.L., Schneider, J. and Carter, S. (1958) Pediatrics 22, 972-99o

13. Marshall, J. (1963) Brain 86, 55-66

14. Masucci, E.F. and Kurtzke, J.F. (1971) J.neurol.Sci. 13, 483-5o1

15. McFarland, H.R. and Heller, G.L. (1966) Arch.Neurol.(Chic.) 14, 196-2o1

16. McLeod, J.G., Walsh, J.C., Prineas, J.W. et al. (1977) J.neurol. Sci. 27, 145-162

17. Oppenheimer, D.R. and Spalding, J.M.K. (1973) J. Neurol. Neurosurg. Psychiat. 36, 979-988

18. Petermann, A.F., Daly, D.D. and Dion, F.R. (1959) Neurology (Minneap.) 9, 533-539

19. Pleasure, D.E., Lovelace,R.E. and Duvoisin, R.C. (1968) Neurology (Minneap.) 18, 1143-1148

2o. Ravin, H. (1967) Acta Neurol. Scand. Suppl. 3o, 43, 9-64

21. Rossi, Livia N., Mumenthaler, M., Lütschg, J. et al. (1976) Neuropädiatrie 7, 42-51

22. Sandu, L. (1974) Lancet 2, 662

23. Siegenthaler, D. and Regli, F. (1966) Schweiz. med. Wschr.96, 781-787

24. Thomas, P.K. (1969) Brain 92, 589-6o6

25. Wiederholt, W.C., Mulder, D.W. and Lambert, E.H. (1964) Proc. Mayo Clin. 39, 427-451

Peripheral Neuropathies
N. Canal and G. Pozza, eds.
© 1978 Elsevier/North-Holland Biomedical Press

ELECTROPHYSIOLOGICAL AND HISTOLOGICAL STUDY IN GUILLAIN-BARRÉ-STROHL
(GBS) SYNDROME

IRENA HAUSMANOWA-PETRUSEWICZ, HANNA JĘDRZEJOWSKA,

BARBARA EMERYK-SZAJEWSKA, KATARZYNA ROWIŃSKA-MARCIŃSKA

Department of Neurology, Medical School, Warsaw, Poland.

ABSTRACT

20 cases of the Guillain-Barré-Strohl syndrome were investigated clinically
and electrophysiologically. 16 cases showed monophasic (acute or subacute)
course of the disease; four cases represented relapsing or recurrent form of
the disease. In six cases the sural nerve biopsy was taken and on the basis
of histological observation it is suggested that all presented cases comprise
one homogenous group in terms of common pathomechanism of myelin destruction.
There was no correlation between clinical symptoms and slowing of motor and
sensory conduction velocity in peripheral nerves. The so-called long nerves
were involved earlier and more markedly than the short. In monophasic cases
however the correlation between conduction velocity changes and histological
findings was found.

INTRODUCTION

The aim of the study was to evaluate the correlation between the clinical,
electrophysiological and histological findings in various forms of GBS syndrome.

MATERIALS AND METHODS

The group consisted of 20 cases; their age ranged from 3 to 53 years. The
course of the disease was monophasic (acute or subacute) in 16 cases, relapsing
in three patients and recurrent in one case. In patients showing recurrent or rel
relapsing course of the disease the number of bouts ranged from three to over
ten. The clinical diagnosis has been based on the commonly accepted criteria.
In two patients with relapsing form of the disease the first episode followed
the course of an acute, monophasic GBS syndrome. In one of the relapsing
cases and in a patient showing recurrent course of the disease the onset of the
illness was similar to that observed in monophasic, subacute form of the disease.
The following applied to the group as a whole:
1. No disease preceding, associated or developed after neuropathy had
   appeared except, in some cases, an inflammatory one.
2. Predominant motor disturbances in form of symmetric involvement of

proximal or proximal and distal limb muscles.

3. Elevated CSF protein level.

For a more objective evaluation of the clinical condition of patients an arbitrary 48-points system of scoring was adopted, according to which the clinical manifestations found in a patient scored each one point or two, depending on intensity of symptom. Clinical and electrophysiological examination were performed in three substages of monophasic form of GBS syndrome:

I - peak of clinical manifestation

II - early improvement, i.e. the first signs of the subsidence of symptoms; and

III - late improvement, usually some months after the onset.

The relapsing and recurrent cases were examined clinically and electrophysiologically many times, during the episodes and between them.

Electrophysiological investigation. The maximum and minimum motor conduction velocities (V_{mot} max and V_{mot} min) and sensory conduction velocity (V_{sen}) were determined in the ulnar and the peroneal nerves; the sensory conduction velocity of the sural nerve and the conduction time in the facial, axillary and musculocutaneous nerves also were determined. Conduction time and distal latency were calculated per 1 cm of nerve length and presented as ms/cm. Motor conduction was investigated by the method described by Hodes et al.[1]; surface electrodes (type 13K62) were used for stimulation and the evoked potentials were picked up with co-axial needle electrodes (type 13K51). Maximum and minimum motor conduction velocities were determined by modificated method of Hopf[2]. The conduction velocity of sensory fibres was measured by the method of Buchtal and Rosenfalck[3]. The conduction time of the facial nerve was measured in the standard manner and that of the axillary and the musculocutaneous nerves was determined by stimulating the brachial plexus at Erb's point and picking up the responses from the deltoid and biceps brachii muscles.

All the investigations were made in a heated room (26°C) with the temperature of the extremities monitored and, if necessary, brought up to 35°C. Normal values were obtained for each nerve from a control group of 20 healthy subjects.

For statistical processing of the data the analysis of variance in non-orthogonal systems of two-way cross classification was applied; Student's test was used for detailed comparisons.

Histological investigation. The sural nerve biopsy was taken in three cases showing monophasic course of the disease, in two cases with relapsing form of disease and in one recurrent case. In two of the monophasic cases the biopsy

was obtained during the substage I (at the peak of clinical manifestation);
in the third monophasic case the biopsy was taken at the substage III (nearly full
recovery). In one of the cases with the relapsing form of the disease the
biopsy was taken during the first bout of the disease, and in the other one it
was done five years after the onset, at the time of a succeeding relapse. In
the case running a recurrent course of the disease the biopsy was obtained
during the third and latest bout.

In examining the sural nerve, conventional routine stains were used, the
axis cylinder diameter was measured in semithin epon sections and teased fiber
preparation as well as electron microscopy were employed. The details of histological methods used in our Department have been described elsewhere[4].

RESULTS

Electrophysiological results. In most patients conduction velocity was
variously slowed in the particular nerves. Efforts at correlating the electrophysiological parameters with the clinical condition of patients as defined by
our scoring system were a failure, which is shown in Fig. 1.

An analysis of the relation between the electrophysiological parameters
and the substage of the disease is shown in Fig. 2 and Fig. 3.

In substage I i.e. at the peak of clinical manifestations motor and
sensory conduction as well as motor latency were altered in a statistically
significant manner in the so-called long nerves (the ulnar, peroneal, and
sural nn.) whereas conduction time in the so-called short nerves (the facial,
axillary, and musculocutaneous nn.) was not. In substage II, the electrophysiological parameters were not improved, in most cases they were even
worse, with conduction slowed still further and distal latency more prolonged.
At this substage there was also a change in the conduction time of short
nerves. In substage III, the parameters in the long nerves becams like in
substage I or even closer to normal.

The changes in the motor conduction of thick and thin fibres (V max and
V min)' were parallel both in the ulnar and peroneal nerves at all the substages
with exception of just one case. It should be noted that there was no correlation between electrophysiological abnormalities and clinical condition.

Comparisons were also made of different nerves in respect of particular
electrophysiological parameters and of different parameters for the same
nerve. Thus the ulnar nerve was compared with the peroneal in regard of
conduction velocity, which was found not to differ substantially between
the two even though the legs were clearly more affected clinically.

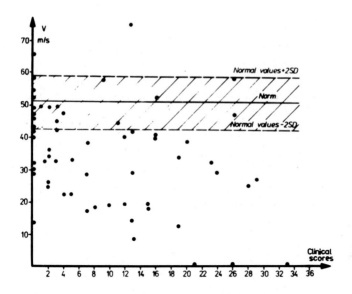

Fig. 1. Motor conduction velocity in peroneal nerve in relation to clinical scores.

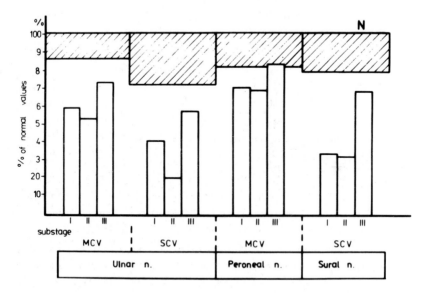

Fig. 2. Conduction velocity at different substages of the disease in 3 long nerves. N – normal values.

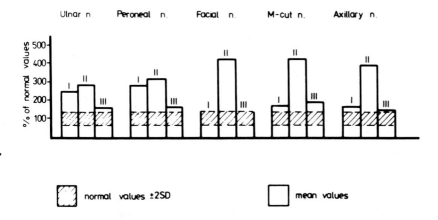

Fig. 3.   Conduction time and latency at different substages of the disease.

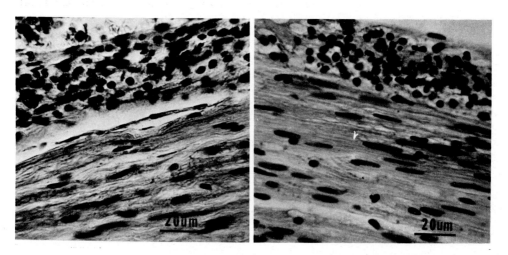

Fig. 4a.   Perivascular mononuclear infiltration in acute, monophasic case (substage I).   Hematoxyline and eosin stain.
Fig. 4b.   Inflammatory infiltration in subacute, monophasic case (substage III). Hematoxyline and eosin stain.

Next, comparisons of motor conduction with the sensory were made between
the deep peroneal and the sural nerve and within the ulnar nerve. The sensory
and motor conduction was similarly changed, even though the clinical sensory
manifestations were rather slight or even altogether imperceptible.

The results obtained in four patients with the relapsing or recurrent form
of the disease need to be presented separately. The conduction value was
low in these patients even during remissions, and was slowed still further after
each succeeding bout. The interrelations between particular electrophysiological
parameters were the same as in the group of monophasic cases.

Histological results. Biopsies of the sural nerve revealed in all six cases
the presence of mononuclear-cell infiltrations and segmental demyelination.
The infiltrations were perivascular and also scattered in the endoneurium
(Fig. 4a, b). In three cases - two monophasic and the one recurrent - the
early stages of demyelination could be observed. Teased-fibre preparations
showed that macrophages can enter the nerve fibers at any point of an internode
(Fig. 5a); demyelination, however, was often seen to begin in the region of a
node of Ranvier (Fig. 5b).

Electron-microscopy showed macrophages penetrating the Schwann cell basal
lamina of seemingly normal fibres (Fig. 6a, b) and beginning to destroy the
myelin (Fig. 6c).

Wallerian-like axonal degeneration and regeneration were in evidence in a
small proportion of fibers in all cases. There was no correlation between
the intensity of segmental demyelination and axonal degeneration.

The most striking histological difference between the monophasic and the
relapsing long-standing cases was proliferation in the latter of endoneurial
collagen. "Onion-bulb" formations were small and infrequently seen.

In two cases there was loss of large myelinated axons. The case in which it
was particularly evident was recurrent and the specimen was taken during
the third and latest episode, 21 months after the onset of the disease (Fig. 7).
Less marked reduction in axon diameter was found in biopsy obtained in the subacute, monophasic illness (see below - patient I.B.).

Some correlation between the electrophysiological and the histological findings were found in cases showing monophasic course of the disease, as it is
shown e.g. in the following cases:

1. Patient Z.G., aged 29, with monophasic, acute course of disease.
Conduction velocity study and sural nerve biopsy were performed in substage I
of the disease. Conduction velocity was relatively little changed and histo-

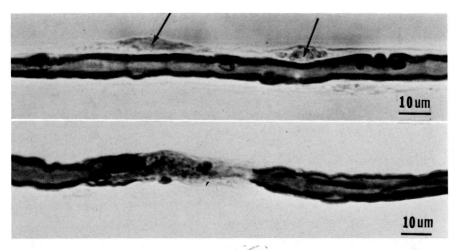

Fig. 5a. Teased preparation. Macrophages (arrows) invading the seemingly normal internode.
Fig. 5b. The demyelinating area in the region of a node of Ranvier.

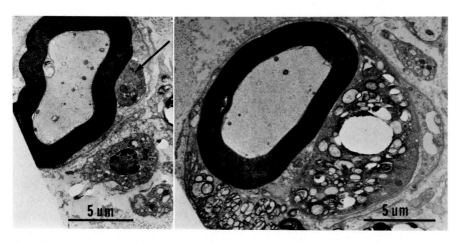

Fig. 6a. Processes of macrophage (arrow) below the basal lamina of Schwann cell.
Fig. 6b. Processes of macrophage has penetrated the basal lamina of Schwann cell. Note the normal structure of Schwann cell, myelin and axis cylinder.

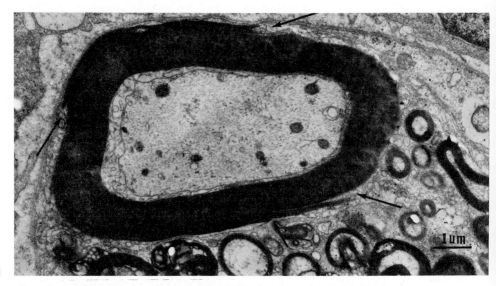

Fig. 6c. The early destruction of myelin by macrophage (arrows).

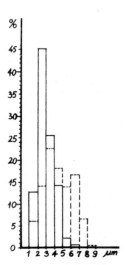

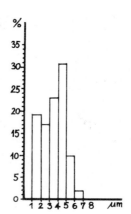

Fig. 7. Case with recurrent form
of disease.

Fig. 8. Case with subacute, monophasic
form of disease (substage III).

The distribution of axon diameters of myelinated fibers. Continuous line-
patients; interrupted line-controls.

logical abnormalities were moderate: 41 per cent of teased fibers showed demyelination and/or remyelination and early stages of myelin destruction were a frequent sight. The remaining 59 per cent of fibres were unaltered and fibre density as well as the histogram of myelinated axon diameters were normal. Similarly to other cases, conduction velocity was slowed in substage II, and became slightly better by the time of the next examination.

2. Patient I.B., aged 3 years. The course of the disease was monophasic and subacute. During substage III slowing of conduction velocity was marked and so were the histological abnormalities revealed by biopsy. Inflammatory infiltrations were conspicuous and as many as 87 per cent of fibers showed demyelination or remyelination. Early stages of myelin destruction were also in evidence. In the diameter distribution of myelinated axons there was a slight shift to the left (Fig. 8). Subsequent check-ups showed a slow improvement of the electrophysiological parameters.

In cases running a relapsing or recurrent course distinct correlation of the electrophysiological parameters with the histological could not be detected.

DISCUSSION

Our study does not show the positive correlation between the clinical condition and changes in the conduction velocity. In monophasic cases however, it was possible to discern a certain rule: during the beginning of the disease, but with the clinical manifestations already at the peak (substage I), the electrophysiological parameters were moderately changed. Afterwards, however, when clinical improvement had already begun (substage II), they not only failed to become better but sometimes even deteriorated. Not until further clinical improvement (substage III) was this trend clearly reversed.

Upon comparison with the results of morphological studies, the sequence of electrophysiological changes seen in our material may be explained by the spreading of the lesion from spinal roots towards the periphery, which is known to occur in most cases of the GBS syndrome [5,6,7]. At the substage II the changes become very evident by using electrophysiological and histological methods. At the same time remyelination begins in the proximal segments and roots gradually abolishing the block and restoring function, thereby giving rise to the first signs of clinical improvement. Further clinical improvement and a gradual normalization of the electrophysiological parameters come much later (substage III), when the reparative processes have probably spread already to the peripheral segments of the nerves.

It is rather difficult to explain the differences in the findings on conduction velocity between the long nerves (ulnar and peroneal nn.) and the so
called short ones (axillary, musculocutaneous, and facial nn.). As has already
been mentioned, conduction was slowed in the long nerves earlier and for longer
time. A possible explanation is perhaps a greater likelihood of demyelination
affecting in the course of the disease a larger number of segments in the long
nerves and therefore leading more rapidly to major changes in conduction[8].

Cases with bouts and remission need to be discussed separately. Some years
ago the recurrent idiopathic polyneuropathy has been considered to be a variant
of acute idiopathic polyneuropathy[5,9,10], whereas nowadays the two are more
often considered as separate varieties[11,12] or even as different nosological
entities[13]. Prineas and McLeod[12] believe that the acute form of GBS syndrome
is a self-limiting auto-alergic reaction directed against peripheral nerves,
whereas in the recurrent and relapsing polyneuropathy we are dealing with a
chronic and periodically exacerbated autoimmune response.

According to our histological findings the monophasic, recurrent and relapsing
cases comprise one homogenous group in terms of common pathomechanisms of myelin
destruction i.e. cell mediated immune demyelination. This was also postulated
by Prineas[11] and Prineas and McLeod[12].

Electrophysiologically, relapsing and recurrent cases are characterized by
conduction velocity that becomes exceptionally low after a few episodes, remains variously reduced during remission and after more numerous episodes
declines very much further, sometimes indicating even a complete block.
This is most probably the consequence of demyelination occurring in the fibers
not completely remyelinated during the stage of remission.

It should be stressed that comparisons of the electrophysiological and
histological data obtained by different authors are not easily made, especially
in regard to the relapsing and recurrent forms of disease. The number and
duration of episodes, intensity of changes during episodes, and their subsidence
during remission explain the differences in the results recorded and complicate
their interpretation.

To judge by our material, there seems to be no correlation between clinical
symptoms and electrophysiological changes. The latter concern both sensory
and motor conduction velocity and are in relapsing and recurrent cases more
evident than in monophasic. However there is some correlation between electrophysiological and histological data especially in monophasic form of the disease.

REFERENCES

1. Hodes, R., Larrabee, M.G., German, W. (1948) Arch. Neurol. Psychiat. (Chic.), 60, 340-365.

2. Hopf, H.C. (1963) Arch. Neurol. (Chic.), 9, 307-312.

3. Buchtal, F., Rosenfalck, A. (1966) Brain Res., 3, 1-122.

4. Jędrzejowska, H. (1977) Acta neuropath. (Berl.), 37, 119-125.

5. Asbury, A.K., Arnason, B.G., Adams, C.D. (1969) Medicine, 48, 173-215.

6. Wiśniewski, H., Terry, R.D., Whitaker, J.N., Cook, S.D., Dowling, P.C. (1969) Acta Neurol. (Chic.) 21, 269-276.

7. Carpenter, S. (1972) J. Neurol. Sci., 15, 125-140.

8. Arnason, B.G.W. (1975) in Peripheral Neuropathy, Dyck, P.J., Thomas, P.K., Lambert, E.H. V.II eds., Sauders Co., Philadelphia, pp. 1110-1148.

9. Marshal, J. (1963) Brain, 86, 55-66.

10. Thomas, P.K., Lascelles, R.G., Hallpike, J.F., Hewer, R.L. (1969), Brain, 92, 589-606.

11. Prineas, J.W. (1971) Acta neuropath. (Berl.) 18, 34-57.

12. Prineas, J.W., McLeod, J.G. (1976) J. Neurol. Sci., 27, 427-458.

13. Dyck, P.J., Lais, A.C., Ohta, M., Bastron, J.A. Okazaki, H. (1975) Mayo Clin. Proc., 50, 621-637.

Peripheral Neuropathies
N. Canal and G. Pozza, eds.
© 1978 Elsevier/North-Holland Biomedical Press

INHERITED AMYLOID POLYNEUROPATHY IN AN ITALIAN FAMILY

BERGAMINI L., SCHIFFER D., DELSEDIME M., FARIELLO R. Jr., FURLAN P.M.,

LACQUANITI F., QUATTROCOLO G. and BECHIS F.

Neurologic Clinic, University of Turin. Turin (Italy)

ABSTRACT

We describe a numerous Italian family affected with an inherited
amyloid polyneuropathy which has clinical features somewhat different from
those of the previously reported types. Sensory-motor neuropathy of both
lower and upper limbs, cranial neuropathy, dysautonomy, cardiopathy and
vitreous opacities were observed. Pathology findings are presented.

INTRODUCTION

Since Andrade[1] first described in 1952 his clinical form in Portugal,
several reports on Hereditary Amyloid Neuropathy (HAN) have been published
in the world.

Three main forms of HAN, Andrade's[1], Rukavina's[2] and Van Allen's[3], are
generally distinguished on the basis of the
prominent involvement of the lower limbs, the upper limbs or both
respectively. Meretoja[4] described a further type with cranial neuropathy.

In this work we present a numerous family affected with HAN.

MATERIAL AND METHODS

Preliminary data on this family have appeared[5,6]; as far as we know ,
this is the first Italian family described with HAN.

The pedigree (fig. 1) includes 93 subjects over five generations. The
total number of certainly afflicted subjects is 30; five other individuals
were uncertainly or mildly affected. Eleven affected subjects (7 males and
7 females) were directly examined.

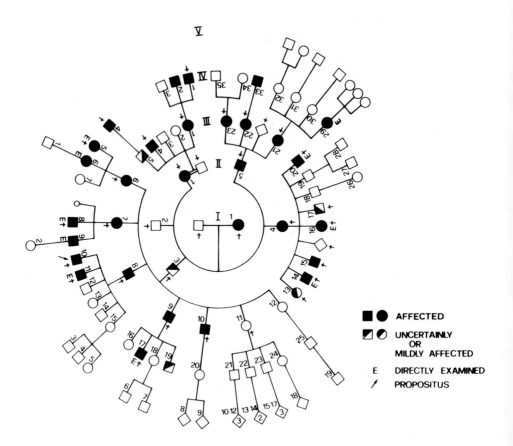

RESULTS

Synthetic data of all the cases directly examined are illustrated in Tab.I.

The onset of the disease was often insidious. Various kinds of dysesthesias (pains, cramps, burning feelings etc.) were in most cases the initial symptoms. Loss of temperature discrimination frequently led to burns. The deep sensibilities were always not much involved. Later on motor dysfunction appeared causing stumbling and steppage. Severe muscle atrophy and flaccid paresis began distally in the limbs and, as the sensory impairment, progressed proximally. Deep reflexes disappeared.

In a lot of cases also cranial nerves were implicated: internal ophthalmoplegia, trigeminal and bulbar nerves palsy were seen.

In the late stages of the illness the patients became tetraparetic and confined to a bed. Marked wasting, painless trophic ulcers were characteristic

CLINICAL SYNOPSIS OF ELEVEN EXAMINED SUBJECTS

Subject no.	III-14	III-16	III-20	IV-5	IV-6	IV-8	IV-9	IV-10	IV-11	IV-17	IV-20
Sex	M	F	M	F	F	M	M	M	M	M	F
Sensory—motor neuropathy	+	+	+	+	+	+	+	+	+	+	+
Pupils abnormalities	+		+		+		+		+		
Facial hypoesthesia		+		+					+		+
Dysphagia and dysarthria		+				+			+		
Trophic ulcers	+	+	+		+		+	+	+	+	
Spontaneos mutilations		+		+							
Disautonomy	+	+	+	+	+	+	+		+	+	
Cardiopathy	+	+	+			+	+	+	+	+	
Vitreous opacities	+			+			+				

of these stages; spontaneous mutilations of toes and fingers occurred
especially in women.

Alternating constipation and diarrhea, double incontinence, impotence, orthostatic hypotension and sweating disturbances were frequent and indicative of
autonomic nervous system involvement. Cardiac ischemia and various kinds of
arrhythmias (right bundle branch and atrio-ventricular block) were particularly
prominent in men. Vitreous opacities could be seen in 3 cases. In only one case
were the kidneys clinically involved.

We possess positive pathologic data of only 2 cases: one complete autopsy
and one sural nerve biopsy. Most of the patients refused any kind of biopsy.

The autopsy revealed at the gross inspection an enlarged, flaccid heart with
mild hydropericardium and arteriosclerotic changes in the coronary arteries and
aorta. Suppurative broncopneumonia was present in both lungs. Gross appearance
of liver, spleen and kidneys was unremarkable. The cerebral hemispheres showed
marked edema and softening areas. The spinal cord was unremarkable externally;
the transverse section revealed atrophy of the posterior columns which

appeared grey and translucent. No thickening could be seen in the peripheral nerves and ganglia.

Congo red stained sections of the various organs were examined with both ordinary light and polarizing microscope. Amyloid was seen diffusely in the heart, liver, spleen and kidneys. It was present in the leptomeninges but not in the substance of the brain. The neurons of the sympathetic and posterior root ganglia were atrophied and rarefied. Amyloid was present in the capsule and in the perivascular spaces of the ganglia. In the roots and the peripheral nerves deposits of amyloid occurred mainly in epineurium but also, although to a lesser extent, beneath perineurium and in endoneurium.

The age of onset of the disease was variable; in one case the illness started at 11 years and in another one at 50 y. But in most cases (25 out of 30) the range was from 22 y. to 38 y. The disease was always progressive and fatal; the duration ranged from 3 to 26 years with an average of 10.4 y.

The disease of our family is inherited in autosomal dominant fashion; this is evident also from the simple inspection of the pedigree. Of course, in order to verify the percentage of the affected and of the healthy people, one must exclude the last generation (V) whose members are too young to exhibit clinical symptoms of the illness.

The phenotypic expression of the gene, as it can be valued from the clinical course, is also sex-related. While, in fact, in women the course of the illness was dominated by the neurodystrophic lesions, in men gastrointestinal and cardiac symptoms were the most prominent.

DISCUSSION

We have summarized in Tab. II the main clinical features of the four types of HAN today recognized (for further data see Andrade[1], Rukavina et al.[2], Van Allen et al.[3] and Meretoja[4] respectively).

All the families reported until now have been classified in one or another of these types. Our family instead can not be fitted exactly into and particular type; seeming rather to imbricate with all of them.

HEREDITARY AMYLOID NEUROPATHIES

	age of onset, yr	death in yr	main neuropathy	other prominent clinical aspects
Andrade type	25 – 35	10 – 12	lower limbs; dysautonomy	cardiopathy
Rukavina type	40 – 50	16 – 35	upper limbs (carpal tunnel syndrome)	vitreous opacities; cardiopathy
van Allen type	30 – 40	10 – 20	lower then upper limbs; dysautonomy	nephropathy; peptic ulcer
Meretoja type	30 – 50	20 – 40	cranial nerves (VII)	lattice corneal dystrophy
our type	25 – 35	5 – 15	cranial nerves (III,V,IX,X); lower and upper limbs; dysautonomy	vitreous opacities; cardiopathy

It shows, in fact, the almost simultaneous involvement of both upper and lower limbs, as in Van Allen type. But unlike this form, in ours cranial nerves are often implicated, while peptic ulcer and nephropathy that are typical features of the family of Van Allen, are absent.

In no case could we observe a classic carpal tunnel syndrome, which is typical of the family of Rukavina. But it is obviously difficult to diagnose this syndrome in the presence of a global involvement of all the nerves of the upper limbs.

Dysautonomy, vitreous opacities, gastrointestinal and cardiac symptoms are similar to those seen in many other families.

Pathology data of our two cases are not dissimilar to those described in most other families; central nervous system is uninvolved whilst peripheral nerves, posterior roots and spinal and autonomic ganglia are extensively infiltrated by amyloid. Amyloid is present not only in the perivascular spaces but also in the interstice of the nerves. Among the other organs heart and kidneys are those in which amyloid is more abundant. It must be noted that its distribution in the nerves and in all other organs appear much more widespread when examined with the polarizing microscope.

Inheritance is autosomal dominant in our family as in all other cases till now reported. But ours is the first kindred in which important differences in the phenotypic extressivity of the gene are sex-related (as already said, in women syringomielic dissociation, neurodystrophic lesions with spontaneous mutilations of the extremities and suppurations of both skin and internal organs dominated the course of the illness; in men, on the contrary, gastro-intestinal and cardiac disturbances prevailed and death was often caused by cardiac failure).

In conclusion, the family described in this report seems to exhibit a form of HAN clinically distinct from all the previous types. More than as a new form, it should be considered, in our opinion, as a transition form linking the formerly reported types and, so, shuffling the cards in the nosography of HAN.

In any case the nosographic limits previously traced out appear uncertain if they are sifted with some criticism.

Although for instance nephropathy is clinically evident only in Van Allen's family (and to a smaller extent in Meretoja's), the kidneys are almost constantly involved by amyloid, as histological examination proves, in most of the other families.

The same can be said for eye involvement by amyloid which gets to different degrees in different HAN forms, going from the progressive blindness determined by the lattice corneal dystrophy of the family of Meretoja to the slight or absent visual deficits associated with the vitreous opacities of the families of Andrade and Rukavina.

Also the differential involvement of the upper limbs in the family of An—drade and in that of Van Allen seems to be quantitative more than qualitative, since in the former the neuropathy begins in the lower limbs and after proceeds to the upper extremities, affecting them less only because the death usually intervenes before.

As already stressed, the carpal tunnel syndrome, apparently a prerogative of Rukavina's type, could be difficult to prove, if it were present, in cases of generalized neuropathy of the upper limbs.

Moreover, the pathological findings are nearly the same in the different types of HAN, thus suggesting that the distribution of the amyloid may be stereotyped even if the clinical aspects may vary from family to family.

Thus, it becomes questionable that the clinical polymorphis of HAN can be explained solely on the basis of a parallel genetic poly-morphism.

It must be noted that about HAN genetics we know little and so many more detailed family studies will need before a well-grounded classification of HAN can be made.

REFERENCES

1) ANDRADE C. (1952) Brain, 75, 408.

2) RUKAVINA, J.G., BLOCK, W.D., JACKSON, C.E., FALLS, H.F., CAREY, J.H. and CURTIS, A.C. (1956), Medicine, 35, 239.

3) VAN ALLEN, M.W., FROHLICH, J.A., and DAVIS, J.R. (1969), Neurology (Minneap.), 19, 10.

4) MERETOJA, J. (1969), Ann. Clin. Res., I, 314.

5) FARIELLO, R.jr., CURTONI, E.S., DELSEDIME, M., MUTANI, R., QUATTROCOLO, G., FARIELLO, R. and FURLAN, P.M. (1971), Arch. Sci. Med., 128, 181.

6) FARIELLO, R., SCHIFFER, D., DELSEDIME, M. and MUTANI, R. (1974), Riv. Pat. Nerv. Ment., 95, I.

Peripheral Neuropathies
N. Canal and G. Pozza, eds.
© 1978 Elsevier/North-Holland Biomedical Press

SUBPERINEURIAL SPACE AND IMMUNOGLOBULIN DEPOSITS IN INFLAMMATORY AND
DYSGLOBULINEMIC NEUROPATHIES

B. SCHOTT [+], G. CHAZOT [+], N. KOPP [++], C. GUILLAUD-BARBARET [++], H. CARRIER [++]
and B. BADY [+]

+ Hopital Neurologique, B.P. Lyon Motchat, 69394 Lyon Cedex 3, France

++ Faculté A. Carrel, Rue G. Paradin, 69008 Lyon,France

ABSTRACT

Immunofluorescence studies were performed on peripheral nerve biopsies in
12 cases of dysglobulinemic neuropathies and 20 cases of *Guillain-Barré* syndrome. Immunoglobulins were frequently identified in the sub-perineurial space.
Electron microscopic studies showed, in some cases, in the sub-perineurial
space, the presence of fibrillary material (ramified and non ramified) suggesting "pre-amyloïd". Immunolabeling with HR peroxydase suggests that the
site of deposit of immunoglobulins and "pre-amyloïd" is the sub-perineurial
space. One might, therefore, discuss of the exact physiopathological role of
sub-perineurial space, conceived either as the site of sequestration of cir-
culating immunoglobulins or as the site of an immunological conflict.

INTRODUCTION

Immuno histochemical techniques and horse-radish peroxydase techniques
applied to nerve biopsies in patients with dysglobulinemia [2,3,4,6] and
inflammatory neuropathies [5] lead us to focus attention on subperineurial
space (S P S) in disease. The immunological signifiance of abnormal deposits
of immunoglobulins (Ig) in S P S and the role played by S P S need to be
discussed.

MATERIALS AND METHODS

Sural nerve biopsy was performed in 20 patients with *Guillain-Barré* syndrome (G.B. syndrome) and in 12 with dysglobulinemia. Fresh frozen sections
were made. Direct labelling method was used with monospecific fluorescein
conjugated anti - IgA, IgG, IgM, C3 sera and anti light chain kappa and lambda
sera (Behring and Hyland Laboratories). The immuno peroxydase technique was
direct labelling with horse-radish peroxydase conjugated anti-sera anti IgA,
IgG, IgM (Pasteur Institute). Standard histological controls were realized
for photonic and electronic microscopy.

RESULTS

We found [7] no immunoglobulin deposits in 11 cases of metabolic and toxic neuropathies whereas in G.B. syndrome and in dysglobulinemia deposits occur in more than 50 % of cases (Fig. 1, 2 and 3). Therefore, it seems highly probable that immunoglobulins play a role in the pathogenesis of these two groups of diseases.

We presently review only cases of G.B. syndrome and dysglobulinemia with a positive fluorescence in S P S (Table I) and discuss its signifiance.

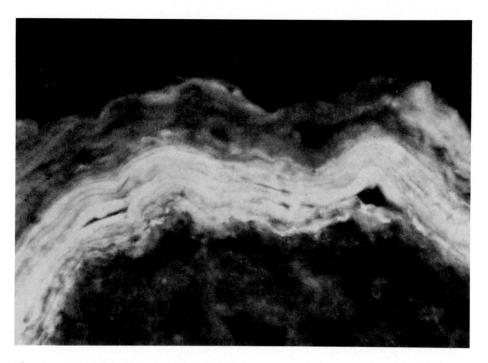

Fig. 1. Subperineurial deposit of IgM in a case of dysglobulinemic neuropathy.
(histofluorescence x 400)

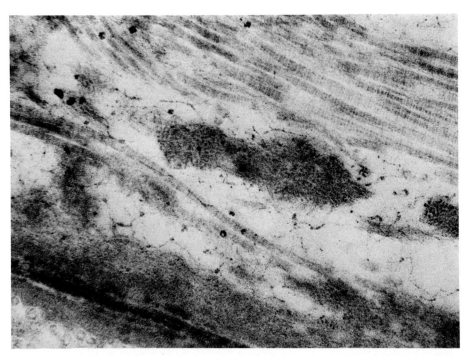

Fig. 2. Ultrastructure of "pre-amyloïd" Fibrillary deposits in subperineurial space. Dysglobulinemic neuropathy (x 2 7000)

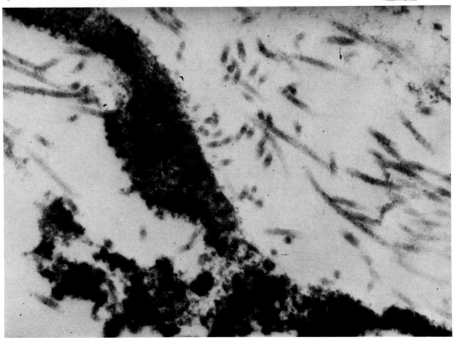

Fig. 3. "Pre-amyloïd" fibrillary deposits labelled with horse-radish peroxydase conjugated antisera anti IgG
Dysglobulinemic neuropathy.

TABLE I : I.F. PATTERNS IN 39 CASES OF GUILLAIN-BARRE SYNDROME AND 16 CASES OF DYSPROTEINEMIC NEUROPATHIES

Pattern 1 : Fluorescent staining in the subperineurial space and into the perineurium.

13 cases of G.B. syndrome	IgM only	(10)
	IgM + IgG	(2)
	IgM + IgG + C$_3$	(1)
3 cases of Dysproteinemia	IgA	(1)
	IgG	(1)
	IgM	(1)

Pattern 2 : Fluorescent staining in the subperineurial space and in the endoneurium.

7 cases of G-B. syndrome	IgG	(7)
9 cases of Dysproteinemic	IgA	(1)
	IgG	(6)
	IgM	(2)

DISCUSSION

The present findings lead us to raise the question of the physiopathological role of S P S in immunological neuropathies. Two main hypothesis can be proposed and discussed.

First hypothesis : passive filtration followed by sequestration of Ig
Several facts and data might be considered as argument in favor of this hypothesis. Molecules without known immunological role(such as fibrinogen and albumin) can be passively transferred from endoneurium (and from epineurium ?) Toward subperineurial space [8]. The passive transfer might depend on an elevation of blood protein concentration ; this possibility exists in dysglobulinemia. The same process of passive filtration might be initiated by a lesion of the "filter" barrier : it is probably true in G-B. syndrome, as suggested by albuminocytological dissociation in C.S.F. It might be of interest, here, to notice the presence of mastocytes in S.P.S.

Second hypothesis : S.P.S. is the site of immunological conflict. Several argument seem to militate in favor of this hypothesis.

- The concentration of Ig does not, apparently, plays a predominant role in several circumstances (some dysglobulinemia with or without clinical neuropathies have a negative immunofluorescence picture ; in G-B. syndrome there is a deposit of Ig without an important increase of immunoglobulins).

- If a simple lesion of the "filter" barrier were to be able to be the only explanation to the disease, one should find a diffusion - not only of IgM (m.w. = 800.000) but also of other Ig of lower m.w. such as IgG (m.w. = 150 000) and IgA (m.w. = 150 000).

- The diseases presently considered imply an immune mechanism : dysglobulinemia is a typical disorder of humoral immunity and it is well known that cellular immunity is implied in G-B. syndrome as well as in experimental polyradiculoneuritis.

- In three cases we found (CARRIER et al.) a deposit that might be an immune preamyloïd substance in S.P.S.

This immunological conflict might be directed against myelin (either normal or modified by a virus) or against basal lamina of perineurial cells. This basal site of conflict is suggested by a modification of basal lamina (particulary clearly seen in electron microscopy) and by the immunofluorescence pictures seen in lupus erythematosus at the dermo-epidermic junction. It is also suggested by deposits shown on the basal lamina in kidney biopsies performed in the course of G-B. syndrome.

CONCLUSION

The presence of Ig in S.P.S. can not be explained only by a process of passive diffusion related to the blood Ig concentration or to achange in membrane permeability. Several arguments are in favor of an immunological conflict in the basal lamina limiting S P S. The visualization of S P S by immunofluorescence is a distinct sign of some neuropathies (G-B. syndrome and dysglobulinemia). It is an argument in favour of an immunopathological process in the genesis of these neuropathies.

REFERENCES

1. CARRIER,H., GUILLAUD-BARBARET,C., CHAZOT,G., BADY,B. and SCHOTT,B. Les neuropathies des gammapathies monoclonales. Immunofluorescence et immunomarquage en microscopie électronique d'immunoglobulines à structure amyloïde. Acta Neuropath. (Berl.) (in press)

2. CHAZOT,G., BERGER,G., BADY,B., DUMAS,R., CREYSSEL,R., TOMMASI,M., SCHOTT,B. and GIRARD,P.F. Neuropathies périphériques au cours des dysglobulinémies malignes. Aspects immunopathologiques. Nouv.Presse Med.,1974, 3, 21, 1355-1358.

3. CHAZOT,G., BERGER,G., CARRIER,H., BARBARET,C., BADY,B., DUMAS,R., CREYSSEL,R., SCHOTT,B. Manifestations neurologiques des gammapathies monoclonales. Formes neurologiques pures. Etude en immunofluorescence. Rev. Neurol.,132, 3, 195-212.

4. IWASHITA,H., ARGYRAKIS,A., LOWITZSCH,K. and SPAAR,F.W. (1974). Polyneuropathy in Waldenström's macroglobulinemia. J. Neurol. Sci.,21,341-354.

5. LUIJTEN, J.A.F.M., BAART DE LA FAILLE-KUYPER,E.H. (1972). The occurence of IgM and complement factors along myelin sheaths of peripheral nerves. An immunohistochemical study of the Guillain-Barré syndrome. J.Neurol. Sci., 15, 219-224.

6. PROPP,R.P., MEANS,E., DEIBEL,R., SHERER,G. and BARRON,K (1975). Waldenström's macroglobulinemia and neuropathy. Neurology (Minneap.) , 1975, 25, 980-988.

7. SCHOTT,B., CARRIER,H., CHAZOT,G., BADY,B. and BARBARET,C. (1977). Immunofluorescence and immune labeling with H.R. peroxidase in the peripheral neuropathies. 11 th World Congress of Neurology. Amsterdam. Excerpta Medica, Amsterdam - Oxford, p.182.

8. VAN LIS,J.M.J., JENNEKENS,F.G.I. (1977). Plasma proteins in human peripheral nerve. J. Neurol. Sci., 34, 329-341.

Peripheral Neuropathies
N. Canal and G. Pozza, eds.
© 1978 Elsevier/North-Holland Biomedical Press

ULTRAMORPHOLOGY OF PERIPHERAL NERVES IN LYSOSOMAL DISEASES

HANS-HILMAR GOEBEL, HANS-GERD LENARD AND ALFRIED KOHLSCHÜTTER
H.H.G.: Div. of Neuropathology - H.G.L. and A.K.: Dept. of Paediatrics, University of Göttingen (West-Germany)

ABSTRACT

Certain lysosomal diseases show accretion of residual bodies in peripheral nerves. The presence in peripheral nerves of neuronal processes, Schwann cells of both myelinated and unmyelinated axons, mesenchymal cells and mural cells of the vasculature broadens the spectrum of sites for lysosomal accumulation. We studied the ultrastructure of peripheral nerves in neuronal ceroid lipofuscinosis, type II glycogenosis, GM_1-gangliosidosis, late infantile, juvenile and adult type metachromatic leukodystrophies, Krabbe's leukodystrophy, mucopolysaccharidoses, and mucolipidoses. Besides accumulation of disease-specific lysosomal residual bodies in various cell types, mild degenerative features of nerves may occasionally be encountered, probably reflecting metabolic damage of Schwann cells, the cell type most frequently and most severely affected when lysosomal diseases involve the peripheral nerve.

INTRODUCTION

Involvement of the peripheral nervous system in lysosomal diseases, a group of autosomal recessively inherited progressive disorders chiefly affecting the nervous system, marked by inborn deficiency of acid hydrolases, is well known in two respects:

1. They affect the neuronal perikarya, located in spinal, autonomic and intestinal ganglia, among which the gangliosidoses and neuronal ceroid-lipofuscinoses are prominent examples, neuronal storage diseases.

2. Others are associated with a breakdown of myelin, leukodystrophies.

Earlier biopsies of cerebral cortex in these lysosomal diseases have now been largely replaced by a diagnostic approach to extracranial sites, such as muscle, liver, skin, peripheral nerves, and lymphocytes. Incorporation into a diagnostic morphological program of peripheral nerves which are obtained by skin and sural nerve biopsies has also yielded ultrastructural data on the pathology of those lysosomal diseases that primarily do not affect myelin.

RESULTS AND CONCLUSIONS

Demyelinating lysosomal disorders, the leukodystrophies, entail Krabbe's disease and the various forms of the sulfatidoses. Both conditions are marked by abnormal electroneurographic data and characteristic light microscopic features, a loss of myelinated axons and PAS-positive and metachromatic material in mesenchymal and Schwann cells.

Ultrastructurally, globoid cell leukodystrophy shows typical membrane-bound needle-like inclusions in Schwann cells and particularly in mesenchymal cells[1]. Similar patterns of distribution of disease-specific residual bodies are found in various forms of the metachromatic leukodystrophies (MLD), the infantile, the juvenile (Fig. 1) and the adult types. They all display the fine structural gamut of residual bodies regarded typical for MLD[2].

GM_1-gangliosidosis, where concerning the nervous system, is usually considered a neuronal storage disease marked by characteristic membranous cytoplasmic bodies and other membrane-bound lamellated lysosomal inclusions[3]. Viscera and even spinal ganglion neurons also contain membrane-bound vacuoles, often harbouring only a few lamellae[3], due to the beta-galactosidase defect that also affects the mucopolysaccharide metabolism. Similar membrane-bound vacuoles are also seen in mesenchymal cells and occasionally in Schwann cells of the peripheral nerve. Abnormal cytosomes seem to be consistently present in GM_1-gangliosidosis as emphasized by ultrastructural findings in the infantile type[4].

The various mucopolysaccharidoses (MPS) and even mucolipidoses themselves may be expected to show electronmicroscopic pathology in the peripheral nervous system (Fig. 2)[5,6]. Again, mesenchymal and Schwann cells are affected as demonstrated even in the mild or adult variant of type VI MPS Maroteaux-Lamy[7].

Niemann-Pick's disease is another lysosomal disorder affecting

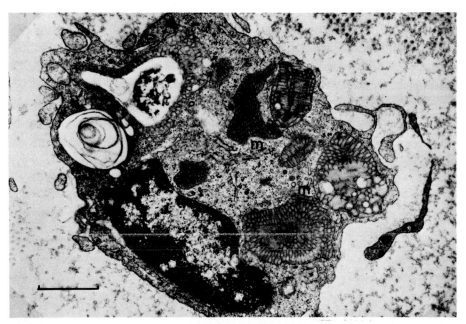

Fig. 1. Multiple membrane bound (m) prismatic type inclusions in mesenchymal cell of sural nerve; juvenile metachromatic leuko-dystrophy.

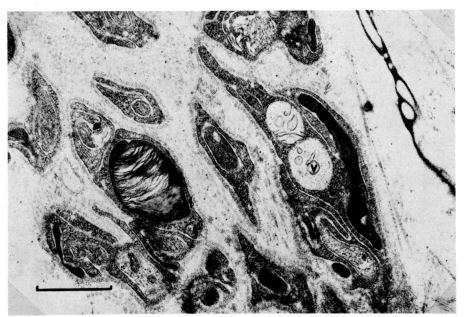

Fig. 2. Lamellated (l) body and clear membrane bound vacuoles (v) in Schwann cell cytoplasm of dermal nerve; mucolipidosis, type III.

the peripheral nerves in that it shows multiform inclusions in Schwann cells[8].

There are other lysosomal entities that display a ubiquitous accretion of lysosomal residual bodies: the infantile type II glycogenosis and the neuronal ceroid-lipofuscinoses.

In Pompe's disease, lysosomal glycogen is present in Schwann cells, mesenchymal cells, mural cells of the vasculature as well as perineural cells (Fig. 3). In addition, extralysosomal glycogen may be encountered in the Schwann cell cytoplasm (Fig. 3)[9], similar to that seen in myofibers. This finding had raised the suggestion of an additional biochemical defect separate from acid maltase deficiency[10]. In contrast to the destruction of myofibers which does not seem to be due to cytoplasmic glycogen aggregation, only minor morphological damage is seen in Schwann cells and their contents, the myelin sheath and its axon. Axonal enlargement, where scantily present, does not show spatial morphological relation to impaired glycogen metabolism[11]. This may reflect a different pathomechanism in glycogen metabolism of myofibers and Schwann cells. In Schwann cells of unmyelinated axons, which normally may harbour lipofuscin granules, lysosomal glycogen and lipofuscin material may appear within the same residual body, whereas lysosomal glycogen is not associated with typical lamellae of pi-granules in Schwann cells of myelinated axons.

In the neuronal ceroid-lipofuscinoses (NCL) mural cells of the vessels, mesenchymal cells and Schwann cells of unmyelinated axons chiefly contain NCL-specific inclusions: curvilinear bodies in infantile NCL and mixed curvilinear-fingerprint bodies (Fig. 4) in juvenile NCL[12]. Schwann cells of unmyelinated axons are much more often affected simulating the frequency of lipofuscin granules in the Schwann cell population of unmyelinated axons under normal conditions. When NCL-specific inclusions were encountered in Schwann cells of myelinated axons, they were often associated with lamellae of pi-granules.

Occasionally, mild degenerative features are associated with Schwann cells and axons, for instance enlargement by mitochondria, dense bodies and proliferated filaments in the latter (Fig. 5). A direct relationship to the lysosomal storage process

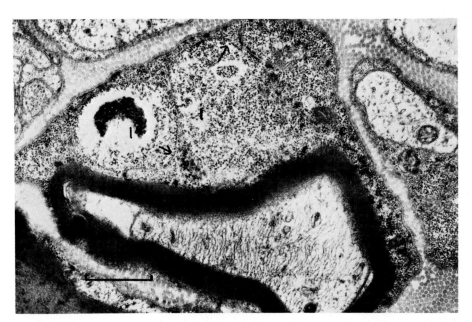

Fig. 3. A Schwann cell of the sural nerve is loaded with membrane bound (arrows) lysosomal (l) and cytoplasmic (c) glycogen;
infantile type II glycogenosis.

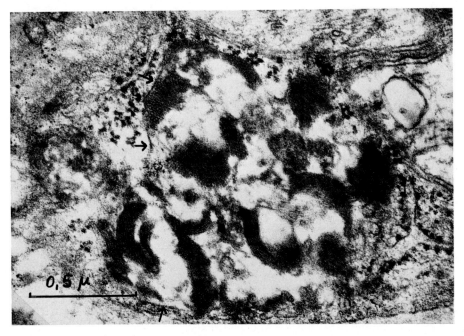

Fig. 4. Membrane bound (arrows) fingerprint body in Schwann cell
of unmyelinated sural axons; juvenile neuronal ceroid-lipofusci-
nosis.

432

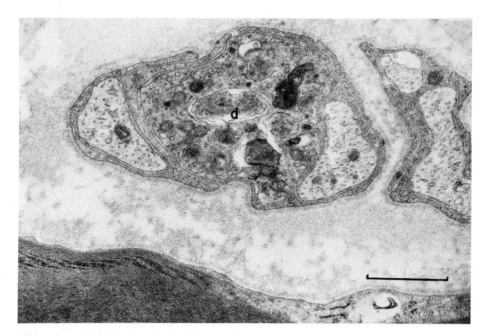

Fig. 5. Degenerating (d) unmyelinated axon in sural nerve of GM_1-gangliosidosis, type II.

is not always apparent but in cases of axonal changes it may be located at the perykaryon level. A preferential loss of unmyelinated fibers has been recorded in Fabry's disease[13] again suggesting the primary lesion to be located at the spinal ganglia level. This may reflect a general principle encountered in peripheral nerves of lysosomal disorders.

ACKNOWLEDGEMENTS

These studies have been supported by the Deutsche Forschungsgemeinschaft, SFB 33. We greatly appreciate the expert technical and photographic contribution to our work by Ms. Rose Kosswig and Mrs. Friedegard Schulz.

REFERENCES

1. Lyon, G., Jardin, L. and Aicardi, J. (1971) J. neurol. Sci., 12, 263-274.

2. Bischoff, A. (1975) in Peripheral Neuropathy P.J. Dyck, P.K. Thomas, E.H. Lambert eds., W.B. Saunders Co. Philadelphia, London, Toronto, pp. 891-913.

3. Patel, V., Goebel, H.H., Watanabe, I. and Zeman, W. (1974) Acta neuropath. (Berl.), 30, 155-173.

4. Tomé,F.M.S. and Fardeau, M. (1976) Path. Europ., 11, 15-25.

5. Swift, T.R. and McDonald, T.F. (1976) Arch. Neurol., 33, 845-846.

6. Lasser, A., Carter, D.M. and Mahoney, M.J. (1975) Arch. Pathol., 99, 173-176.

7. Pilz, H., von Figura, K. and Goebel, H.H. (1978) Ann. Neurol., in press.

8. Gumbinas, M., Larsen, M. and Mei Liu, H. (1975) Neurology (Minneap), 25, 107-113.

9. Araoz, C., Sun, C.N., Shenefelt, R. and White, H.J. (1974) Neurology (Minneap), 24, 739-742.

10. Hug, G. (1976) Birth Defects: Original Article Series, 12, No 6, pp 145-175.

11. Goebel, H.H., Lenard, H.G., Kohlschütter, A. and Pilz, H. (1977) Ann. Neurol., 2, 111-115.

12. Goebel, H.H., Zeman, W. and Pilz, H. (1976) J. Neurol., 213 295-303.

13. Ohnishi, A. and Dyck, P.J. (1974) Arch. Neurol., 31, 120-127.

Peripheral Neuropathies
N. Canal and G. Pozza, eds.
© 1978 Elsevier/North-Holland Biomedical Press

HEREDITARY SPHEROCYTOSIS IN PERONEAL MUSCULAR ATROPHY

C. ANGELINI, M. ARMANI, S. LÜCKE, and N. BRESOLIN
C.A., M.A. and N.B.: Neurological Clinic, University of Pado-
va.
S.L.: CNR Center of Muscle Biology and Physiopathology.

ABSTRACT

We observed the association between congenital spherocytosis
and hereditary motr sensory neuropathy (HMSN) type 1, in one
family. In view of this previous unreported association between
two dominant autosomal traits we investigated how and why both
syndromes occur in one kinship.

INTRODUCTION

Peroneal muscular atrophy has been classified according to
clinical, genetic and electrophysiological and pathological
studies[1,2,3].

The association with spastic paraplegia, and optic atrophy
is known, we observed in one kinship the association of a dominant
autosomal HMSN type 1 congenital hemolitic anemia.

MATERIALS AND METHODS

Case history. The patient, a 39 year old man, came to our clinic
for a progressive distal muscular weakness that resulted in
walking difficulty. At the age of 9 years he showed a severe
hemolytic crisis that was found to be due to the presence a
congenital spherocytosis. At the age of 15 years he underwent
splenectomy which improved his symptoms, although he presented
intermittent fever. On neurological examination he had bilateral
pes cavus, atrophy in the distal limb muscles, areflexia of lower
and upper extremities, apallesthesia in the affected limbs.
The conduction velocities of the motor fibers of the median nerves
were 24,4 m/sec. Laboratory data showed 5.100.000 RBC with
numerous erythrocytes, other routine tests were negative. The
phosphorylation with P^{32} of band II spectrin, isolated by pre-
parative sodium dodecyl sulfate polyacrylamide slab gel electro-

phoresis of erythrocyte ghosts was decreased.

Family history. A genetic tree (Fig. 1) showed four relatives with pes cavus. Our patient's mother had pes cavus and the conduction velocities of the motor fibers of the ulnar nerves were 25 m/sec. The patient's mother also had a severe iron deficienty anemia that after i.v. iron treatment showed the presence of spheroidocytes. The spherocitic trait in the mother was confirmed, after treatment, by a decreased resistence of RBC to hemolysis in hypotonic saline solution. The patient underwent a muscle biopsy of gastrocnemius muscle and a sural nerve biopsy according to Dyck's and Lofgren's technique[4].

RESULTS

The light microscopy of the frozen sections, processed for routine alkaline ATPase, showed a picture characterized by the presence of fibers type grouping and a marked atrophy of scattered fibers. The electron microscopy picture of the nerve showed an evident decrease of the large myelinated fibers with fragmentation and vacuoles formation in the myelin (Fig. 2). Further, we noticed the presence of single demyelinated nerve fibers with Schwann cells apposed, intermingled with collagen pockets. In several areas we found the presence of onion bulbs (Fig. 3). We concluded that the ultrastructural pathology of the biopsy was that of hypertrophyc neuropathy classified according to clinical data as hereditary motor and sensory neuropathy type 1. Thus this patient had an association of HMSN and a Minkowski-Chauffard's hemolytic anemia. We found aspects of the above described association in the patient's mother too. Anomalies of erythrocytes have been reported in Duchenne muscular dystrophy[5] and myotonic dystrophy[6] with morphological and several biochemical changes. In these diseases a diffuse membrane abnormality is hypothized.[7-9] In our family the association of peroneal muscular atrophy and spherocytosis may be part of a common membrane abnormality or due to the casual association of two separate genetic entities.

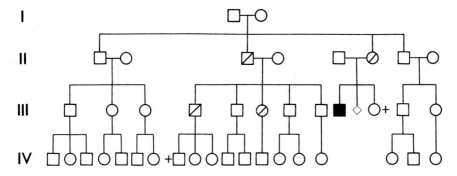

Fig.1: Genealogical tree of the family. Hatched square is our pa-
       tient. Square and round figures with a transversal line
       are the patient's relatives with pes cavus.

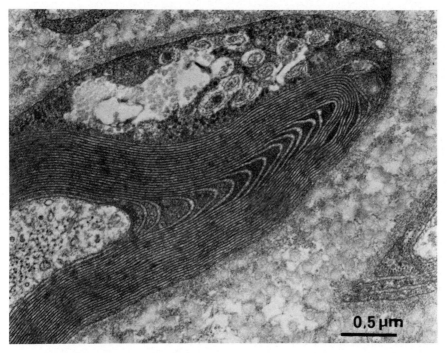

Fig.2: Nerve biopsy of HMSN type 1. Anormality of a large myelina-
       ted fiber, note vacuoles containing glycogen and vescicles
       with convoluted membranes.

438

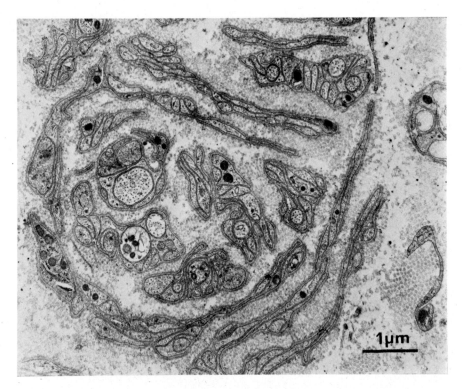

Fiġ.3: Nerve biopsy of HMSN type 1. The electron micrograph
shows demyelinated axons in the centre of an onion bulb
formation.

SUMMARY

A patient with an hereditary form of spherocytic anemia (Min-
kowki-Chauffard's disease) developed at the age of 39 years progressive weakness, asthenia and amyotrophy of upper and lower
extremites. On EMG the conduction velocities of median and ulnar
nerves were extremly low (24,4 m/sec). On muscle biopsy neurogenic atrophy with type 1 prevalence grouping of muscle fibers
was seen. On sural nerve biopsy we observed a marked decrease
of large myelinated fibers, residual fibers presented abnormal

Schwann cells with vacuoles containing glycogen and vescicles with convoluted membranes.

Anomalies of erythrocytes have been observed in Duchenne muscular distrophy an myotonic dystrophy but not in association with peroneal muscular atrophy. In this family it is suggestive to think to a possible diffuse membrane abnormality.

ACKNOWLEDGEMENTS

This work was supported by a grant from Muscular Dystrophy Association.

REFERENCE
1. Dyck, P.J., Lambert, E.H.,(1968) Lower motor and primary sensory neuron diseases with peroneal muscular atrophy. I. Neurologic, genetic and electrophysiologic findings in hereditary polyneuropathies. Arch. Neurol. (Chic.), 18, 603-618.
2. Dyck, P.J.,(1975) in Peripheral Neuropathy, Dyck, P.J., Thomas, P.K., Lambert, E.H., eds., W.B. Saunders Company, London, Toronto, pp. 825-867.
3. Madrid, R., Bradley, W.G., Davis, C.J.F., (1977) The peroneal muscular atrophy syndrome - clinical, genetic, electrophysiological and nerve biopsy studies, Part 2 (Observations on pathological changes in sural nerve biopsies), J. Neurol. Sci., 32, 91-122.
4. Dyck, P.J., Lofgren, E.P., (1966) Method of fascicular biopsy of human peripheral nerve for electrophysiologic and histologic study, Mayo Clinic Proc., 41, 778-784.
5. Roses, A.D., Roses, M.J., Miller, S.A., Hull, K.L., Appel, S.H., (1976) Carrier detection in Duchenne muscular dystrophy, New England Journal of Medicine, 294, 193-198.
6. Roses, A.D., Appel, S.H., (1973) Protein kinase activity in erythrocyte ghosts of patients with myotonic muscular dystrophy, Proc. Natl. Acad. Sci. USA, 70, 1855-1859.
7. Mokri, B., Engel, A.G., (1975) Duchenne Dystrophy: electron microscopic findings pointing to a basic or early abnormality in the plasma membrane of the muscle fiber, Neurology, 25, 1111-1120.

8. Schotland, D.L., (1977) in Pathogenesis of human muscular
   dystrophies, Rowland, L.P. ed., Excerpta Medica, Amsterdam-
   Oxford, pp. 562-569.
9. Roses, A.D., (1977) in Pathogenesis od human muscular
   dystrophies, Rowland, L.P. ed., Excerpta Medica, Amsterdam-
   Oxford, pp. 648-658.

Peripheral Neuropathies
N. Canal and G. Pozza, eds.
© 1978 Elsevier/North-Holland Biomedical Press

PERONEAL MUSCULAR ATROPHY (PMA) WITH POSTURAL TREMOR.

P. MARTINELLI, P. PAZZAGLIA, P. MONTAGNA, P. TINUPER, G. MORETTO,
N. RIZZUTO and E. LUGARESI
Institute of Neurology, University of Bologna and Institute of
Neurology University of Verona - Italy

ABSTRACT

The authors report clinical, electrophysiological and pathological findings in 7 patients affected by peroneal muscular atrophy
and postural tremor. Tremor in all patients showed similar features
to essential tremor. Changes in sural nerve biopsies were typical
either for neuronal or hypertrophic type of PMA.

INTRODUCTION

Postural tremor (PT) in peroneal muscular atrophy (PMA) was first
described by Raymond [1]. In 1906 Marie [2] stressed the occurrence of
these clinical features in two brothers; in one of them Boveri [3]
showed abundance of "onion bulb" formations in peripheral nerves.
Four out of seven patients described by Roussy & Lévy [4] had also
PT of the upper limbs.

Numerous authors have hitherto reported on the occurrence of PT
in PMA [5, 6, 7, 8, 9]. Some authors also provided data about pathological findings: in most of the patients, changes were typical
for the hypertrophic type of PMA [5, 8, 9].

However, in a case reported by Delwaide & Schoenen [7] non hypertrophic axonal degeneration was present. Patients showing tremor
of the hands and PMA were grouped by Buchthal and Behse [10] as
"neuronal plus" patients: biopsy and electrophysiological findings
were typical for the neuronal type of PMA.

It is our aim to report here 7 patients in whom PMA was associated with PT, and to relate clinical findings to pathological

changes as obtained by sural nerve biopsy.

PATIENTS AND METHODS.

Seven patients were investigated. The main clinical findings are summarized in Table I.

Concentric needle EMG examination of muscles of upper and lower extremities was performed in all patients and motor nerve conduction velocity (MNCV) determined. Tremor in upper limbs was recorded by surface electrodes and by quartz accelerometers placed on the distal phalanx of index finger.

A biopsy of sural nerve was carried out in each patient: one portion of the specimens was fixed in 2.5% gluteraldehyde in 0.1 M phosphate buffer at pH 7.40, post-fixed in Dalton chromeosmium and processed for EM investigation. The remainder was similarly fixed and then placed into glycerin for teasing.

TABLE I

CLINICAL FINDINGS

Case N.	1	2	3	4	5	6	7
Sex	M	M	M	M	M	M	M
Age at onset of PMA (years)	30	6	45	42	43	?	10
Age at onset of PT (years)	37	20	46	43	43	9	10
PMA in family	0	?	0	0	0	?	+
PT in family	0	0	0	0	0	0	+
Pes cavus	+	+	+	+	+	+	+
Deep reflexes Upper limbs	+	++	+	0	$\pm$	+	$\pm$
Lower limbs	0	0	$\pm$	0	$\pm$	0	0
Distal sensory loss	+	+	+	+	+	+	+
Hypertrophic nerves	0	0	0	++	0	0	0

RESULTS

In all patients routine EMG examination showed neurogenic atrophy in distal muscles of upper and lower extremities. MNCV values and characters of tremor are shown in Table II. Postural tremor was mainly evident in upper limbs; cases 3 and 4 had also PT of lower limbs. All patients received phenobarbitone (PB), 1 mg/Kg body weight as treatment for tremor; one also received propranolol (120 mg daily) and two timolol (15 mg daily). PB resulted in a decrease in amplitude of PT in all patients; propranolol and timolol had the same effect of PB.

Findings in sural nerve biopsies are reported in Table III and in Fig. 1

TABLE II

ELECTROPHYSIOLOGICAL FINDINGS: CHARACTERS OF TREMOR AND MOTOR NERVE CONDUCTION VELOCITY (MNCV)

Case n.	At rest	TREMOR Postural Frequency (Hz)	Mean amplitude (g)	M N C V (m./s.)
1	0	6.50	0.43	R.Ulnar: 35 R. Peroneal: 32
2	0	6.50	0.60	L. Median: 46 R. Peroneal: ∅
3	0	4.10	1.10	R. Median: 44 R. Peroneal: 37
4	0	4.50	1.90	L. Median: 28 R. Ulnar: 22 R. Peroneal: ∅
5	0	5.80	0.20	R. Median: 48 R. Peroneal: 40
6	0	4.00	0.80	R. Median: 40 R. Peroneal: 30
7	0	6.25	0.49	R. Peroneal: 44

∅ : absence of evoked muscle action potential.

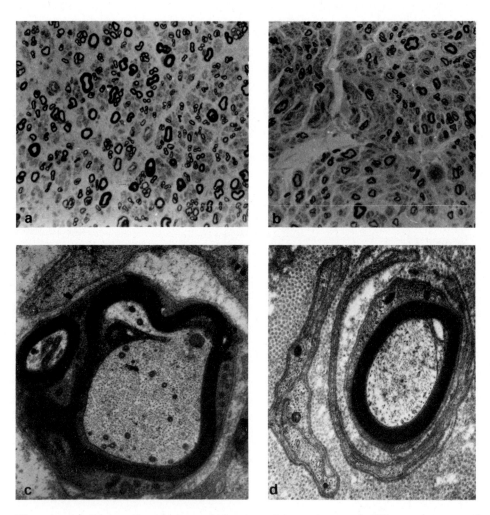

Fig. 1: a) Nerve fascicles without evident loss of fibers (neuronal type of PMA) 380 x. b) Severe loss of myelinated fibers with onion bulbs (hypertrophic type of PMA) 380 x. c) A remyelinated axon is encompassed by Schwann cell processes, 6000 x. d) Concentric proliferation of Schwann cell processes, forming an onion bulb, 8000 x.

TABLE III

NERVE BIOPSY FINDINGS.

	Loss of fibers	Wallerian degeneration	Segmental demyelination	Onion bulbs	Clusters
Case 1	severe	no	much	numerous	no
Case 2	severe	no	much	numerous	no
Case 3	moderate	no	no	no	no
Case 4	moderate	rare	no	simple type	no
Case 5	slight	rare	no	no	no
Case 6	moderate	no	no	no	yes
Case 7	slight	rare	no	no	no

Quantitative evaluation of nerve fascicles is under study.

DISCUSSION

Clinical and electrophysiological data in our patients are in keeping with features currently observed in PMA [11]. The low incidence of family history is probably related to the fact that direct examination of kinship was sometimes impossible.

PT showed clinical and electrophysiological characters similar to those described in essential tremor [12]. Also in regard to therapy PT in PMA behaved like essential tremor since it was reduced by beta-blockers and by PB [13,14].

As to pathology, 3 of our patients had a hypertrophic type of PMA (cases 1, 2 and 4), and 4 a neuronal type. These findings thus allow the consideration that no pathological changes are specific for PMA associated with PT.

REFERENCES

1. Raymond F. (1900). Leçons sur les Maladies du Systême Nerveux, G. Doin, Paris, Vol. 3 pp. 346-365; Vol. 6, pp. 203-227.

2. Marie P. (1906). Rev. Neurol., 14: 557-559.

3. Boveri P. (1910). Sem. méd. Paris, 13: 145-150.

4. Roussy G. & Lévy G. (1926). Rev. Neurol., 2: 427-450.

5. Salisachs P. & Lapresle J. (1973). Rev. Neurol., 129: 119-125.

6. Thomas P.K., Calne D.B. and Stewart G. (1974). Ann. Hum. Genet., Lond., 38: 111-153.

7. Delwaide P.J. & Schoenen J. (1976). J. Neurol. Sci., 27: 59-69.

8. Endtz L.J., Bots G.T.M., Goor C. et Frenay J. (1976), Rev. Neurol., 132, 2, 99-111.

9. Salisachs P. (1976). J. neurol. Sci, 28: 17-40.

10. Buchthal F. & Behse G. (1977). Brain, 100: 41-66.

11. Dyck P.J., Thomas P.K. and Lambert E.H. (1975). Peripheral Neuropathy, Vol. 2, pp. 834-855.

12. Shahani B. & Young R.R. (1976). J. Neurol. Neurosurg. Psych., 39: 772-783.

13. Winkler G.F. & Young R.R. (1974). New Engl. J. of Med., 290: 984-988.

14. Pazzaglia P., Baruzzi A., Martinelli P., Sacquegna T., Forti A., D'Alessandro R., Frank G., Lugaresi E. (1977). XX Congresso S.I.N., Roma, 24-26 November 1977.

MISCELLANEOUS

Peripheral Neuropathies
N. Canal and G. Pozza, eds.
© 1978 Elsevier/North-Holland Biomedical Press

FILAMENTOUS INCLUSIONS IN SCHWANN CELL NUCLEI

F.M.S. TOMÉ, M. FARDEAU and H. COLLIN

Research Group on Neuromuscular Biology and Pathology (INSERM U.153 and
CNRS ER.107), 17, rue du Fer à Moulin, 75005-Paris (France)

ABSTRACT

Intranuclear rodlets in Schwann cells were frequently observed in two cases

of polyneuropathy without any evident aetiological relationship. However, a

complete demyelination of the nerves biopsied was common to both cases. In the

other cell types of the nerve and muscle were seen nuclear bodies but not in-

tranuclear rodlets.

INTRODUCTION

Intranuclear filamentous inclusions have been observed in many cell types,

particularly neurones and glial cells (see [1,2,3]). To our knowledge they have

not been reported within Schwann cell nuclei. We have found them in this loca-

tion and with high frequence in two cases of polyneuropathy.

MATERIAL AND METHODS

Case 1 : E.C., a man of 52, who had a severe motor and sensory polyneuropathy which started 10 months before a biopsy of the nerve and muscle was taken.
He had been diagnosed as having a chronic lymphoid leukemia 1 year before the
onset of the symptoms of polyneuropathy. He was given chlorambucil and he improved temporarily of the general condition but died of the leukemia 2 years and
3 months after the diagnosis had been made.

Case 2 : S.Z., an algerian girl aged 9 1/2 years, who presented talipes
equinovarus, associated with weakness and wasting of the leg and hand muscles.
Tendon reflexes were absent. Impairment of the cutaneous and position sensibility was not evident to her clinician. Nerve hypertrophy was not found. EMG
showed a neurogenic pattern. Motor conduction velocity of the median nerve was
36 m/sec. Evoked sensory potentials were not found in median nerve. Several
investigations, including serum CPK and phytanic acid in the urine, were normal.

A nerve biopsy was performed in the superficial peroneal nerve in case 1 and
in the sural nerve in case 2. The nerve samples were fixed in glutaraldehyde,
post-fixed in osmium tetroxide and embedded by the Spurr's method.

From both cases a biopsy of the peroneus brevis muscle was also taken and
study by histochemistry and electron microscopy according to the techniques
used in our laboratory.

RESULTS

Nerve Biopsies. Case 1 : The nerve was completely demyelinated and the num-

ber of unmyelinated axons reduced (density : $31,000/mm^2$). Collagen tissue was abundant.Phagocytes were rare and infiltration by leukemic cells did not occur.

The Schwann cells had an active cytoplasm, rich in filaments, and contained often myelin debris. They presented numerous closely applied processes. Their nuclei presented frequently filamentous inclusions. In longitudinal sections of the nerve the Schwann cell nuclei were elongated and the inclusions consisted in rodlets (up to 3.3 μm long and 0.1 μm wide) formed by parallel filaments (60-80 Å thick) with a center to center spacing of about 125 Å (Fig. 1). In transverse sections the rodlets consisted in collections of up to 33 "dots" and were found in about 10 % of the nuclei of a given section.

The rodlets run parallely or obliquely to the long axis of the nucleus and are eccentrically located. They never reached the nuclear membrane and were independant of the nucleolus. They were often surrounded by a narrow clear zone. At the extrimities of the rodlets the filaments became indistinct and appeared to be lost in a fine fibrillary material.

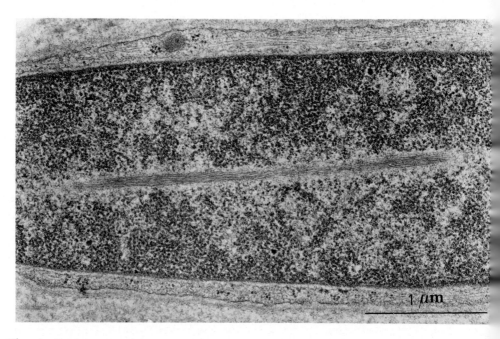

Fig. 1. Case 1 : Longitudinal section of the nerve. The Schwann cell nucleus contains a rodlet formed by parallel filamentous. x 33,000.

Some Schwann cell nuclei presented nuclear bodies of varying type but they were not seen coexisting with the rodlets in the same nucleus. Nuclear bodies were also seen in perineurial, interstitial and endothelial cells. Filamentous inclusions were searched but not found in all these cells.

Case 2 : The nerve was also completely demyelinated and most of the changes were common to case 1. The main differences were a greater reduction in the number of unmyelinated axons and a higher frequence of intranuclear inclusions (in about 20 % of the nuclei transverse sections) in this case. The longest rodlet was 4.4 μm long and 0.12 μm wide. In transverse sections the largest one had 0.3 μm of diameter and was formed by about 200 filaments (Fig. 2). The diameter of the filaments was identical to that of case 1.

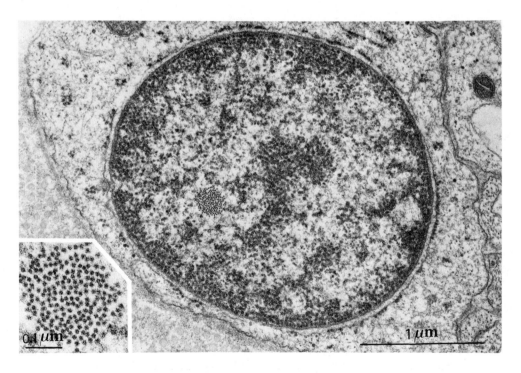

Fig. 2. Case 2 : Transverse section of the nerve. A large collection of filaments, corresponding to a transversely cut rodlet, lies within the Schwann cell nuclei. x 34,000. Inset : High power of this rodlet showing distinctly the filaments. x 100,000.

A particular change of case 2 was the presence of numerous long-spacing col-lagen fibrils amongst the collagen bundles of the endoneurium.

Muscle Biopsies. In both cases the changes were those of denervation atrophy. In the intramuscular nerves (case 2) were seen a few Schwann cells but rodlets were not found neither in their nuclei nor in other cells of muscle.

DISCUSSION

The intranuclear rodlets here reported are identical to the filamentous type of rodlet described by Seïte et al.[1] in sympathetic neurons and to those found by other authors in various cells in normal and pathological conditions. Their proteinaceous composition have been demonstrated[1,4]; they do not contain RNA or DNA.[4] Most authors regard them as a normal cell organelle. However their occurrence has a marked individual variation.[5] An increase in their number by electrical stimulation and cyclic AMP was reported by Seïte et al.[5] who suggested that the formation of the rodlets is related to "the general level of neuronal activity".

In our own material, intranuclear rodlets have been found only in two nerve biopsies and were confined to Schwann cell nuclei. In this location they have not been described so far. The preference given by neuropathologists to transverse rather than to longitudinal sections may be partially responsable for missing them. The completely different origin of the polyneuropathy in the two patients does not allow to invoke a common aetiological factor in the formation of the rodlets. However in both biopsies there was common pathological changes, namely complete loss of myelinated fibres and increased activity of the Schwann cells which may be related to the presence of the rodlets.

ACKNOWLEDGEMENTS

We are indebted to Drs. J.C. Brouet and C. Roy who referred the patients.

REFERENCES

1. Seïte,R., Escaig,J., and Couineau,S. (1971) J. Ultrastruct.Res. 37, 449-478.
2. Clattenburg, R.E., Singh, R.P. and Montemurro, D.G. (1972) J. Ultrastruct. Res. 39, 549-555.
3. Lafarga, M. and Palacios, G. (1977) Experientia 33, 1368-1369.
4. Masurovsky, E.B., Benitez, H.H., Kim, S.U. and Murray, M.R. (1970) J. Cell Biol. 44, 172-191.
5. Seïte, R., Leonetti, J., Luciani-Vuillet, J. and Vio, M. (1977) Brain Research, 124, 41-51.

Peripheral Neuropathies
N. Canal and G. Pozza, eds.
© 1978 Elsevier/North-Holland Biomedical Press

GANGLIOSIDES IN DENERVATION : AN EXPERIMENTAL AND CLINICAL STUDY

Maria G. ALBIZZATI, Sirio BASSI, Cesare CERRI, Lodovico FRATTOLA and Gianni MEOLA

Neurological Department, University of Milano (Italy)

INTRODUCTION

Our work aims at evaluating the effect of brain cortex ganglio-sides (°) treatment on the development of the damage to a periphe-ral nerve. This research is justified by observations proving that under various experimental conditions, gangliosides are promoting a nerve regeneration and a tissue reinnervation process[1,2].

Our study has been carried on along an experimental and clinical course. By the formes we have been investigating the alterations determinated by gangliosides on the biochemical changes induced in a rat muscle by denervation by cooling[3]. As metabolic marker we have investigated adenylate cyclase (A-C), guanylate cyclase (G-C) and cyclic nucleotides phosphodiesterase (PDE) enzymes that are altered in the denervated muscle[4-11].

MATERIALS AND METHODS

The criodegeneration of soleus and EDL nerves was performed on female Sprague-Dawley rats weighing 220-250 gr, subdivided into 3 groups of six animals. The first group included normal rats; the 2nd lesioned animals and the third rats criodegenerated and treated with gangliosides. The treatment was 50 mg/Kg of brain cortex gangliosides, injected every day e.p. for 10 - 15 - 20 days.

(°) FIDIA Research Laboratories, Abano Terme (Italy)

454

TABLE 1. Cyclic nucleotides enzymes in soleus and EDL muscles.

	Days	SOLEUS			EDL		
		Controls	Cooling	Cooling + treatment	Controls	Cooling	Cooling + treatment
Adenylate cyclase °	10	17.1 ± 2.3	33.1 ± 4.1*	27.3 ± 3.9*	15.6 ± 2.1	27.6 ± 4.2*	23.1 ± 3.2*
	15	17.9 ± 1.9	37.9 ± 5.2*	31.1 ± 2.4*	14.3 ± 1.2	34.7 ± 3.9*	26.9 ± 1.9*
	20	18.3 ± 2.4	41.1 ± 3.8*	24.1 ± 3.6	15.8 ± 1.8	35.9 ± 4.3*	19.8 ± 2.9
cAMP-PDE °°	10	38.4 ± 4.1	47.2 ± 5.1	51.1 ± 5.4*	32.1 ± 2.7	39.2 ± 3.2*	41.7 ± 3.0*
	15	39.3 ± 2.7	56.1 ± 4.9*	53.3 ± 5.7*	32.8 ± 2.9	46.3 ± 5.2*	43.7 ± 3.9*
	20	38.1 ± 2.9	60.4 ± 7.4*	42.1 ± 5.3	31.3 ± 1.9	50.3 ± 6.3*	36.7 ± 3.8
Guanylate cyclase °	10	7.8 ± 0.6	11.4 ± 0.9*	12.1 ± 1.1*	6.4 ± 0.3	10.2 ± 0.5*	9.4 ± 0.7*
	15	8.0 ± 0.7	17.5 ± 2.3*	13.2 ± 1.3*	5.8 ± 0.3	12.8 ± 0.9*	10.2 ± 0.9*
	20	7.3 ± 0.6	18.9 ± 2.2*	8.2 ± 0.9	5.9 ± 0.2	14.2 ± 0.9*	6.9 ± 0.4
cGMP-PDE °°	10	43.7 ± 5.1	52.1 ± 6.1	50.7 ± 4.9	34.9 ± 2.0	41.1 ± 4.9	42.3 ± 1.1*
	15	42.1 ± 1.9	56.1 ± 4.7*	55.4 ± 5.8*	32.5 ± 2.8	49.8 ± 5.1*	42.9 ± 4.7
	20	42.5 ± 3.7	72.3 ± 6.3*	41.3 ± 3.2	34.2 ± 2.7	53.3 ± 5.9*	29.6 ± 2.4

° = p mol cyclic nucleotide formed/1 mg Pr/1'; °° = n mol substrate hydrolized/1 mg Pr/10'
(mean of 6 determinations performed in triplicate ± S.E.; * = p < 0.01

After the drawing, the muscle tissues were frozen in liquid nitrogen and then homogenized in 6 vol of 0.25 M sucrose containing 10 mM Tris-HCl buffer (pH 8.0) and centrifuged for 15 min at 1500 x g (a.v.). The supernatant was employed as enzyme crude homogenate preparation. Composition of the trials for enzymatic determinations was one showed in the various methods.

The A-C was determined according to Canal et al[8]; the G-C was measured by the method of Cerri et al[11]; the cyclic adenosine-3',5'-monophosphate (cAMP)-PDE and cyclic guanosine-3',5'-monophosphate (cGMP)-PDE was determined as indicated by Filburn and Karn[12]. Noncollagenous protein concentration was determined according to Lowry et al[13] after alkali digestion[14].

The data significance was evaluated by the Student's t test.

Clinic survey was carried out on 20 subjects suffering from toxic-lacking polineuropathy and in 8 cases of spinal muscular atrophy.

The EMG study was performed on the beginning and the end of therapy composing od 100 mg gangliosides daily for 30 following days. With the exception of anti-diabetes therapy, no other drug was administered. Motor conduction velocities (ulnar, median and peroneal) (V.d.C.) and S.A.P.s (ulnar, median and sural) were the examined parameters. On ulnar nerve a wrist repetitive stimulation at 2-5-20 Hz was performed. In the patients affected by spinal muscular atrophy F-wave velocity was considered too.

At the end of every week therapy, usual blood routine tests and anti-gangliosides antibodies test always were within normal range.

RESULTS

In the normal muscle the enzyme activities are higher in the soleus muscle than in the EDL. After cooling, in the untreated-rats muscles an increase in PDE and cyclase enzymes activities was observed (Table 1). This increase in activity was already present at tenth day, but it joined the maximum rise at twentieth($p < 0.01$)

and it was higher for A-C and for G-C than for cyclic nucleotides
PDE. In the gangliosides-treated rats, after a beginning increase
in enzymatic activity, like that of untreated-animals, enzymatic
activities come back to values close to controls at 20th day from
denervation.

In the patients examined the motor V.d.C. and sensitive potentials have shown, at the completion of the month of treatment, a
very moderate increase. In 5 cases, repetitive stimulation has
evidenced a decrease of MAP, however non-significant (less than
10 per cent) and non-modified by the treatment.
The F-wave speed, in patients suffering from spinal amiotrophy,
has remained unchanged as well.

Table 2 shows the amplitude variations of the potential summo-
ned at supermaximum stimulation (MAP).

TABLE 2

MAP amplitude variations (mV) (negative phase) at supramaximal
stimulation.

	Before treatment		After treatment*	
	ulnar	median	ulnar	median
Diabetic (10) neuropathy	5.0 ± 0.7	5.3 ± 0.6	$8.5 \pm 0.4°$	$8.7 \pm 0.4°$
Ethylic (10) neuropathy	4.2 ± 0.6	4.8 ± 0.5	$9.4 \pm 0.3°$	$9.1 \pm 0.8°$

In brackets: number of cases.

Values expressed as mean $\pm$ S.E.

* = 100 mg daily for 30 following days.

° = $p < 0.01$

As may be observed, the rate of such response varied in the diabetic form from 5 mV to 8.5 mV for the ulnar nerve and from 5.3 mV
to 8.7 mV for the median nerve. In toxi-ethylic form it varied
respectively from 4.2 to 9.4 for ulnar and from 4.8 to 9.1 for the
median nerve.

DISCUSSION

Our test observations are evidencing that in the homogenate of muscle denervated by cooling, A-C, G-C and PDE enzyme activities are increased on the 15th and 20th day from the lesion. On the other hand, the ganglioside-treated rats, 20 days after the lesion showed a reverse of enzymatic activities towards normal range.

Although the role of cyclic nucleotides in skeletal muscle has not been weel established, increasing evidences[4-11] support their role in the mediation of the influences by the nerve on muscle. It could be assumed that the lack of neuronal influence might induce some denervation supersensitivity effects[2,4,5,7,9]. According to this hypothesis, the progressive decrease in the enzyme activity related to the cyclic nucleotides in the ganglioside-treated animals, would indicate a parallel decrease of the supersensitivity phenomenon, due to the reinnervation processes.

As far as clinical results are concerned, we are of the opinion that the increase of the motor V.d.C. and of the SAPs should not - owing to its moderate extent - be attributed to a pharmacological action, but rather to a possible spontaneous evolution of the disease. The F-wave velocity in cases of spinal amiotrophy proved unchanged[15].

These data seem to exclude any interference by gangliosides both at peripheral nervous trunk and at spinal cell levels. However, the drug has shown a substantial effect in modifying the MAP amplitude. The results tally with some test observations, both electrophysiological and biochemical: the former let us suppose an ganglioside influence on the reinnervation process; the latter show the substance to be present in its top concentration near the nervous terminations, where it promotes the formation of acetylcholine-sensitive extrajunctional loci and synaptic excitability[1,2].

The possibility that the gangliosides action should materialize mainly at the neuromuscular junction had led us to effect a repetitive nerve stimulation in order to evidence a possible alteration of myastheniform reactions in the course of polyneuropathies.

Unfortunately, this electrophysiological event was not detect in our patients.

We propose to carry on an additional study for evaluating the effect of the ganglioside-treatment on the MAP drop in a more specific pathology, like e.g. in myasthenia.

REFERENCES

1. Obata, K. and Oide, M. (1977) Nature, 266, 369-371.

2. Ceccarelli, B., Aporti, F. and Finesso, M. (1976) in Ganglioside Function, Porcellati, G., Ceccarelli, B. and Tettamanti, T. eds., Plenum Press, New York, pp. 275-294.

3. Takano, B. (1976) Exp. Brain Res., 26, 343-354.

4. Greengard, P. and Kebabian, J.W. (1974) Fed. Proc., 34, 1059-1067.

5. Standaert, K.F., Dretchen, K.L., Skirboll, L.R. and Morghenroth, W.M. (1976) J. Pharmacol. Exper. Ther., 199, 553-564.

6. Festoff, B.W., Oliver, K.L., Reddy, B.N. (1977) J. Membr. Biol. 32, 331-343.

7. Mawatari, S. and Rowland, L.P. (1974) Arch. Neurol., 30, 95-102.

8. Canal, N., Smirne, S. and Frattola, L. (1975) J. Neurol., 208, 259-265.

9. Novom, C. and Lewinstein, C. (1977) Neurology, 27, 869-874.

10. Pacifici, G.M., Pellegrion, C., Maffei, C. and Beconcini, D. (1978) in Molecular Biology and Pharmacology of Cyclic Nucleotides, Folco, G. and Paoletti, R. eds., Elsevier, Amsterdam, pp. 297-300.

11. Cerri, C., Canal, N. and Frattola, L. (1978) J. Neurol. Neurosurg. Psych. (in press).

12. Filburn, C.R. and Karn, J. (1973) Anal. Biochem., 52, 505-516.

13. Lowry, O.H., Rosebrough, N.J., Farr, A.L. and Randall, R.J. (1951) J. Biol. Chem., 193, 265-279.

14. Lillienthal, J.L., Zierlor K.L., Folk, B.P. (1950) J. Bill. Chem., 185, 501-518.

15. Albizzati, M.G., Bassi, S., Passerini, D. and Crespi, V. (1976) Acta Neurol. Scand., 54, 269-277.

Peripheral Neuropathies
N. Canal and G. Pozza, eds.
© 1978 Elsevier/North-Holland Biomedical Press

CLINICAL AND NEUROPHYSIOLOGICAL FINDINGS IN 47 LONG -TERM SURVI-
VORS OF CHILDHOOD MALIGNANCIES TREATED WITH VARIOUS DOSES OF
VINCRISTINE

LOWITZSCH,K*, P.GUTJAHR**, and H.OTTES**
Departments of Neurology*(Head:H.C.Hopf,M.D.) and Paediatrics**
(Head:J.Spranger,M.D.),University of Mainz, FRG

ABSTRACT

96 long-term survivors of cancer in childhood were reexamined
after succesful therapy.In 49 who had not been treated with
VINCRISTINE (VCR) reflex status and motor conduction velocities
were normal.In contrast,47- after treatment with VCR-had loss of
deep tendon reflexes in a high rate and a prolongation of sensory
CV independent of the
1. total cumulative dose of VCR,
2. application mode according to different treatment regimen,
3. time interval since the last injections of the drug,
4. age of children at onset of therapy.

INTRODUCTION

Neuropathy is a well-known side-effect of VINCRISTINE (VCR)-
treatment[1-8].Sandler[3] and co-workers demonstrated in 1969 the
appearance of neurological signs already at doses of 4 mg after
a two months treatment in 60% of their patients.Lateron,Casey[7]
and co-workers found a very strong correlation between the development of different neurological symptoms and signs and the total dose given during a treatment period in adults.In children,
however,up to now there are very few observations on the side-
effects of this drug[5].

So far,no investigations have been initiated concerning the
question,wether or not and to what extent VCR neuropathy is of
importance as a late side-effect of cancer treatment.

Therefore, in a series of 96 children,5 to 15 years of age,and
suffering from various malignant tumours a clinical and neurophysiological examination was performed after VCR treatment had
been finished.

460

PATIENTS

96 children with malignant tumours and 22 controls were examined.Clinical diagnosis and reflexdata are set up in table 1.
47 had been treated with VCR and 49 had had tumour treatment without the use of VCR.

TABLE 1

CLINICAL DIAGNOSIS AND DEEP TENDON REFLEXES IN 96 LONG-TERM SURVIVORS.
Group 1● to 5●:47 children after VCR treatment.
Group 6● and 7●:49 children with tumour treatment without the use of VCR.

Group	N	Clinical diagnosis	Loss of deep tendon reflexes (Achilles)	(all)
1●	15	Acute lymphoblastic leukaemia	3/15	2/15
2●	9	Malignant non-Hodgkin's lymphoma	5/9	3/9
3●	6	Solid tumours (extracranial): (neuroblastoma (2),Rhabdomyosarcoma (2),Ewing sarcoma (2)	6/6	5/6
4●	7	CNS tumours:(medulloblastoma (5) ependymoma (2)	4/7	2/7
5●	10	Others:(teratoma (1),retino-blastoma (1),Osteo-sarcoma (2),ca-testis (2),hypernephroma (1),others (3)	6/10	6/10
6●	28	CNS tumours:(cerebellar astrocytoma (9),craniopharyngioma (5), optic nerve glioma (4),others (10)	0/28	0/28
7●	21	Solid tumours (extracranial): (Wilms tumour (13),others (8)	0/21	0/21

The total dosage of VCR in the treated groups 1● to 5● varied between 6 and 76 mg x m^{-2},the duration of the treatment between 4 weeks and 2 years,and the time interval after the last injection between 1 week and 6 years (table 2).

22 age matched sound children were set up as controls.

METHODS

In all patients and controls deep tendon reflexes and - as far
as possible because of cooperation problems - sensibility status
was performed.Moreover,motor conduction velocity of the tibial
nerve was tested in group 1 • to 7 • and sensory conduction velocity of the median nerve in the subgroups 1■,3■,4■ as well as in
the controls (table 2).

Motor conduction velocity was calculated from latencies of surface recorded map's elicited by supramaximal shocks applied proximally and distally to the nerve trunc.

Sensory conduction velocity was determined from latency of the
first positive deflection of the compound nap picked up at the
wrist via surface electrodes.Supramaximal stimulation was performed orthodromically at index finger nerves.Temperature was
measured on the index finger as well as on the wrist using a ther-
mistor element.The measured sensory conduction velocity was adjusted to 35°C tissue temperatur according to a temperature dependence of 1.3 m/s per 1°C alteration[9].

RESULTS

Clinical findings. Loss of deep tendon reflexes was most prominent in group 3• and 5• concerning patients with extracranial
tumours and high VCR dosages (table 1).Furthermore,in groups 2•
and 4• Achilles reflexes were absent in about 2/3 indicating
peripheral neuropathy.The lowest rate was found in group 1• which
consists of patients treated for acute lymphoblastic leukaemia
with 4-6 VCR doses only.In contrast to these findings no child
treated for a malignant tumour without the use of VCR had diminished tendon reflexes.

Sensibility status could be performed in 12 tumour children
after VCR therapy.Inspite of a careful examination including
several modalities no disturbances could be detected.

Motor conduction velocity (tibial nerve).Motor conduction velocity of the tibial nerve was measured in 47 children after VCR
therapy (group 1• to 5•;table 1 and 2),in 49 children without VCR
therapy (group 6• and 7•table 1 and 2) and in 22 age matched con-
trols.Neither in children treated with VCR but those in group 2•
nor in children without VCR therapy the values were significantly
prolonged (table 2;fig.1).Possibly,in group 2• malignant

TABLE 2

PARAMETERS OF VCR TREATMENT AND MEAN CONDUCTION VELOCITIES (CV).

For the different clinical groups 1● to 7● see table 1. (1■), (3■), (4■): subgroups for sensory CV in the median nerve, adjustet to 35°C tissue temperature.

Group	N	Total dosage of VCR (mg x m^{-2})	Duration of treatment (weeks/years)	Interval after last injection (weeks/years)	Motor CV● tibial nerve (m/s; $\bar{x}$±1SD)	t-test (p<)	Sensory CV■ median nerve '35°C' (m/s; $\bar{x}$±1SD)	t-test (p<)
1●	15	6 - 9	4 - 6 w	2 - 6 y	47.2 ± 2.4	n.s.		
2●	9	22.5 - 25.5	2 y	8 w-1;6y	44.2 ± 2.7	0.01		
(1■)	(17)	(6 - 25)	(4w-2y)	(4w-4;2y)			49.2 ± 2.9	0.01
3●	6	60 - 72	2 y	8 w-2 y	46.4 ± 1.4	n.s.		
(3■)	(8)	(27 - 72)	(1/2-2y)	(1w-2y)			52.5 ± 4.2	0.01
4●	7	60 - 76	2 y	4 w-3 y	45.0 ± 3.1	n.s.		
(4■)	(6)	(15 - 45)	(1 - 2y)	(2w-2;6y)			51.2 ± 2.2	0.01
5●	10	10 - 75	(6w-2y)	8 w-3 y	48.3 ± 4.1	n.s.		
1●to5● (■3,4■)	47 (31)	>6 - 76	4w-2y	1 w-6 y	46.4 ± 3.3	n.s.	50.7 ± 3.2	0.01
6●	28	Ø	Ø	Ø	47.5 ± 4.2	n.s.		
7●	21	Ø	Ø	Ø	47.6 ± 4.3	n.s.		
6●to7●	49	Ø	Ø	Ø	47.6 ± 4.3	n.s.		
Controls 22 (21)		Ø Ø	Ø Ø	Ø Ø	48.5 ± 4.3	-	58.2 ± 3.6	-

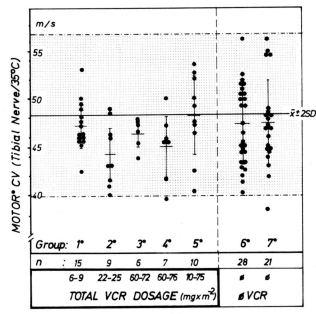

Fig.1. Histograms of motor conduction velocities (tibial nerve) for groups 1● to 7● (s.table 1).Mean values and standard deviations are indicated. Stippled area:95% confidence limits for the control group.Cumulative VCR dosages in mg x m^{-2} at the bottom.

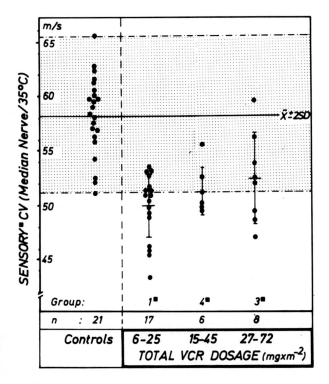

Fig.2. Histograms of sensory conduction velocities (median nerve,adjusted to 35^{6}C tissue temperature)for groups 1■, 3■,and 4■ (s.table 1). Otherwise see fig.1.

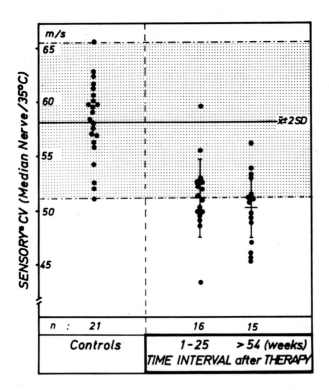

Fig.3. Sensory con-
duction velocity
(median nerve) and
time interval after
VCR treatment in
weeks.Otherwise see
fig. 1 and 2.

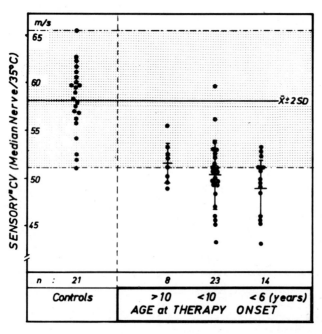

Fig.4. Sensory con-
duction velocity
(median nerve) and
age at onset of
VCR therapy.Other-
wise see fig. 1 and
2.

non-Hodgkin's lymphoma itself may prolong conduction **velocity as a**
paraneoblastic syndrom [10-11].

<u>Sensory conduction velocity (median nerve)</u>.Sensory conduction
velocity of the median nerve was measured in 31 children after
VCR therapy (group 1■,3■,4■,table 2) and in 21 age matched con-
trols.The values were adjusted to 35°C tissue temperature.

Independant of the cumulative VCR dosage a significant prolongation of sensory conduction velocity could be observed in all
groups tested (fig 2).

Morever,if two groups with different time intervals after the
last VCR injection are set up,no significant difference can be
demonstrated (table 2;fig.3).

Recently,if subgroups of different ages at therapy onset are
established,a slight tendency of velocity decreasing with lower
ages can be observed (fig.4).However,an increase of conduction
velocity with increasing age is well-known in children [12-13] and
therefore not relevant for the VCR side effects.

CONCLUSIONS

Our findings demonstrate that signs of VCR-neuropathy are present also in long-term survivors of childhood malignancies.They
may persist even after end of treatment.Until now,however,these
findings do not appear to be of clinical importance for the
children haven survived cancer.

REFERENCES

1. Moress,G.R.,D'Agostino,A.N.and Jarcho,L.W.(1967)Arch.Neurol.
   16,377-384
2. Gottschalk,P.G.,Dyck,P.J.and Kiely,J.M.(1968)Neurology 18,875
3. Sandler,S.G.,Tobin,W.,Henderson,E.S.(1969)Neurology 19,367-374
4. McLeod,J.G.and Penny,R.(1969)J.Neurol.Neurosurg.Psychiat.32,297
5. Bradley,W.G.,Lassmann,L.P.,Pearce,G.W.and Walton,J.N.(1970)
   J.Neurol.Sci.10,107-128
6. Daun,H.and Hartwich,G.(1971)Fortschr.Neurol.Psychiat.39,151-165
7. Casey,E.B.,Jellife,LeQuesne and Milleit (1973)Brain 96,69-86
8. Caccia,M.R.Comotti,Ubiali and Lucchetti (1977)J.Neurol.216,2126
9. Lowitzsch,K.,Hopf and Galand (1977),J.Neurol.216,181-188
10.Wells,C.E.and Silver (1957)Ann.Intern.Med. 46,439
11.Hymann,C.B.et al.(1965),Blood, 25, 1
12.Mortier,W.(1977) Z.EEG-EMG 8,36
13.Schulte,F.J.,Michaelis,R.,Linke and Nolte(1968)Pediatrics 41

Peripheral Neuropathies
N. Canal and G. Pozza, eds.
© 1978 Elsevier/North-Holland Biomedical Press

INVOLVEMENT OF PERIPHERAL NERVOUS MECHANISMS IN THE "REMOTE EFFECTS" OF CANCER ON SKELETAL MUSCLES? A LIGHT MICROSCOPIC STUDY ON AUTOPSY MATERIAL

HORST PETER SCHMITT
Institute of Neuropathology, University of Heidelberg,
Im Neuenheimer Feld 220-221, D-6900 Heidelberg 1 (GFR)

ABSTRACT

Three different muscles each from 112 autopsy cases with malignant tumours were studied. 15 % showed a marked small-group and 2 % a large-group atrophy. In these cases a loss of myelinated nerve fibres could often be demonstrated in the intramuscular nerve twigs and in the deep peroneal and ischiadic nerves. Some target fibres and central chromatolysis of some anterior horn neurons of the spinal cord completed the picture of neurogenic involvement in the changes of the voluntary muscles.

INTRODUCTION

Under the term "carcinomatous neuromyopathy"[3] a number of different remote effects of cancer on the central and peripheral nervous system as well as on the skeletal muscles have been summarized, such as limbic and bulbar encephalitis, PMLE, cerebellar and subacute spinocerebellar degeneration, ALS, subacute necrotizing myelopathy, and dermato- and polymyositis*.Despite their important rôle in the general discussion they are rare events. The problem has recently been reviewed by Scarlato[13].

Among 6100 autopsy cases from the Institute of Pathology of the University of Heidelberg since 1973 including 2000 tumour cases, only one limbic encephalitis and three cases of PMLE had been observed. No poly- or dermatomyositis had occurred. Sensory or motor neuropathies had not been clinically reported. This demonstrates that the reported incidence of the mentioned paraneoplastic disorders of 1 to 6.6 %[2,4,5,9,16] is probably overestimated, although in our material peripheral neuropathies sometimes may have been clinically missed and thus remained autoptically unidentified.

---

*) and necrotizing myopathy a.sensory and sensorimotor neurop.

Apart from the disorders of the nervous system mentioned above, another kind of changes has repeatedly been described in the skeletal muscles of victims of malignant tumours, such as scattered single fibre atrophy and grouped atrophy[7,9,10-12,19]. These changes are likely to occur more frequently than the other diseases mentioned above, although an assess of their incidence is still missing.

MATERIAL AND METHODS

From 112 randomly selected tumour cases, including 60 males and 52 females with an average age of 60.5 years, ranging from 16 to 89 years, specimens of three muscles each (deltoideus, rectus femoris and tibialis anterior), the deep peroneal nerves, and in some cases the ischiadic nerves were obtained on autopsy, fixed in 10 % formalin and embedded in paraffin. 7/u and sometimes 50/u thick sections were stained with H.E., Sudan Black B, according to Masson-Goldner and to Bodian's axon stain. The peripheral nerves were in addition stained according to Klüver-Barrera. In four cases the spinal cords were also examined. In none of the cases had a sensorimotor neuropathy clinically been substantiated.

RESULTS

In the light microscope 19 of the 112 cases (=17 %) exhibited a markedly grouped fibre atrophy in the three examined muscles, the atrophy being of the small-group type in 17 (=15 %) and of the large-group type in 2 (=1.8 %) cases (Fig. 1 B-D). The grouped atrophy was usually combined with a moderate to marked scattered single fibre atrophy, which exclusively was prominent in additional 22 (=31 %) cases, always already showing a tendency for grouping. The average age in both groups (60.8 and 61.3 years) did not significantly differ from the mean age of the total sample. In 6 cases very scanty target and targetoid fibres were found (Fig. 1 C, inset). In 44 cases (=39 %) the scattered or grouped fibre atrophy was developed to a moderate degree.

In the 19 cases with grouped atrophy often degeneration of single nerve fibres with demyelination were observed in the deep peroneal and the ischiadic nerves, being clearly distinguishable from postmortal or traction artifacts (Fig.1 H-M). Occasionally severe axonal swellings with formation of retraction bowls

(Fig.1 N)together with the occurrence of single anterior horn neurons exhibiting central chromatolysis in one of the examined spinal cords (Fig.1 E) pointed towards an axonal type of nerve fibre
degeneration. Small intramuscular nerve twigs sometimes showed a
loss of myelinated nerve fibres (Fig.1 F,O), partially with acute
demyelination figures. The condition of the intramuscular axonal
branchings was difficult to judge with the employed methods, because often axonal swellings were not clearly distinguishable
from postmortal artifacts. Sometimes, however, spherical axonal
swellings as well as less frequent droplet-like desintegrations
were very suggestive of being intravital (Fig.1 G,P). In some
cases the terminal axons at the motor end-plates showed a patchy
enlargement, partially accompanied by fragmentation, the whole
picture looking like elk antlers (Fig. 1 Q, inset). Occasionally
there seemed to be an increased ramification of terminal axons
(Fig.1 Q) and some motor end-plates looked "naked", the terminal
and subterminal axon branches being completely missing.

COMMENTS

The findings of a marked small-group atrophy in 15 % and of a
large-group atrophy in about 2 % of cases with malignant tumours
are very suggestive of an involvement of neurogenic disturbances
in the muscular changes, especially if one considers the occasional occurrence of target and targetoid fibres.

The demonstration of single degenerated nerve fibres, probably
of the axonal degeneration type, in some ischiadic and the deep
peroneal nerves of the 19 cases with grouped fibre atropy, which
are in a good aggreement with the findings of other investigators
[5,10,17-20] are not capable to explain the muscular changes in all
these cases. Axonal degeneration of a single extramuscular nerve
fibre should result in the atrophy of a large group of muscle
fibres (see Fig.1 A) because in the long limb muscles between
100 and 200 muscle fibres are said to belong to one motor unit[1].
Thus, only in the cases with large-group atrophy, which must not
necessarily be of spinal origin, the single nerve fibre degeneration might be regarded as consistent with the muscular changes.
Correspondingly in one related spinal cord central chromatolysis
of single anterior horn cells was observed as an indication of
distal axonal damage.

Small-group atrophy, if neurogenic at all, could only result
from damage of the most distant parts of the peripheral nerves,
e.g. the intramuscular twigs, the terminal axons or the motor
end-plates. In this dimension it is very difficult to substantiate axonal changes by means of the employed methods and on autopsy material. On one hand the intramuscular nerve twigs are not
evenly distributed and even in large specimens often only few
twigs are suitable for judgement. So it is impossible to obtain
a complete evaluation sufficient for quantitative correlation
with the muscular findings. However, in some of the cases it was
possible to demonstrate small intramuscular nerve branches,which
were very suggestive of a loss of myelinated fibres (Fig.1 F,O),
and sometimes dystrophic spherical axonal swellings as well as
scanty droplet-like degeneration figures were found (Fig.1 G,N,P).
Here the limits of light microscopy and of the employed methods
are almost reached. The separation of real intramuscular axonal
damage from artifacts is very difficult and a slight total loss
of single preterminal and terminal axons is almost impossible to
substantiate.

The same difficulties were true for the judgement of the condition of the motor end-plates, especially as the intravital methylene blue method of Coërs could not supravitally be applied to

---

Fig. 1. Synopsis of the findings in muscles and nerves of autopsy
cases with malignant tumours: A) Origination of small- and large-
group fibre atrophy and the site of the nervous lesions (see text)
B) large-group atrophy in the TA* of A 1179/75 (bronchus carcinoma) and small-group atrophy (C,D) in the MD* of A 1353/73 (clito-
ris carcinoma) and A 1165/73 (Hodgkin sarcoma); inset: target
fibre. E) Central chromatolysis of motor neurons in the lumbar
spinal cord as they should be expected according to Aa (normal
neuron on the left - A 363/78, bronchus carcinoma). F,G,O) Intramuscular nerve twigs with a loss of myelinated nerve fibres and
axonal swellings (G →) (A 411/75, lymphosarcoma, SBB*, Bodian,
x400 orig. magnif.). H-M) Single fibre demyelination in the deep
peroneal and ischiadic nerves (411/75 and 1179/75, SBB, x400);
N) Axon picture corresponding to M: retraction bowls; P) spherical
and cylindrical swellings of an intramuscular preterminal axon
(A 1165/73, MD, Bodian, x1000 orig. magnif.). Q) Motor end-plate
being very suggestive of an overarborization of terminal axons
(A 1165/73, RF*, x1000 orig. magnif.); inset: elk antlers-like
enlargement of a terminal axon at the end-plate A 638/74, x1000).
*) TA = tibialis anterior, MD = m. deltoideus, RF = rectus femo-
ris, SBB = Sudan Black B

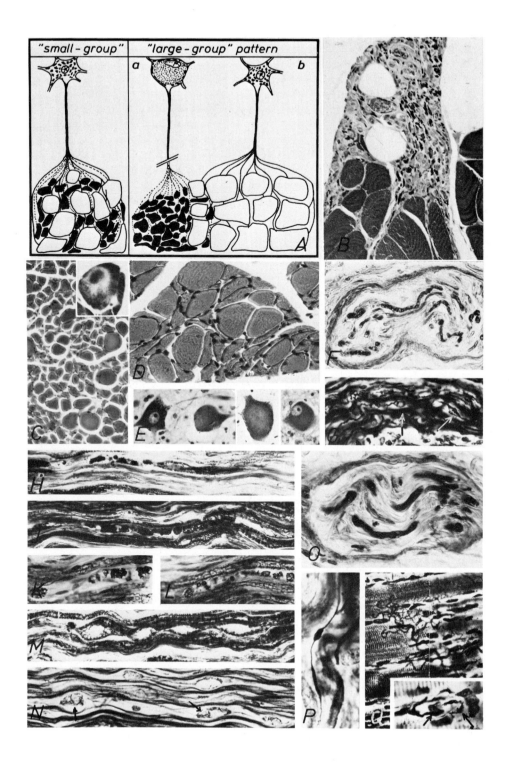

the at least 12 to 24 hours old autopsy material. Despite some
elk antlers-like degeneration figures, sometimes with fragmentations, could be found in the terminal axons, being very suggestive
of intravital changes.

Harriman[7] did not observe changes of the terminal axons by
applying the Coërs method to biopsies of patients with carcino-
mas. He ascribed the single and small-group fibre atrophy to
cachexia. "Cachexia", however, is not a unique nosologic entity
but the result of a very complex interaction of metabolic disturbances, and thus cannot cause any changes in the voluntary
muscles. These must be due to the metabolic deterioration which
occurs with chronic diseases.

Contrary to Harriman Coërs and Woolf and coworkers[10,19,20] were
able to demonstrate in the muscles of patients with malignant
tumours changes of the terminal axons and the motor end-plates
including spherical swellings, droplet-like desintegration, and
increased ramifications of the terminal axons with an augmentation
of the number of end-plates. These findings are in a good aggreement with the present findings and with the postulate concerning
the origin of small-group atrophy (Fig.1 A). Finally, electromyographical investigations on carcinomatous patients[6] revealed
further indications of very distal neurogenic lesions in the
muscles.

Comparing the types of tumours in the cases with markedly grouped muscle atrophy and those without, no statistically significant differences were found. Thus, no special type of tumour is
likely to preferentially produce the atrophic changes under
discussion. Besides, a previous study[15] revealed that small-group
fibre atrophy occurs in various diseases such as diabetes, uremia,
cardiovascular disorders, and alcoholic neuromyopathy, thus indicating that the phenomenon is very unspecific and rather a result
of general metabolic disturbances in chronically wasting disorders than due to a specific action of malignant tumours. This,
however, does not mean that the changes in the skeletal muscles
are entirely independent from the malignomas. In malignant diseases the tumours just mediate general metabolic impairment and
other mechanisms[15], which may in the same way be elicited by
various chronic disorders.

TABLE 1

TYPES OF TUMOURS IN THE PRESENT MATERIAL

		all cases	atrophy cases
1. Carcinomas:	lung	30	7
	intestinal (liver,gall,pancr.,oesoph.)	30	5
	breast and uro-genital tract	24	5
	others (partially unidentified)	11	2
2. Sarcomas:	(lymphatic,Hodgkin,Leukemia, others)	15	–
3. Teratomas and Glioblastomas:		2	–

$$n = 112 \quad = 19$$

REFERENCES

1. Adams, R.D. (1975) In: Diseases of Muscle. Hargerstown, Maryl. Harper & Row, Pbl., 3rd Ed., p. 54

2. Baumberger, K., Mumenthaler, M. (1971) Schweiz. med. Wschr. 101, 452-460

3. Brain, R., Henson, R.A. (1958)Lancet 2, 971-974

4. Croft, P.B., Wilkinson, M. (1965) Brain 88, 427-434

5. Croft, P.B., Urich, H., Wilkinson, M. (1967) Brain 90, 31-66

6. Edström, L., Kugelberg, E. (1968) J. Neurol., Neurosurg., Psychiat. 31, 424-433

7. Harriman, D.F.G. (1965) In: Proc. Vth int. Congr. Neuropath. Amsterdam: Excerpta Medica, Int. Congr. Ser. 100, 677-683

8. Henson, R.A. (1970) In: D. Williams (Ed.) Modern Trends in Neurology, 5, 209

9. Henson, R.A. (1974) In: J.N. Walton (Ed.) Disorders of Voluntary Muscle. Edinburgh: Ch. Livingstone, 3rd Ed., pp.760-774

10. Hildebrand, J., Coërs, C. (1967) Brain 90, 67-83

11. Marin, O.S.M., Denny-Brown, D. (1962) Amer. J. Path. 41,23-29

12. Rebeiz, J.J., Moore, M.J., Holden, E.M., Adams, R.D. (1972) Acta neuropath. (Berl.) 22, 127-144

13. Scarlato, G. (1978) Akt. Neurol. 5, 15-21

14. Scelsi, R., Pinelli, P. (1977) Acta neuropath. (Berl.) 38,103

15. Schmitt, H.P. (1978) Acta neuropath. (Berl) in press

16. Shy, G.M., Silverstein, J. (1965) Brain 88, 515-528

17. Walsh, J.C. (1971) Arch. Neurol. (Chic.) 25, 404-414

18. Webster,H. de F., Schröder,J.M., Asbury, A.K., Adams, R.D. (1967) J. Neuropath. exp. Neurol. 26, 276-299

19. Woolf, A.L. (1965) In: Proc. Vth int. Congr. Neuropath., Amsterdam: Excerpta Medica, Int. Congr. Ser. 100, 641-647

20. Woolf, A.L., Coërs, C. (1974) In: J.N. Walton (Ed.) Disorders of Voluntary Muscle. Edinburgh: Ch.Livingstone,pp. 274-309

Peripheral Neuropathies
N. Canal and G. Pozza, eds.
© 1978 Elsevier/North-Holland Biomedical Press

AUTONOMIC DYSFUNCTION AND MYOKYMIA IN GOLD NEUROPATHY

M.MEYER, M.HAECKI, W.ZIEGLER, W.FORSTER and H.H.SCHILLER

M.M. and H.H.S: Dept. of Neurology, M.H., W.Z. and W.F.:
Dept. of Internal Medicine, University Hospital, 8091 Zürich,
Switzerland

ABSTRACT

Two cases of adverse effects of gold therapy are reported, concerning hypertension, postural hypotension, tachycardia, sweating
and myokymia. This symptomatology resembles a syndrome, first
observed by Morvan, 1890, which was reported in association with
gold therapy and mercury poisoning but may be caused by other
toxic agents too. Data on electromyography and plasma catechola-
mines during physiologic and pharmacologic tests point to a
metabolic disturbance in the peripheral effector-receptor interactions of the sympathetic and the motor nervous system.

Neurologic and neuropsychiatric side-effects of gold therapy
occur rarely. Their reported incidence varies between 0,5 and
15% (1,2). According to Endtz (3), who reviewed 72 cases of gold
neuropathy in 1958, neurologic side effects of gold therapy can
be differentiated into 4 groups, namely a syndrome of symmetrical
peripheral predominantly motor neuropathy, a group with severe
burning pain, an enzephalopathy with mental symptoms and organic psychosis and a group with a variety of sporadic cases. This
present report is based on recent observation of two cases, manifesting an involvement of the vegetative nervous system.

Case 1. A 29 years old male patient with rheumatoid arthritis
was treated with a total dose of 1190 mg of gold sodium thio-
malate given over 12 weeks. Initial adverse symptoms were a diffuse dizziness, occurring only in the upright position and a
hypertension of 180/120 mmHg. These symptoms were followed by
a tachycardia without respiratory arrythmia, a generalised myo-

kymia, excessive sweating and an exfoliative dermatitis. The
upright position and walking could not be tested because blood
pressure (BP) in standing position was not measurable. The CSF
showed an increase of the proteins. In addition, the patient
developed mental symptoms and an organic psychosis with halluzi-
nations. 20 weeks after onset, most of the observed signs and
symptoms had disappeared, with the exception of the absent
respiratory arrythmia.

Case 2. A 31 years old female patient with rheumatoid arthritis
was treated with gold-sodium-thiomalate. After 14 weeks and a
total dose of 1400 mg, she showed generalised myokymia, excessive sweating, hypertension of 170/120 mmHg, transient slight
postural hypotension and tachycardia. The neurologic examination
failed to show additional deficiencies. This patient did not
develop mental symptoms. Clinical remission of the symptomatology started 5 weeks after onset.

ELECTROMYOGRAPHIC INVESTIGATIONS

The undulating, spontaneous muscular contractions, called
myokymia, were caused by recurrent duplets, triplets and multi-
plets and were identified by this pattern as the Denny-Brown
and Foley type (fig. 1a). The interval between the motor unit of
a multiplet was in the range of 10 to 30 msec. The myokymia persisted in the tibial anterior muscle during total block of the
peroneal nerve (fig. 1b), but was stopped by the action of
succinylcholine, which caused an absolutly silent EMG (fig. 1c).
The motor compound potential after a single supramaximal stimulus was followed by additional after-discharges (fig. 1d). The
silent period of the T- and H-reflex was present (fig. 1e), but
sometimes superimposed by the characteristic motor unit discharges (fig. 1f). During sleep the myokymia did not stop.
Phenytoin reduced the frequency of the discharges, Diazepam had
no effect.

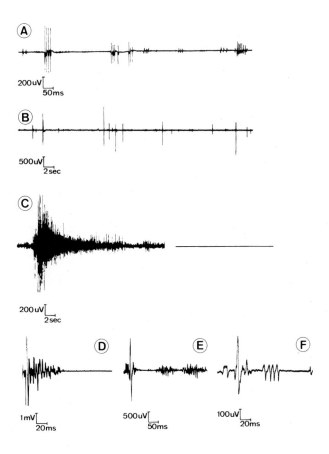

Fig. 1. Electromyographic tracings recorded from case 2. They
are discussed in the text.

TABLE I

BLOOD PRESSURE, HEART RATE, PLASMA-NOREPINEPHRINE (NE) AND - EPINEPHRINE (E) CONCENTRATION RESPONSE TO POSTURAL CHANGE AND TO THE COLD PRESSOR TEST (CPT)

	blood pressure mmHg	heart rate beats/min	NE pg/ml	E
Case I horizontal	145/115	116	529	40
upright after 2 min	98/78	116	1400	72
CPT after 1 min	152/123	115	911	54
Case II horizontal	171/106	80	1766	113
upright after 2 min	169/110		1332	75
CPT after 1 min	192/95		1568	113

TABLE II

EFFECT OF TYRAMINE AND OF PHENTOLAMINE ON BLOOD PRESSURE, HEART RATE AND PLASMA CONCENTRATION OF NOREPINEPHRINE (NE) AND EPINEPHRINE (E)

	blood pressure mmHg	heart rate beats/min	NE pg/ml	E
Case I horizontal	140/100	108	550	116
0,1/kg Tyramine i.v.				
after 2 min	151/103	80	431	95
0,1/kg Phentolamine i.v.				
after 3 min	146/95	112	814	84
Case II horizontal	171/106	80	1766	113
0,1/kg Tyramine i.v.				
after 2 min	190/94		1237	79
0,1/kg Phentolamine i.v.				
after 3 min	204/90	100	1800	87

PHYSIOLOGICAL AND PHARMACOLOGICAL INVESTIGATIONS

Response to postural change. To test the integrity of the baroreceptor reflex arc, some parameters of the cardio-vascular
responses of the two patients to postural change from the supine
to the upright position are measured (table I). The concentration
of norepinephrine (NE) in the recumbent position is slightly
above the normal range (normal=under 500 pg/ml) in case 1 and
pathologically high in case 2. Despite the pronounced postural
hypotension in case 1, the NE-level is rising. The postural
change in this case leads to a normal action of the baroreceptor
reflex, which results in a release of NE by the postganglionic
nerve endings. Nevertheless BP decreases, suggesting a disturbed
function of the alpha-receptors.

Response to the cold pressor test. In the cold pressor condition only the efferent adrenergic fibres to the arterioles are
tested. The normal reaction to the cold pressor test consists
in a rise in BP. This normal reaction surprisingly was seen in
both patients, with a concomitant rise in NE in case 1, suggesting
that efferent sympathetic pathways are functioning (table I).

Effect of Tyramine. The effect of intravenously applied Tyramine, a precoursor of NE, which releases stored NE at the sympathetic nerve endings is shown on table II. The action of Tyramine leads normally to a rise in NE and consequently in BP.
However, there is no increase in plasma concentration of NE although a certain rise in BP is observable (false transmitter
action?). This fact may suggest an additional pathological condition of the adrenergic nerve endings.

Effect of Phentolamine. Phentolamine, an alpha-receptor-
blocker should cause a decrease of BP. In both cases there is an
abnormal reaction. The alpha-receptors don't react to this
blocking agent.

DISCUSSION

The similar clinical presentation of the two cases suggests
that myokymia combined with sweating, hypertension, tachycardia
and other signs of autonomic nervous system dysfunction may represent a unique and specific sign of gold toxicity. As early

as 1890, the French physician Morvan described 5 cases with an
almost identical symptomatology, and in the French literature similar observations have been published from time to time. The
syndrome has been associated with gold therapy and with mercury
poisoning, it has been called "chorée fibrillaire de Morvan" (4).
In the German (5) and Anlo-Saxon literature (6) the term myokymia
is used for the same muscular contractions. and this symptom is
mostly combined with excessive sweating and with other signs of
autonomic dysfunctions. Autonomic dysfunction of predominantly
cardio-vascular characteristic is known in other heavy metal
intoxications, like lead and thallium poisoning.

A great part of the symptomatology in our cases can be explained
by a disturbance of the sympathetic postganglionic adrenergic
and cholinergic and the alpha-motor nerve endings. We suggest an
additional lesion of the alpha-adrenergic receptors. This situation may lead to a reactive hyperactivity of the sympathetic
system, reflected by the raised plasma-NE. The raised plasma-NE
may contribute to the hypertension.

ACKNOWLEDGEMENTS
We gratefully acknowledge the expert technical assistance of
Ms E.Fahrnbühl. This study was supported in parts by the
EMDO foundation.

REFERENCES
1. Hartfall, S.J., Garland, H.G. and Goldie, W. (1937) Lancet 2,
   838-842.
2. Sundelin, F. (1941) Acta Med. Scan., Suppl. 115, pp. 1-291.
3. Endtz, L.J. (1958? Rev. neurol. 99, pp. 395-410
4. Roger, H., Alliez, J. and Roger J. (1953) Rev. neurol.,
   88, pp. 164-173
5. Schultze, F. (1895) Dtsch. Z. Nervenheilk., 6, pp- 65-70
6. Gardner-Medwin, D. and Walton. J.N. (1969) Lancet 1,
pp. 127-130

Peripheral Neuropathies
N. Canal and G. Pozza, eds.
© 1978 Elsevier/North-Holland Biomedical Press

COLLAGEN MEASUREMENT IN HYPOEXTENSIBILITY OF THE SOLEUS MUSCLE 6 TO 9 DAYS
AFTER LOCAL INJECTION OF TETANUS TOXIN

A.HAYAT, J.MIGNOT and C.TARDIEU

A.Hayat and C.Tardieu: FRA 18 INSERM, Hôpital Raymond Poincaré, 92380 GARCHES F.

J.Mignot: Hôpital Ambroise Paré, 9 avenue Ch. de Gaulle, 92100 BOULOGNE F.

ABSTRACT

Gordon-Sweets staining for reticulin was used to measure the total connective tissue of the hypoextensible soleus muscle and the contralateral muscle
in the same guinea-pig. No significant difference was found between the two
solei.

INTRODUCTION

In neurological disorders like cerebral palsy and stroke one of the clinically assessed factor is the reduced elasticity of the muscle (hypoextensibility).

It has been demonstrated that following a period of immobilization (6days)
in the shortened position, guinea-pigs soleus looses sarcomeres (5%) along
the length of the isolated muscle fibres [1].

While it has been possible to produce a short term (4 to 7 days) reduction of sarcomeres (40%) by local injection of tetanus toxin[1]; the associated hypoextensibility was investigated through possible changes in the
connective tissue.

MATERIALS AND METHODS

Experimental animals. 16 guinea-pigs were selected and used in this study.
Weights on average 600 g and sizes allow satisfactory measurements when
conventional length-tension curves are established. 6 animals were used
for the passive tension-extension curves. 5 animals were used for total
connective tissue evaluation, among them 3 were also used for perimysial
evaluation. 5 animals were used for endomysial measurement.

Tetanus toxin. Purified tetanus toxin [2] obtained from Pasteur Institut
(Paris) was dissolved in 1 ml pepton solution. Appropriate dose was selected to generate a local tetanus confined to the muscle of one hind limb.

Clinical assessment. 6 to 9 days after the injection, the hind limb is
always in extension. Before the animal was killed a section of the tendon

of the quadriceps and of the sciatic nerve makes possible a complete flexion of the knee and a clinical assessment of the soleus hypoextensibility without interference of muscle contractions.

Length-tension curves. A comparison was made between the injected side soleus to the contralateral muscle. Animals were deeply anesthetized by intraperitoneal pentobarbitone(40 mg/kg). Sciatic nerve was sectioned at a high level in the thigh. Guinea-pig was placed ventral side down and tibia firmly affixed to the frame of the holding apparatus. Through a reference marked on the soleus, measurement of muscle lengthening related to different ankle angles was performed. Passive tension was measu ed for the different degrees of muscle stretch.

Histological methods. Animals were killed by intracardiac injection of pentobarbitone. Then the whole legs were removed from the animals and pinned on a wooden board. The two ankle angles being identical. Then wooden board was moved to formol (15%). The same ankle angles fixation allows an equal length of the muscles and homogenous comparison of related width in connective tissue - 12 μ m sections of the soleus were taken at equal lengths from the tibio-calcaneal insertions for each muscle - 15 serial transversal cuts in the median plane were made and stained using the Gordon-Sweets method for reticulin identification.

Morphometric measurements. Sections were photographed under a Leitz microscope and developped under a special exposure of the positive film. Then classical morphometric methods were used: corresponding areas of surface cells and connective tissue were cut out and weighted. For each muscle section (6.3 mm^2) an area of about one tenth was selected at random. This area was different from one muscle to the other, thus absolute comparisons are not possible between muscles. Total amount of connective tissue was evaluated for areas including more than 400 cells for each muscle. Weighted connective tissue and muscle cells were compared, allowing calculation of ratios of total connective tissue per muscle cell areas. Independant evaluation of perimysial and endomisyal tissue was performed. In endomysial evaluation density per μ m all along the periphery of the cell was evaluated.

RESULTS

Clinical assessment of the muscle hypoextensibility was performed. The measured ankle angle was between 100° and 125° instead of 30° for the contralateral hind limb.

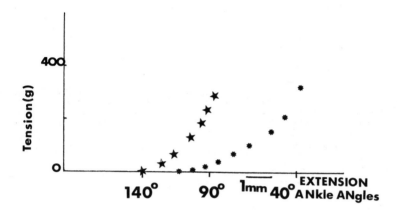

Fig. 1. Passive tension-extension curve for tetanized muscles (★) and contralateral one (＊). Extension is within the physiological articular range.

Figure 1 shows passive tension-extension curve of local tetanized soleus compared to the contralateral muscle. For tetanized soleus a given tension is recorded for a shorter muscle length than for the contralateral side. Tension increases more rapidly with extension for tetanized soleus.

In serial sections of the soleus muscle, silver impregnation was specific for reticulin of the connective tissue which is probably related to collagen type III.

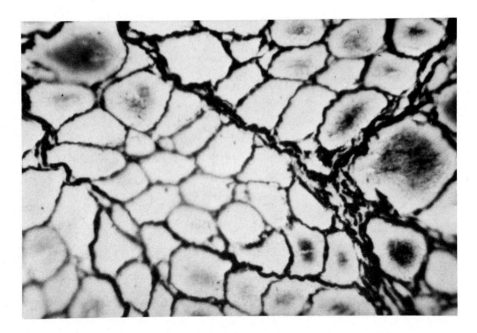

Fig. 2. Connective tissue of tetanized muscle stained according to Gordon-Sweets silver impregnation. Note the possible remodelling of the perimysial level.

Figure 3 shows the distribution of cell areas in μm^2 for tetanized and contralateral side. More then 500 cells were measured and distributed in four classes ranging from less than 470 μm^2 to more than 931 μm^2 cell areas. While a gaussian distribution is demonstrated for the contralateral side, hypertrophic tendancy occured for tetanized cells.

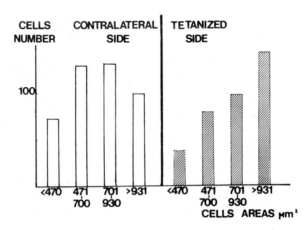

Fig. 3. Histogram distribution of cell areas for contralateral and tetanized soleus muscles.

Related areas of connective tissue and muscle cells were measured in Table I for tetanized (T) and contralateral (C) soleus muscles. When ratios of the total connective tissue over the corresponding muscle cell areas were compared, difference between tetanized and contralateral soleus was not significant.

TABLE I

CONNECTIVE TISSUE

GUINEA PIGS	CONNECT. TISSUE		MUSCLE CELLS		RATIO	CONN. MUSC.
	C.	T.	C.	T.	C.	T.
39	3.89	9.90	12.55	22.18	0.31	0.45
42	8.20	4.02	22.99	12.71	0.36	0.32
267	4.98	4.55	19.71	22.28	0.25	0.20
269	6.67	5.78	23.69	30.88	0.28	0.19
270	5.85	5.18	26.55	20.02	0.21	0.25
					m:0.28	m:0.28
					$\pm$ 0.02	$\pm$ 0.05

Table I. Total connective tissue evaluated as a ratio of endo and perimysial surface related to muscle cell areas.

Since the tetanized soleus underwent hypertrophy and lost cells, histogram distribution of the cells was not comparable between tetanized and contralateral soleus, thus absolute endomysial tissue cannot be reported to cell surface. For this reason, it was decided to measure endomysial density by μ m cell along the periphery of each cell. 0.47 ± 0.07 was obtained for the tetanized soleus and 0.48 ± 0.06 for contralateral soleus. In a few cases it was found in some muscles areas that perimysial density of connective tissue was increased in the tetanized soleus compared to the contralateral muscle.

DISCUSSION

It is rather intriguing that no difference was found between ratios of connective tissue over muscle cell areas between tetanized and contralateral soleus. This finding is more remarkable by the relative increase in muscle cell areas due to hypertrophy in tetanized soleus muscles. Anyhow this increase may be balanced by the relative lost in muscle cells.

Bailey[3] reported immunofluorescent study on the collagen types of the striated muscle. According to the author, Gordon-Sweets reticulin identification seems to be correlated with type III collagen associated with glycoproteins - it is suggested that in the present study, types I and V collagens were not identified. To explain hypoextensibility of tetanized muscle, different modifications of connective tissue may be invoqued: changes in width, length or structure. This study suggests an absence of modification in total width of endo and perimysial connective tissue, though some remodelling of the perimysium was somehow observed. Scanning examination, collagenolytic activity as well as cross-links and GAG's distribution must be evaluated in the future to face other modifications of connective tissue related to muscle hypoextensibility.

REFERENCES

1. Huet de la Tour,E. et al. (1978) Submitted to J.of Neurol. Sciences.
2. Bizzini,B. et al. (1969) Ann. Inst. Pasteur 116, 686-712.
3. Dvance,V.C. et al. (1977) FEBS letters vol.79, N°2, pp.248-252.

Peripheral Neuropathies
N. Canal and G. Pozza, eds.
© 1978 Elsevier/North-Holland Biomedical Press

STUDY OF THE EFFECT OF GANGLIOSIDES ON EXPERIMENTAL CARBON DI
PHIDE NEUROPATHY.

C.BULGHERONI, M.MARONI, A.COLOMBI, L.COTRONEO, V.FOA', R.GILIOLI, E.R
TA, D.PELUCCHETTI[*] E.BOTTACCHI[*] and A.VOLTA

Clinica del Lavoro "L.Devoto" dell'Università - Milano - Italy

Istituto Neurologico "C.Besta" - Milano - Italy [*]

INTRODUCTION

The nervous system is considered the target organ in carbon disulphide (CS_2) intoxication both for central and peripheral structures.[1-12] Several studies have shown a slowing of the maximal and slow fibres motor conduction velocities of peripheral nerves in subjects with CS_2 poisoning [6,7,11,12,13]. Experimental studies have shown a slowing of motor nerve conduction velocity in rats and rabbits during long -term CS_2 exposure [13,14,15].

Object of our study is to confirm a possible protective action of bovine cerebral cortex gangliosides on CS_2 experimental neuropathy in the rat. In the present communication, preliminary results of our study are reported concerning the evaluation of protective effect of gangliosides during the period of induction of the CS_2 peripheral neuropathy.

MATERIALS AND METHODS

Forty joung adult male White Star rats (weighting in average 350 gr) were subdivided at random in five groups with the same number of animals:

group 1: was exposed to CS_2 and not treated;

group 2: was exposed to CS_2 and treated with daily i.p. dose of 10 mg/kg of ganglio sides (3 ‰ in physiological solution);

group 3: was exposed to CS_2 and treated with daily i.p. dose of 0.5 mg/kg of gangliosides (0.15 ‰ in physiological solution);

group 4: was exposed to CS_2 and treated with daily i.p. dose of 0.5 mg/kg of vitamin B_1 and 1 mg/kg of vitamin B_6 (0.45 ‰ in physiological solution);

group 5: was neither treated nor exposed to CS_2 and served as control.

The CS_2 exposure was obtained by an air-conditioned Rochester's inhalation chamber of 8 m^3 of volume. The desired concentration of CS_2 in air resulted from diluting a concentrated flow of air-CS_2 (obtained by a Drechsel apparatus) in the principal airflow of the chamber. The actual concentration in the chamber was verified daily with

...od (colorimetric analysis).

...ls were exposed at a CS_2 mean concentration of 550 ppm for 12 weeks, 5 ...r 5 days/week. All the animals received conventional food and water ad

...luation of the degree of peripheral nerve impairment was performed in ...mals by electromyographic examination of the sciatic nerve and gastro- ...muscle: the rest activity, the maximal and slow fibres motor conduction ... (MCV and SFCV respectively) by the desynchronization method [16] were ... using a DISA 1501 instrument. Room temperature as well as skin temperature ...actically constant.

...neurophysiological studies were coupled with morphological investigations by ...of light and electron microscopy. However these studies are still in course and ...s will not be presented here.

...he control tests were performed at pre-exposure period and then at 4th, 8th and ...week.

RESULTS

The mortality during the experiment was quite different in the five groups: it was ...bout 15 % in non-treated rats and about 30 % in all treated groups; no control rats died.

The mean weight gains of the treated groups were respectively 24 gr for the high-dose-ganglioside group, 58 gr for the low-dose-ganglioside group and 51 gr for the vitamin-group, whereas non-treated rats had a mean weight decrease of 24 gr and control rats a mean weight increase of 165 gr.

During the exposure to CS_2 some rats looked drowsy in all the groups. No marked impairment of movements was observed in the animals during the experiment, but from the 10th - 11th week of exposure some rats of the non-treated and vitamin -treated groups demonstred slight difficulty on posterior limbs in standing and walking.

The results of neurophysiological examinations are summarized in Table 1 and Fig. 1, in Table 2 and Fig. 2, where the behavior of respectively MCV and SFCV are reported. The statistical comparison among groups was performed using the one tailed t Student test on the means of individual variations from the pre-exposure values.

With respect to MCV (Table 1 and Fig. 1) the results indicate an important decrease in non-treated rats (Group 1) that is evident from the 4th week and attains the lowest value on the 12th week. In the vitamin-treated rats (group 4) the MCV had a similar but less marked behavior, so that at 12th week the mean of individual decrease significantly differs from that of non-treated rats. The high-dose-ganglioside-treated animals (group 2) did not suffer any decrease in MCV for the first eight week, thus differing in a

TABLE 1. BEHAVIOR OF MAXIMAL MOTOR CONDUCTION VELOCITY OF SCIATIC NERVE OF RATS DURING
EXPOSURE TO CARBON DISULPHIDE.

GROUP	PRE-EXPOSURE TIME MCV (m/sec)	AFTER 4 WEEKS MCV-individual variations from pre-exposure values	AFTER 8 WEEKS MCV-individual variations from pre-exposure values	AFTER 12 WEEKS MCV-individual variations from pre-exposure values
GROUP 1 mean (±sd) n°	52.8 (± 4.0) 8	− 11.2 (± 10.9) 8	− 13.9 (± 6.1) 7	− 16.2 (± 4.0) 7
GROUP 2 mean (±sd) n° significancy-level versus group 1*	52.0 (± 3.1) 8 −	+ 1.3 (± 6.3) 8 P < 0.01	+ 0.2 (± 8.6) 7 P < 0.01	− 11.9 (± 3.4) 5 P > 0.05
GROUP 3 mean (±sd) n° significancy-level versus group 1*	46.6 (± 3.5) 8 −	− 5.8 (± 9.5) 8 P > 0.05	− 1.2 (± 8.8) 6 P < 0.01	− 0.1 (± 9.4) 6 P < 0.0025
GROUP 4 mean (±sd) n° significancy-level versus group 1*	49.9 (± 4.5) 8 −	− 3.5 (± 8.5) 8 P > 0.05	not measured	− 10.1 (± 5.9) 5 P > 0.05

* statistical analysis performed by "t Student" test on means of individual variations.

n° = number of treated subjects.

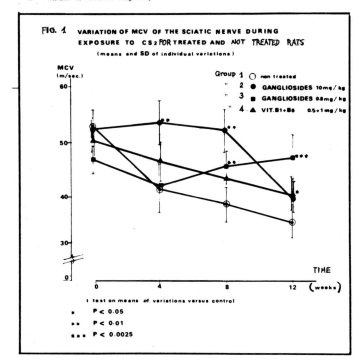

FIG. 1 VARIATION OF MCV OF THE SCIATIC NERVE DURING
EXPOSURE TO CS2 FOR TREATED AND NOT TREATED RATS
(means and SD of individual variations)

MCV (m/sec.)

Group 1 ○ non treated
" 2 ● GANGLIOSIDES 10mg/kg
" 3 ■ GANGLIOSIDES 0.5mg/kg
" 4 ▲ VIT.B1+B6 0.5+1mg/kg

TIME (weeks)

t test on means of variations versus control

•   P < 0.05
•• P < 0.01
••• P < 0.0025

significant way from non-treated rats; thereafter they showed a rapid decrease of MCV, similar to the of non-treated group.

The low-dose-ganglioside-treated rats (group 3), after an initial drop of the MCV, reached the pre-exposure level from the 8th week and then mantained this level with high-significantly difference from non-treated animals and vitamin-treated animals also.

The same trend of decrease, as expected, was seen in non-treated rats also for what concerns the SFCV (Table 2 and Fig. 2). At the end of the experiment the SFCV in this group was about half the pre-exposure level.

As observed for MCV, the vitamin-treated group showed a similar behavior, while significantly different results were obtained for ganglioside-treated groups.

In the high-dose treated, the decrease of SFCV was well defined only at 12th week, when the SFCV equalled the non-treated rats levels. On the contrary, in low -dose-ganglioside animals the SFCV decreased rapidly in the first weeks and slightly in the last weeks so that the total decrease was not so marked as in the non-treated rats.

The non-exposed animals (group 5) were tested at pre-exposure time and then after 12 weeks: the MCV and SFCV mean values were respectively 54.5 ($\pm$ 2.7) and 46.3 ($\pm$ 3.7) in the first control and 52.6 ($\pm$ 3.5) and 46.3 ($\pm$ 2.8) in the last control.

It is also noteworthy that in recording rest muscle activity at the 12th week, nearly all non-treated and vitamin treated rats showed a great deal of fibrillation, while the rest activity was less marked in the high-dose-ganglioside group and was absent in the low-dose rats.

DISCUSSION

The CS_2-induced polineuropathy is one of the most investigated toxic neural lesions,and shows several clinical and pathological findings in common with many other toxic occupational neuropathies.

In the early stage of the poisoning the most apparent clinical feature is the slowing of the conduction velocity of the involved nerves. This occurs without morphological evidence of myelin sheaths degeneration, while subcellular fine structures of axons are fairly disrupted, thus indicating probably the site of primary lesion in the axon filament[17,18].

The preliminary results of our study on the protective effect of gangliosides are encouraging and seem to confirm the therapeutic effectiveness of this drug in this area also. In fact with the administration of gangliosides in high doses (10 mg/kg), we have noted even from the first weeks of exposure to CS_2 a marked tendency of the maximal and slow fibres conduction velocities to remain unchanged. After 2 months, this protection was completely lost, being so far the grounds for this phenomenon unknown.

TABLE 2. BEHAVIOR OF SLOW FIBRES MOTOR CONDUCTION VELOCITY OF SCIATIC NERVE OF RATS DURING EXPOSURE TO CARBON DISULPHIDE.

G R O U P	PRE-EXPOSURE TIME SFCV (m/sec)	AFTER 4 WEEKS SFCV-individual variations from pre-exposure values	AFTER 8 WEEKS SFCV-individual variations from pre-exposure values	AFTER 12 WEEKS SFCV-individual variations from pre-exposure values
GROUP 1 mean (±sd) n°	43.9 (± 5.4) 8	− 9.6 (± 6.7) 8	− 12.4 (± 8.6) 7	− 18.2 (± 4.9) 7
GROUP 2 mean (±sd) n° significancy-level versus group 1*	46.0 (± 3.5) 8	− 1.6 (± 8.6) 8 P < 0.05	− 3.3 (± 7.9) 7 P < 0.05	− 16.5 (± 3.3) 4** P > 0.05
GROUP 3 mean (±sd) n° significancy-level versus group 1*	41.2 (± 4.0) 8	− 10.3 (± 7.8) 8 P > 0.05	− 6.3 (± 7.6) 6 P > 0.05	− 12.8 (±3.9) 6 P < 0.05
GROUP 4 mean (±sd) n° significancy-level versus group 1*	42.8 (± 5.1) 8	− 9.0 (± 11.5) 8 P > 0.05	not measured	− 12.6 (± 5.7) 5 P > 0.05

* statistical analysis performed by "t Student" test on means of individual variations.
n° = number of treated subjects.
** SFCV was undetectable in one of the analysed subjects.

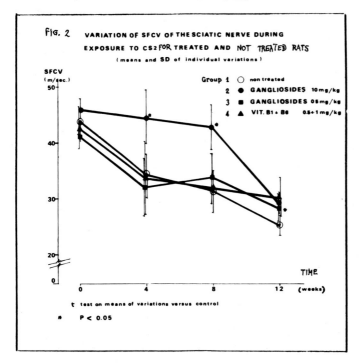

FIG. 2 VARIATION OF SFCV OF THE SCIATIC NERVE DURING EXPOSURE TO CS2 FOR TREATED AND NOT TREATED RATS
(means and SD of individual variations)

Group 1 ○ non treated
2 ● GANGLIOSIDES 10 mg/kg
3 ■ GANGLIOSIDES 05 mg/kg
4 ▲ VIT. B1 + B6 0.5 + 1 mg/kg

SFCV (m/sec.)

TIME (weeks)

t test on means of variations versus control
* P < 0.05

The administration of gangliosides in lower doses (0.5 mg/kg), like those commonly used in human therapy, results less rapidly in a protective effect, as if some time were needed for the drug to reach therapeutic concentration in tissues or to manifest its effect. However in this case the protective effect is long-lasting and the low-dose-ganglioside-treated animals are the only experimental group that showed no fibrillation at electromyographic recording after 12 weeks of exposure.

Since our results are only preliminary, it is too early to debate pharmacological ipothesys, but as from now these ensues suggest the need for extensive research in this field.

REFERENCES

1. Vigliani, E.C. and Cazzullo (1950) Med.Lav. 41, 49

2. Vigliani, E.C. (1954) Brit.J.Industr.Med. 11, 235

3. Nunziante Cesaro, A. (1954) Fol. Med., 37, 466

4. Maugeri (1971) Med. Lav., 62, 398

5. Navarro Martinez and Farina, G. (1969) Med. Lav. 59, 11

6. Marm, P., Lilis, R., Laucranjan, I., Ionescu, S. and Vasilescu, I. (1970) Med. Lav. 61, 102

7. Seppalainen, A.M., Tolenen, M., Karli, P., Hanninen, H. and Hernberg, S. (1972) Work-Environm. Hlth 9, 71

8. Foà, V. and Gilioli, R. (1974) Atti XVIII Congresso Soc.Ital.di Neurologia, Roma 5-8/12/1973, Riv.Pat.Nervosa e Mentale, 2,1

9. Knave, B., Kalmodin-Edman, B.,Person, H.E. and Goldberg, J.M. (1974) Work - Environm. Hlth 11, 49

10. Seppalainen, A.M. and Tolonen, M. (1974) Work-Environm. Hlth 11, 145

11. Vasilescu, C. (1972) Rev.Roum.Neurol. 9, 63

12. Gilioli, R., Bulgheroni, C., Bertazzi, P.A., Cirla, A.M., Tommasini, M., Cassitto, M.G. and Jacovone, M.T. (1978) Med.Lav. 69, 130

13. Lukas, E. (1970) Med. Lav. 61, 302

14. Seppalainen, A.M. and Linnoila, I. (1975) Scand.J.Work-Environm. Hlth 1, 178

15. Seppalainen, A.M. and Linnaila, I. (1976) Neuropath.Appl.Neurobiol. 2, 209

16. Cosi, N. (1966) Conferenza di aggiornamento della Soc.Ital. di Elettroencefalografia e neurofisiologia, Chianciano, 7-9 ottobre.

17. Linnoila, I., Haltia, M., Seppalainen, A.M. and Palo, J. (1974) VIIth International Congress of Neuropathology, Budapest 1-7 september

18. Juntunen, J., Haltia, M. and Linnoila, I. (1974) Acta Neuropath. 29, 361.

Peripheral Neuropathies
N. Canal and G. Pozza, eds.
© 1978 Elsevier/North-Holland Biomedical Press

PERIPHERAL NERVE CHANGES IN REFSUM'S DISEASE BEFORE AND AFTER TREATMENT

ELFRIEDE SLUGA

Neurological Institute, Schwarzspanierstr. 17, Vienna (Austria)

HERMANN LENZ

Neurological Department, Hospital Barmherzige Brüder, Rudigierstr. 11-30, Linz (Austria)

INTRODUCTION

Refsum's disease is one of the rare neurological maladies with a known metabolic defect.

Refsum described in 1945[25] a condition which he called heredopathia atactica polyneuritiformis[26], first observed in 5 cases of two unrelated families. He delineated the clinical syndrome with the cardinal features consisting of chronic polyneuropathy, cerebellar ataxia, retinitis pigmentosa, hemeralopia and increased cerebrospinal fluid protein. Less constant signs can be associated, including ichthyosis, cardiomyopathy, lens opacities and skeletal abnormalities[27, 28]. 58 cases have been reported in 30 years[27], an indication that the disease is not a frequent one.

But it is an important one insofar as biochemical abnormalities are well known in detail and give a model for the possible development of a metabolic neuropathy. Refsum himself suggested already that the disease is akin to a lipidosis, but it was Klenk and Kahlke (1963)[15] who produced the first proof. They reported the presence of abnormal concentrations of a branched 20 C fatty acid, the phytanic acid (3, 7, 11, 15 - tetramethylhexadecanoic acid) in blood and tissue of a Refsum's patient. And this substance has been regularly identified in subsequent cases. Phytanic acid is present in normal persons in blood as well as in tissues but only in traces in a rather undetectable amount[2], e.g. in serum below 0, 5% of the total fatty acids. The augmentation of phytanic acid in serum to values up to 30% and more is the first diagnostic data in cases clinically supposed to be Refsum's disease.

Phytanic acid accumulation in tissues is proved for peripheral nerve, brain, liver, kidney and heart muscle[23, 1, 11]. And in peripheral nerve the myelin-lipid fractions contain considerable amounts of this acid[18], in higher concentrations than in central nervous system[13,16]. The cause of the phytanic acid accumulation is a defect in the oxydative pathway of its degradation[33, 34].

The initial step of α -oxydation is blocked by an α -hydroxylase deficiency [19, 14, 31]. Phytanic acid originates in the diet alone, it is not synthesized endogenously and is quickly formed from phytol out of chlorophyll-containing substances[33, 34]. Phytol-low diet was the therapeutic consequence of these data[7].

In contrast to these nearly complete biochemical data, examinations of the pathological tissue changes are relatively rare, mostly concerning nervous tissue[24, 3, 4, 11, 10]. The hypertrophic neuropathy in peripheral nerves, first described by Cammermeyer[3] is consistently present and often documented even in electron microscopy[5, 8, 9, 10, 11]. Lipid deposits in meningeal tissue and basal ganglia are observed[4]. But the relation between the biochemical abnormalities and the pathological findings remains still poorly explained[27, 36], especially for the most prominent finding of hypertrophic neuropathy and its fiber lesion, already supposed by Cammermeyer as a demyelinating one.

To give further data to the evolution of hypertrophic neuropathy and its changes in the course of dietary treatment is the topic of our present studies. We had the opportunity of a long-term observation in one of the two cases of Refsum's disease in Austria, and we could carry out two nerve-biopsies, one in a period of acute relapse and a second 2 years after a dietary treatment.

CASE REPORT

Our case was a 46 year old woman, daughter of consanguineous parents. Since childhood she was a little clumsy. But not before the age of 30, after the delivery of her second child did she notice symptoms. Anosmia, hemeralopia and visual field disturbances appeared. At the age of 39 she had concentrically constricted visual fields and the first neurological examination revealed pes cavus, a slight loss of power distally in the limbs, absent tendon jerks for the Achilles reflex and distal impairment of all modalities of sensations in all four limbs - signs of a sensory-motor polyneuropathy. Ataxia of the gait was present and the first mis-diagnosis was a Heredoataxia Friedreich. During the next 6 years the condition remained without considerable changes. At the age of 46, some months before readmission, a new attack occurred with deterioration especially of the motor disabilities in the lower limbs. At admission considerable troubles of walking were prominent, consisting of ataxia and paresis. Ataxia in the upper limb was mild as well as a scanning speech. Anosmia was unchanged, visual fields concentrically constricted to 5 $^{\circ}$. Now the retinitis pigmentosa was realised and prompted together with the polyneuropathy and the cerebellar signs to the diagnostic suspicion of Refsum's disease.

Examinations revealed an extinction in the electroretinogram, lesions of the inner ear and skeletal abnormalities with shortening of the metatarsal bones 4 and 5. No palpable enlargement of peripheral nerves was clinically present. Nerve conduction velocity (NCV) was unmeasurable in both fibular nerves and had 17 m/sec. In the median nerve. CSF had a normal cell number, but an elevation of proteins to 180 mg% at this time. Finally phytanic acid in serum (examination: B. Molzer/H. Bernheimer) was highly augmented to 27% of the total fatty acids.

Diagnosis of Refsum's disease was confirmed. Worsening went on during the hospitalisation time.

FIRST NERVE BIOPSY FINDINGS

In this period of an acute relapse, still untreated, we performed the first sural-nerve biopsy.

In light microscopy there was a severe reduction of myelinated fibers (fig. 1 and 2). Quantitatively the reduction was expressed in a total number of less than 1000 fibers/mm^2 (750), against normal values of 4.000 to 8.000 fibers (fig. 3). In higher magnification it was to be seen that only small myelinated fibers were still preserved (fig. 2). This observation is in good agreement with the histometric findings; only fibers of small diameters esp. from 2 - 6 mμ were present (fig. 3). Only some of the small myelinated fibers were surrounded by onion bulbs, some were still devoid of them (fig. 2). Schwann cells were increased and often loaden with droplet-like structures (fig. 2). In electron microscopy the severe reduction of myelinated fibers was to confirm (fig. 4, 6). A considerable amount of collagen fibers was all over present (fig. 4, 6, 7). Some onion bulbs were clearly to delineate, mostly around small, still well myelinated fibers (fig. 4), but sometimes also around a fiber with an unproportional thin myelin sheath (fig. 5). Bulbs with centrally located Schwann cells esp. with Büngner-band-formation were not evident and in the processus of the bulbs unmyelinated fibers were not (fig. 4) or only very rare present. But unmyelinated fiber-groups were numerous present, appearing unchanged in their original structure and order (fig. 4).

The most impressive findings in this first sural-nerve biopsy was the presence of a considerable number of myelinated fibers in d e m y e l i n a - t i o n (fig. 6, 7).

Changes of the myelin appeared over the whole thickness of the sheath (fig. 6), most often, or over a part of it, then always involving the axon-near inner group of the myelin-lamellae, while the more circumferential mem-

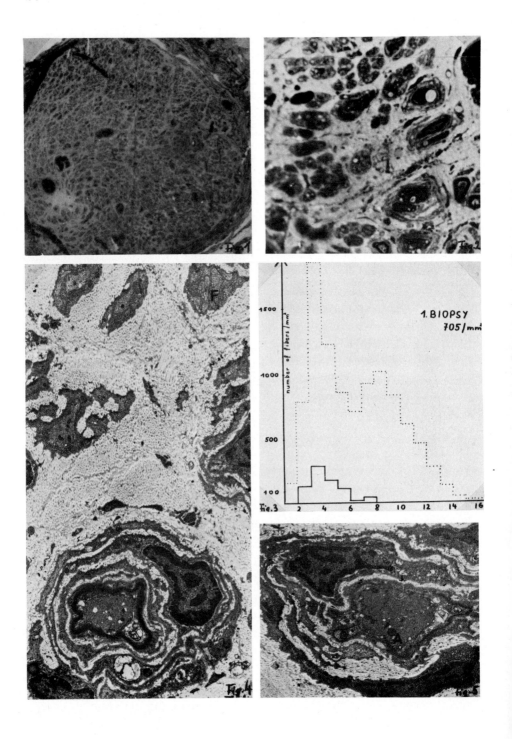

1. BIOPSY
705/mm²

branes persisted (fig. 7). In the area of the changed myelin lamellae an irregular network of "vesicles" and membranes were present (fig. 8, 9, 6, 7). These areas impressive in low magnification more by their "vesicular" appearence (fig. 6, 7) may give rise to the findings in light microscopy of droplet-loaden Schwann cells (fig. 2). In higher magnification these demyelinating-zones consisted all over of numerous delamellated membranes, most often single, sometimes in small groups (fig. 8-12). In between spaces were present, mostly empty, which seemed as if surrounded by the delamellated membranous structures, conditions giving rise to the "vesicular-like" appearance (fig. 8-12).

Membrane groups had different periodicities - solitary and only in axon-distant zones myelin-like (fig. 8, 12), but more often membranes without alternating lamellae were present (fig. 10, 12, 15). These equithick membrane-groups had sometimes distances of still 150 $\overset{o}{A}$ (fig. 10), but much more frequently small groups of more closely packed membranes with a distance of 40 - 60 Å were to be seen (fig. 10, 13, 15). Blind loops of membranes were there in between (fig. 10), but more often these structures could be observed in demyelinating zones of only partially involved myelinated fibers (fig. 13, 14). Here the innermost lamellae of the still compact myelin in the transition-zone against the demyelinating area formed loops (fig. 14 inset, 14, 13) while against the axolemma in the demyelinated area the "membrane-surrounded vesicles" appeared (fig. 13), structures resulting from numerous delamellated membranes, mostly single ones. A progressive development from looping of just demyelinating membranes to "vesicular" appearing formations of membranes resp. membrane-fragments seems apparently, obvious as consequence of the

First sural nerve biopsy: Fig. 1 - 15.

Fig. 1   Subtotal loss of myelinated fibers in a sural nerve fascicle.
x 46

Fig. 2   Reduction of myelinated fibers.
Only smaller-diameter fibers are preserved. Onion bulb formation.
Schwann cell cytoplasm droplet-loaden.
x 295

Fig. 3   Histometric findings of myelinated fibers in first biopsy.
Reduction of the total number to 705 against normal values of
4.000 - 8.000.
Only small calibrated fibers esp. 6-2 mµ are represented.

Fig. 4   Severe myelinated fiber reduction.
Onion bulbs; around a myelinated fiber.
Unmyelinated fibers - F
Increase in collagen.
x 5520

Fig. 5   Onion bulb formation around an unproportional thin myelinated fiber.
A - axon
x 5520

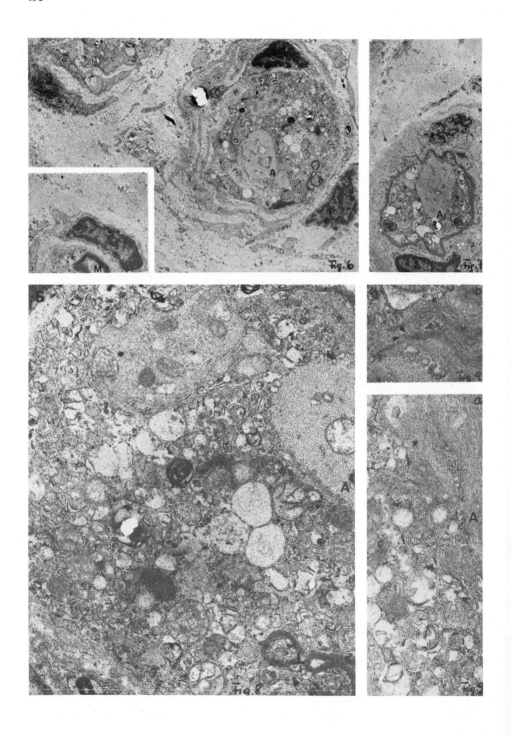

delamellation of myelin, the predominant phenomenon in the present demyelination .

In the zones of "going over" myelin sheaths to demyelination also several
splitted groups of periodicity-changed membranes appeared sometimes (fig.15).

But in these demyelinating fibers the still persisting myelin sheaths were
not completely unchanged. In a lot of small areas of these myelin sheaths
changes in periodicity appeared (fig. 13-15). Spots of uni-equi-distant membranes were present, with a periodicity of 40 - 60 Å, as observed in demyelinated areas (fig. 13, 14). The basic structural changes of this shift of periodicity was the appearance of two dark lines between each major dense line of the
involved region (fig. 13a, 14a).

Axons in demyelinating fibers were well preserved (fig. 6-8). Axon changes
with an increase in mitochondria or vesicular structures were sometimes to
be seen, but no recent desintegrative changes were manifest.

Summarizing the findings of the first sural-nerve biopsy the syndrome of a
hypertrophic neuropathy was to delineate. The examined stage of neuropathy
consisted of moderate onion bulb formation, of considerable "old" removed

---

Fig. 6   Demyelinating fiber
          -demyelination over the whole thickness of the sheath, "vesicular"
          appearence.
          Severe myelinated fiber reduction, only one small myelinated
          fiber - M is present. A - axon
          Increase in collagen.
          x 5520

Fig. 7   Demyelinating fiber
          -only partial demyelination, inner lamellae are involved, circum-
          ferential membranes are preserved. A - axon
          Increase in collagen.
          x 5520

Fig. 8   Demyelinating fiber.
          Detail: "vesicular" appearing area -
          -consisted of an irregular network of delamellated membranes and
          "vesicular-like" spaces, predominantly empty.
          Numerous membranes appear single, membrane groups are scanty,
          solitary myelin-like = L
          A - axon, S - nucleus of a surrounding Schwann cell.
          x 22,910

Fig. 9   Demyelinating fiber.
          Detail a: "vesicular" appearing area, with an irregular network of
          delamellated membranes and spaces. A - axon
          Detail b: Residuals of myelin-membranes in delamellation
          x 22,910

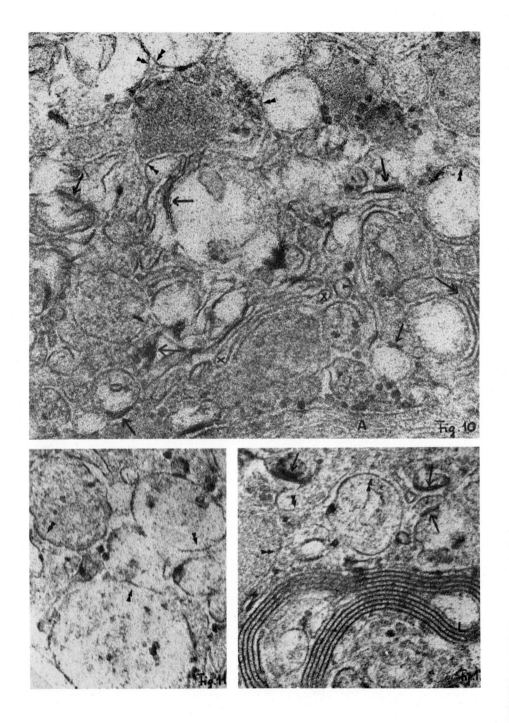

Fig. 10

Fig. 11

fiber changes expressed in the high reduction of myelinated fibers and of numerous most impressive, very recent, just "going on" changes in myelinated
fibers. These recent fiber changes were pure demyelinations, extensive -
mostly over the whole thickness of the sheath, with myelin-membrane delamellation mostly of single ones, consecutive complex "vesicular-like" arrangement with fragmentations and with changes in periodicity, the latter even in
spot-like distribution on still preserved parts of the myelin-sheaths. Regenerative phenomena like Büngner-bands, axon-sprouting or recent remyelination
were not to reveal. Disproportional thin myelin sheath and their onion bulbs
indicate some performed remyelinating phenomena.

FURTHER COURSE

Immediately after verification of the diagnosis a dietary treatment was initiated in our patient. Details and diagrams are published elsewhere[16b].
Therapy was done over a time of 2 1/2 years. 14 months the diet of Steinberg
and co-workers[35] was used, a diet low in phytol. During this treatment it was
necessary to do plasmapheresis in the 6th month after beginning and to change
the oil in the 9th month of therapy. After 1 year and 2 months Steinberg's diet
was changed to Stokke's prescription[36], a fat free diet.

In the clinical course deterioration was going on over more than 1 year,
especially pronounced after plasmapheresis. The patient became unable to
walk alone, difficulties in moving the right hand appeared as well as intensification of sensibility-disturbances and ataxia. Body weight became reduced.
Clinical remission began after about 1,5 year.

Fig. 10   Detail of the "vesicular-like" demyelinating area.
           Numerous delamellated membranes appearing as:
           1. single membrane structures often arranged around empty
           spaces "vesicle-like" -↓
           2. membrane groups a. rarely with myelin-membrane distances
           but without their periodicity - ↑↓ b. often as equithick mem-
           branes with 40-60 Å distance - |
           Blind loops - X   A = axon
           x 80,040

Fig. 11   Detail of the "vesicular-like" demyelinating area - inner, axon -
           near zone. Numerous delamellated single membranes -↓ with
           larger "vesicular" spaces
           x 80,040

Fig. 12   Detail of the "vesicular-like" demyelinating area - outer zone.
           Some delamellated single membranes -↓↓ , several membrane
           groups with small distances of 40-60Å - ↑ and a solitary mem-
           brane group with myelin periodicity, in delamellation - L
           x 80,040

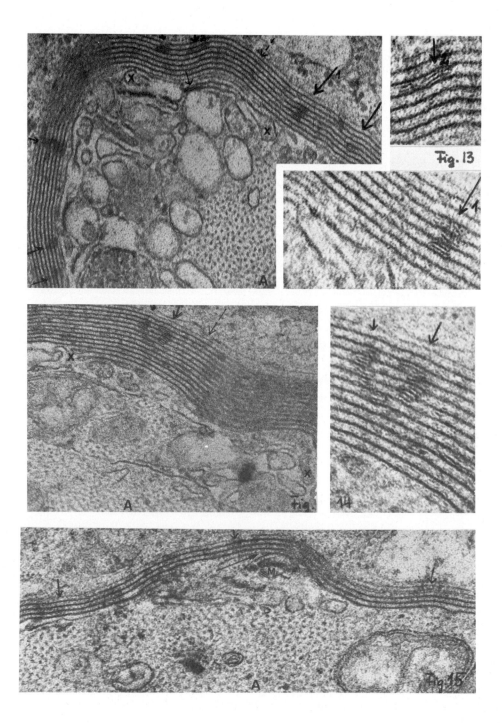

Fig. 13

Fig. 14

Fig. 15

CSF-protein increased in the first 3 months to 280 mg%.
NCV in ulnar nerve reduced to unmeasurable values during the first year
while phytanic acid levels remained unchanged.
After a year slowly increasing NCV and slowly decreasing levels of phytanic
acid appeared.
The best therapeutic result was gained 1 year and 10 months after the be-
ginning of the dietary treatment.
Phytanic acid in serum was reduced to 14%.
NCV in ulnar nerve had regained 22 m/sec and protein in CSF had again its
initial value of 180 mg %.
Clinically the patient was again able to walk alone, even over longer distances,
motor ability of the hands and sensibility, except vibration, were restituted.
Ataxia was decreased and body weight increased.

This was the moment we decided to re-examine peripheral nerve changes.

SECOND NERVE BIOPSY FINDINGS

The second sural-nerve biopsy was done in a moment of the course of the
disease when clinical improvement was stabilised over weeks to months, when
nerve conduction velocity had again measurable values and when phytanic acid
was reduced to more than half of the initial value, but still far away from
normal. In light microscopy, already in low magnification, a considerable increase in myelinated fibers was to be seen (fig. 16). Histometric examinations
revealed the total number increased from 750 to 1. 700 myelinated fibers/mm^2,

---

Fig. 13   Partially demyelinating fiber. Blind loops - X and "vesicle-like"
formations in delamellated membranes between axon - A and persisting compact myelin sheath. Periodicity changes in numerous
spots of the compact myelin sheath - ↑
x 80,040
Inset: Periodicity changes due to two dark line appearing locally
between major dense lines
x 240,120

Fig. 14   Partially demyelinating fiber with blind loop formation - X at the
inner myelin lamellae and changes in periodicity of the still compact myelin - ↑
x 80,040   A - Axon
Inset: Periodicity changes due to two dark lines appearing between
major dense lines
x 240,120

Fig. 15   Partially demyelinating fiber. Delamellation and splitting of the
innermost lamellae - ↑ with appearing of periodicity changed
splitted membrane groups - M. Local periodicity changes in the
still compact myelin sheath - ↑
x 51,520   A - axon

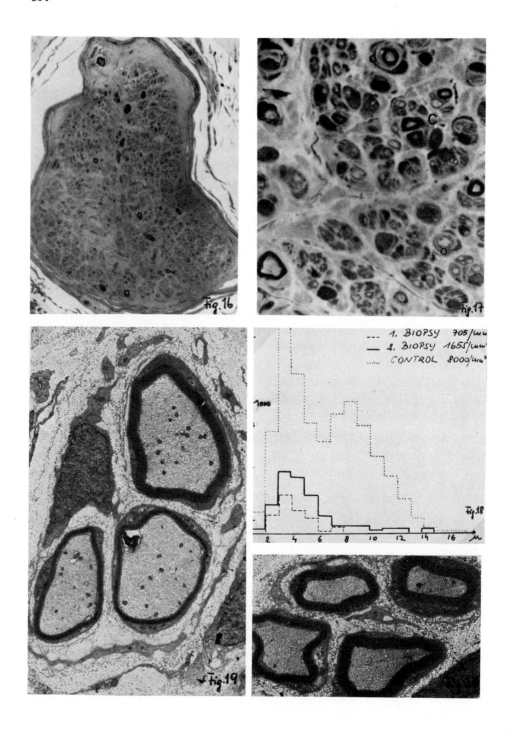

Fig. 16

Fig. 17

Fig. 18

1. BIOPSY   705/mm
2. BIOPSY 1655/mm
CONTROL 8000/mm²

Fig. 19

mostly participating were the fiber groups of 4 - 6 mµ diameter (fig. 18). In higher magnifications of semithin section the augmented myelinated fibers appeared in small groups - "cluster-like", or in onion bulbs (fig. 17).

In electron microscopy a lot of cluster formations were the most impressive findings (fig. 19, 20). Onion bulbs were more numerous but still only with few layers of the concentrically arranged processus (fig. 21-23). Center of the onion bulbs were predominantly myelinated fibers, mostly remyelinating (fig. 21, 24). While the inner part of the sheath consisted still of loose myelin, compact myelin was already formed in the outer parts (fig. 24). Often those fibers had at the outer circumference irregular myelin-bodies or myelin loops (fig. 22, 23, 25). But no myelin degradation nor changes in structure or periodicity of the myelin lamellae were apparent (fig. 26). Several myelin fibers with thick and throughout compact lamellae were present too (fig. 27).

Unmyelinated fibers were numerous, band-like arrangement appeared sometimes (fig. 28). Collagen fibers were still increased (fig. 19-23, 27). Summarizing the findings of the second sural-nerve biopsy hypertrophic neuropathy was still to delineate. But now the syndrom consisted of no recent, acute changes but of numerous regenerative phenomena. Clusters, remyelinations, onion bulbs and rare band-like formations indicated a strong reparative process with axon regeneration and remyelination, ending lastely in a considerable increase of myelinated fibers, proved even through quantitative data.

DISCUSSION

Comparative examinations of peripheral nerve-changes in Refsum's disease before and after treatmant, during relapse and remission are not known in literature. Several nerve biopsies are investigated in Refsum's disease, light

---

Second sural nerve biopsy: Fig. 16 - 25

Fig. 16   Some myelinated fibers in a sural nerve fascicle - increase in myelinated fibers against the first biopsy.
x 46

Fig. 17   Increased myelinated fibers appearing in onion bulbs - O, or in small groups "cluster-like" - c
x 295

Fig. 18   Comparative histometric findings of myelinated fibers. Total number increased from 705 to 1.655. The fiber size spectrum is much more enlarged, from 14 - 2 mµ

Fig. 19   Clusters of myelinated fibers
x 5520

Fig. 20   Clusters of myelinated fibers
x 5520

506

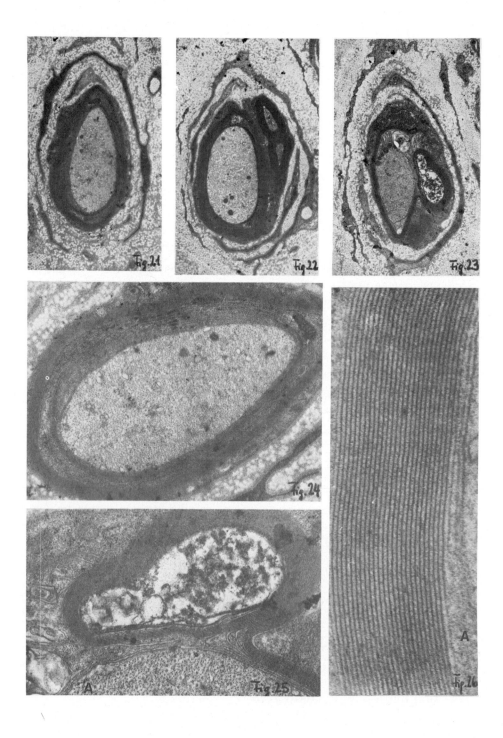

microscopically[23, 40, 21, 12, 10, 39] and with ultrastructural findings[5, 8, 9, 11, 10]. Myelinated fiber reduction, onion bulb formations and endoneural fibrosis gave evidence of the neuropathy, hypertrophic type. Only in light microscopy demyelinations were described[40, 21, 39], while in none of the electron microscopic examinations the process of demyelination was present and no fiber-teasing with proof of segmental demyelination is known[10]. Unproportional thin myelin sheaths[9, 10], wallerian degeneration[11] and numerous unmyelinated axons in the layer of the bulbs[9, 10, 11] are documented as fiber changes in Refsum's neuropathy. The similarity to other hypertrophic neuropathies esp. to Dejerine-Sottas is emphasized. Lipid-inclusions and paracristalline inclusions in mitochondria are constantly described[8, 9, 11, 10]. The possibility of an intra-mitochondrial localisation of the metabolic defect in Refsum's disease is discussed[10]. But the evolution of the observed fiber changes and the problem of reversibility resp. regeneration after a sufficient treatment was not yet observed.

No helpful data were coming from experiments, because Refsum's disease is not reproducible by feeding phytanic acid: only toxic effects appear[32]. Also in tissue cultures only toxic effects are described esp. for nerve cells[6]. In human pathology only one case had 2 biopsies in different stages of the disease[40, 9]. But the findings, done on different levels of resolution, were not compared[16a, 9].

The comparative examinations in our case of Refsum's disease resulted in some contributory findings to these problems of evolution and course of peripheral nerve changes. Recent pathological changes in relapse are exclusively demyelinating and the demyelination is an extensive one, most often over the

---

Fig. 21-23 Onion bulb formations, consisting only of few concentrically
arranged layers
21 - around a remyelinating fiber
x 5520
22 - around a fiber with myelin ovoids
x 5520
23 - around a fiber with an irregular contour
x 5520

Fig. 24 Remyelinating fiber. Loose myelin lamellae in the inner part of the
sheath, compact myelin in the outer zones
x 13,800

Fig. 25 Myelinated fiber with irregular sheath contours. A - axon
x 22,910

Fig. 26 Myelin sheath. Detail: Unchanged periodicity and structure. A -axon
x 22,910

508

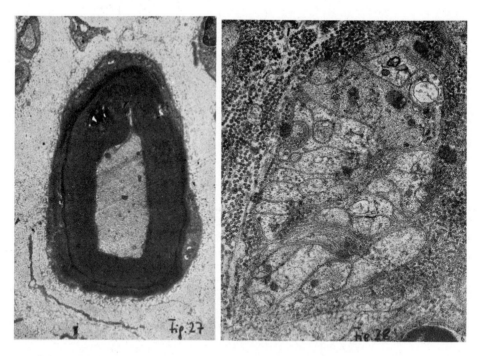

Fig. 27   Myelinated fiber with a proportional thick sheath
x 5,520

Fig. 28   Unmyelinated axons in band-formation
x 13,800

whole thickness of the sheath. Remyelination and regeneration appear plentiful in remission, when phytanic acid level is lowered but still highly abnormal.
No recent pathological changes esp. no demyelination is going on in this period, an observation which indicates the importance of quantitative conditions
for the tissue changes.

In detail, our first biopsy gave evidence that in an already pre-altered
nerve with considerable fiber deficit, "new", recent pathological changes can
take place, consisting of demyelination of still myelinated fibers. The demyelinating fibers were without storage material, but the demyelination was a
peculiar one. Not the whole pattern of the unspecific myelin-degradation products as e.g. in wallerian degeneration was present. Only blind loop-forma-
tion, delamellation of membranes, mostly single, sometimes few but then often
changed in periodicity, and "vesicular" arrangement of the delamellated,
splitted membranes with fragmentation appeared. Especially no membran-

structured myelin-ovoids resp. -bodies of the early stage, or membran-contai-
ning dense bodies appeared. None of the observed demyelinating membrane
changes are per se special e. g. blind loops are found in M. S.[37], shift of membrane distances, splitting or even delamellation are common in the degradation of all demyelinations.But the all over predominance of delamellation mostly
of single membranes or small groups, frequently periodicity-changed, indicates
a myelin-membrane involvement of a peculiar instability.

These demyelination findings gave some possibilities of explanation. Are
they only corresponding to a moment of an unspecific kind of demyelination,
related e. g. to a time factor of an acute relapse with rapid demyelination without evolution of all stages of degradation ? Or are the findings related to the
particularity of Refsum's disease ? For the last possibility the appearance of
periodicity changes in still preserved myelin of demyelinating fibers could be
a strong support. Changes in periodicity are rare in structural intact myelin
[22, 29, 30] and the appearance of additional structures, like the two dense lines
in our case, argue against a pure toxic effect.

The relation between biochemical abnormalities and pathological changes of
Refsum's disease esp. myelin sheaths is discussed for toxic phenomena or incorporation of phytanic acid[27, 36].

Incorporation of phytanic acid in myelin lipids is a concept of O'Brien's
theory of membrane instability in Refsum's disease[18]. Molecular packing is
the dominant factor of membrane stability, including length, straightness and
saturation of fatty acids as stabilizing factor[20]. Incorporation and accumulation of a branched fatty acid would have a "pronounced disrupting effect due
to steric hindrance of molecular packing"[20, 27] and the changement in the
highly ordered and strongly proportional chemical topography of membranes
can explain the consecutive instability.

This kind of myelin membrane involvement would be in good agreement with
the observed ultrastructural findings in myelin of our case.The particular delamellating type of demyelination seems a good expression of the consequence
of instable membranes.And the periodicity changes in myelin of just demyelinating fibers indicate membrane changes or shifts in the highest accumulating
membranes, just before demyelination. A close relationship between quantity
of stored fatty acid and pathological changes of myelin involvement is to
suppose.

This explains some findings of the second biopsy too. Although phytanic
acid is still present with 14 % of the total fatty acids in serum, no more structural myelin changes are present. On the contrary an extensive remyelination
activity has taken place, expressed in numerous remyelinated fibers with regular myelin periodicity. Only the relatively frequent appearance of myelin

ovoids or irregular contours of the sheaths may indicate some irregularities
in incipient remyelination. It seems that the schwann cells are capable of
remyelinating their axons in a milieu low but not free of phytanic acid. Axonal
changes were rare in the acute-stage biopsy, no desintegration took place at
this time, augmentation of some organelles is a known phenomenon accompanying demyelinating neuropathies. But axon degenerations have to take place
not only for the fiber reduction, but also to the appeared regeneration phenomena with cluster- and band-formations. Axon degenerations seem to be a
secondary phenomenon to the extensive demyelination, and axon regeneration
took place as well as remyelinations in patients with still augmented phytanic
acid levels.

That remyelination and regeneration are mostly due to the effects of the dietary treatment and its biochemical consequences is to delineate out of the
first biopsy which had no evidence of such reparative signs, and was from a
nerve exposed already to a long and changing course of the disease.

Summarizing the discussed data, demyelination is the basic pathological
change in Refsum's disease, strongly argued as the consequence of accumulated phytanic acid in myelin lipid bilayer with instability of membranes. Periodicity changes indicate pre-stage of demyelination and first structural
signs of high amounted accumulation, whose increasing values result   in a
demyelination of a delamellating type. Decreasing but still considerable pathological values of the accumulated phytanic acid had no more demyelinating
activity, on the contrary plentiful remyelination and regeneration appear, the
morphological basis of an efficient remission.

REFERENCES
1. Alexander, W. (1966) J. Neurol. Neurosurg. Psychiat. 29, 412-416.
2. Avigan, J. (1966) Biochem. biophys. Acta 116, 391-394.
3. Cammermeyer, J. (1956) J. Neuropath. exp. Neurol. 15, 340-361
4. Cammermeyer, J. (1975) in Handb. of Clinc. Neurol. Vol. 21, North Holland
   Publishing Company, pp. 231-261.
5. Dereux, J. et Gruner, J. E. (1963) R. Neurol. 109, 564-
6. Dubois-Dalcq, M. D. et al. (1972) J. Neuropath. exp. Neurol. 31, 645-667.
7. Eldjarn, L. et al. (1966) Lancet 1, 691-693.
8. Fardeau, M. and Engel, W. K. (1969) J. Neuropath. exp. Neuro. 28, 278-294.
9. Fardeau, M. et al. (1970) Rev. Neurol. 122, 185-196
10. Fardeau, M. (1975) in Peripheral Neuropathy Vol. II, chap. 42, Dyck,
   Thomas, Lambert eds., Saunders Comp., pp. 881-887.
11. Flament-Durant, J. (1971) Path. europ. 6, 172-191.

12.Fryer, D.G. et al. (1971) Neurology 21, 162-167.

13.Hansen, R.P. (1965) Biochem. Biophys. Acta 106, 304-310.

14.Herndon, J.H.Jr. et al. (1969) J.Clin.Invest.48, 1017-1032.

15.Klenk, E. and Kahlke, W. (1963) Hoppe-Seylers z. Physiol. Chem, 333, 133-139.

16a. Lapresle, J. et Salisachs (1969) in Wolf L.M. et al. Rev. Neurol. 120, p. 89.

16b. Lenz, H. et al. (1978) in press.

17.Lundberg, A. et al. (1972) Europ. Neurol. 8, 309-324.

18.Mc Brinn, M. and O'Brien, J.S. (1968) J. Lip. Res. 9, 552-561.

19.Mize, C.E. et al. (1969) J. Clin. Invest. 48, 1033-1040.

20.O'Brien, J. (1967) J. Theoret. Biol. 15, 307-324.

21.Quinlain, C.D. and Martin, E.A. (1970) J. Neurol. Neurosurg. Psychiat. 33, 817-823.

22.Raine, C. and Bornstein, M.D. (1976) Lab. Invest. 391-401.

23.Rake, M. and Saunders, M. (1966) J. Neurol. Neurosurg. Psychiat. 29, 417-422.

24.Reese, H. and Bareta, J. (1950) J. Neuropath. exp. Neurol. 9, 385-395.

25.Refsum, S. (1945) Nord. Med. 28, 2682-2685.

26.Refsum, S. (1946) Acta psych. neurol. scand., suppl. 38.

27.Refsum, S. (1975) in Handb. Neurol. Vol. 21, Chap. 10, North Holland Publishing Company, pp. 181-229.

28.Refsum, S. (1975) in Peripheral Neuropathy, Vol. II, chap. 42, Dyck, Thomas, Lambert eds., Saunders Company, pp. 868-872.

29.Sluga, E. (1970) Wr. Klin. Wschr. 82, 667.

30.Sluga, E. (1974) in Polyneuropathien. Typen und Differenzierung. Ergebnisse bioptischer Untersuchungen, Springer Verlag, pp. 31-53.

31.Steinberg, D. (1978) in Metabolic basis of inherited disease. Stanbury-Wyngaarden-Fredrickson. McGraw-Hill Book Company, Chap. 33, pp. 688-706.

32.Steinberg, D. et al. (1966) J. Lip. Res. 7, 684-691.

33. Steinberg, D. et al. (1965) Biochem. biophys. res. Commun. 19, 783-789.

34. Steinberg, D. et al. (1966) J. clin. Invest. 45, 1076-1077.

35. Steinberg, D. et al. (1970) Arch. Int. Med. 125, 75-87.

36. Stokke, O. and Eldjarn, L. (1975) in Peripheral Neuropathy, Vol. II, eds: Dyck, Thomas, Lambert, pp. 873-890.

37. Suzuki, K. et al. (1969) Lab. Invest. 20, 444-454.

38. Try, K. et al. (1972) Europ. Neurol. 8, 301-309.

39. Thümler, R. et al. (1977) Dtsch. med. Wschr. 102, 1454-1457.

40. Wolf, L.M. et al. (1969) Rev. Neurol. 120, 89-95.

AUTHOR INDEX